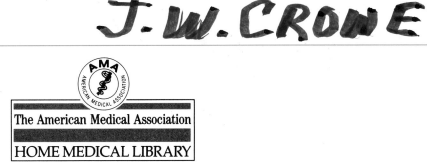

The American Medical Association

HOME MEDICAL LIBRARY

# KNOW YOUR DRUGS AND MEDICATIONS

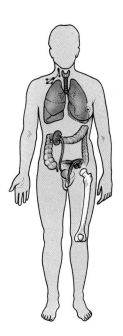

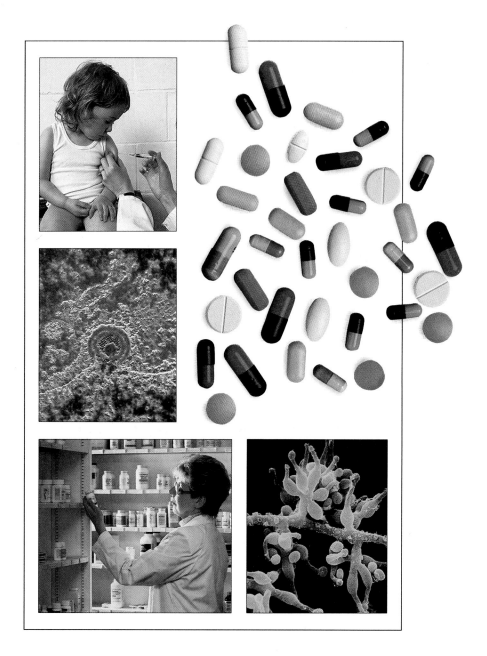

# THE AMERICAN
# MEDICAL ASSOCIATION

# KNOW YOUR DRUGS AND MEDICATIONS

Medical Editor
CHARLES B. CLAYMAN, MD

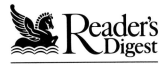

THE READER'S DIGEST ASSOCIATION, INC.
Pleasantville, New York/Montreal

The information in this book reflects current medical knowledge. The
recommendations and information are appropriate in most cases;
however, they are not a substitute for medical diagnosis. For specific
information concerning your personal medical condition, the AMA
suggests that you consult a physician.

The names of organizations, products, or alternative therapies appearing
in this book are given for informational purposes only. Their inclusion
does not imply AMA endorsement, nor does the omission of any
organization, product, or alternative therapy indicate AMA approval.

The AMA Home Medical Library is distinct from and unrelated to the
series of health books published by Random House, Inc., in conjunction
with the American Medical Association under the names "The AMA Home
Reference Library" and "The AMA Home Health Library."

**Library of Congress Cataloging in Publication Data**

Know your drugs and medications / medical editor, Charles B. Clayman.
        p. cm. — (The American Medical Association home medical
library)
  At head of title: The American Medical Association.
  Includes indexes.
  ISBN 0-89577-386-4
  1. Pharmacology—Popular works. 2. Drugs—Popular works.
I. Clayman, Charles B. II. American Medical Association.
III. Series.
RM301. 15. K58 1991
615'. 1—dc20

                                                        90-26984

# FOREWORD

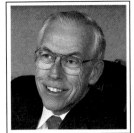

Medicinal drugs and vaccines have played a vital role in the conquest of disease. During the 20th century, drugs have contributed substantially to an increase in life expectancy and an improved quality of life for people with chronic diseases. Advances in immunization have also resulted in more effective protection against infectious diseases. This volume of the AMA Home Medical Library provides you with an overview of many medications so that you can understand their effects and use them safely. It explains the discovery and development of drugs, the different classifications of drugs, how drugs work in your body, and medical conditions for which drug therapy is currently the treatment of choice. A special chapter is devoted to helping you make the most appropriate choice among over-the-counter medications.

Despite the remarkable rise in the number of medications available and the extraordinary success of drug treatment, some people remain concerned about possible harmful effects of drug treatment. Although all drugs in the US are manufactured to rigorous safety standards, drugs are powerful substances and must be used with care. The benefits from drug treatment are, on the whole, far greater than the drawbacks.

In developed countries, people spend an average of between 1 and 2 percent of their income on medications and vitamin and mineral supplements. Drugs are not a "cure-all" for disease; you can often achieve the greatest benefits from drug treatment by also adopting a healthy life-style and eating a nutritious, well-balanced diet. Scientists and researchers have made great advances in developing more effective and safe drugs – from the days when most drugs were obtained from plants and minerals to today, when sophisticated techniques are used to produce drugs in a laboratory. The search for more effective drugs continues, and the future is challenging.

**JAMES S. TODD, MD**
Executive Vice President
American Medical Association

# CONTENTS

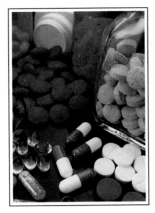

# CHAPTER ONE

# DRUGS PAST, PRESENT, AND FUTURE

INTRODUCTION

THE STORY OF DRUGS

THE PHARMACEUTICAL INDUSTRY

UNTIL THE BEGINNING of the 20th century, most drugs were obtained from plants and from a few minerals or metallic elements such as mercury and arsenic. Today, most new medications are made in synthetic form in a laboratory. In the last 40 years or so, vaccines have eliminated smallpox and reduced the incidence of polio; antibiotics and antibacterials have greatly reduced the incidence of and deaths from infectious diseases. Medications have played a major role in improving the quality of life of people with a variety of chronic diseases. Statistics on cerebrovascular disease (strokes and related conditions) in the US over the past 50 years indicate that nearly a half million deaths have been prevented and as many as 6 million nonfatal strokes have been avoided by the long-term use of medications that effectively lower blood pressure.

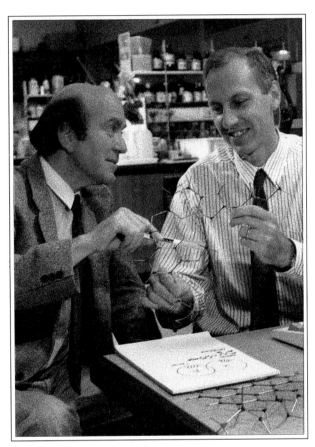

While no one denies the contribution that advances in medicine have made to better health, many people are concerned about the potentially harmful effects of some medications. However, these drawbacks seem insignificant when compared to the benefits derived from the proper use of drugs and the harm caused by motor vehicles, cigarettes, and alcohol. Americans spend about 1 to 2 percent of their money every year on medicines, vitamins, minerals, and other health supplements. Critics of the pharmaceutical industry often point to the rising cost of prescription drugs. Taking the rate of inflation into account, the average cost of moving a new chemical through the drug development and approval process doubled between 1980 and 1990. This chapter follows the discovery and development of drugs from ancient times to the present and beyond. The first section begins with the discovery of the medicinal effects of the opium poppy and the deadly nightshade plant. It then reviews the chemical revolution, from the development of aspirin and the first antibacterial drugs up to the latest tailor-made and genetically engineered drugs. The second section reviews today's pharmaceutical industry and includes a description of the steps involved in the development, testing, and marketing of a new drug. It also discusses governmental regulations and the need for extensive testing of a drug before it is approved for general use.

Scientists and researchers continue to search for new drugs that are more effective and have fewer side effects. For diseases such as AIDS and certain forms of cancer, for which there are few useful drugs currently available, the search is challenging.

# THE STORY OF DRUGS

The origins of today's pharmaceutical industry can be traced back many centuries. In ancient times, people found that certain plants and minerals could alleviate some of their ills, and a primitive tradition of drug treatment began to evolve from these haphazard discoveries. The remarkable achievements of modern medicine are part of that continuing process of evolution that began long ago.

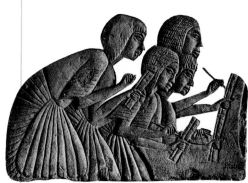

**Ancient Egypt**
*Archaeologists have deciphered papyrus documents recounting that the medical practitioners of ancient Egypt used substances such as belladonna and peppermint that are still being used in medicine today.*

## QUININE

Quinine is derived from the bark of the South American cinchona tree. Long recognized by the natives of Peru as a remedy for malaria, cinchona bark was brought to Spain in the 17th century. In time, scientists isolated its active ingredient, the alkaloid quinine, and accurate and effective dosages for the treatment of malaria were determined. Until well into the 20th century, quinine was the only drug available specifically for malaria; it is still used to treat strains of malaria that have become resistant to newer drugs.

## THE DAWN OF MEDICINE

The ancient Egyptians used opium to relieve pain and castor oil to kill parasitic worms. Arab physicians in the 12th century treated goiter patients with burned sponges – a rational treatment, as it turns out, because of the iodine content of the sponges. Medical practi-

**Parent of modern pharmacy**
*Paracelsus, a Swiss physician and alchemist, introduced many new substances into medical use.*

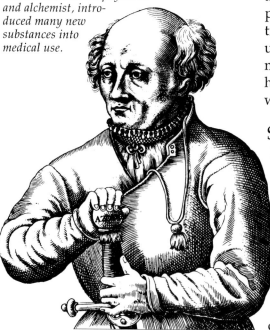

tioners in ancient Greece and Rome used crude extracts of the deadly nightshade plant (belladonna) for its sedative and colic-relieving properties. However, along with these now-validated remedies were many others of little or absolutely no scientific merit. As late as 1700, apothecaries – the forerunners of today's pharmacists – were still dispensing a traditional elixir (sweet medicinal liquid, often containing alcohol) that was a mixture of powdered lion's heart, dried human brains, gold, witch hazel, earthworms, and Egyptian onions.

### Scientific observation

For many centuries the body of medical knowledge regarding both diseases and their treatment contained as much fiction as fact. It was not until the 16th century that scientific observation of the effects of medical treatment began, initiated by the medical practitioner Philippus Paracelsus (1493-1541). Paracelsus believed in much of the alchemy and occultism that were characteristic of his time, but he also recognized that a knowledge of chemistry was a fundamental element in the effective practice of medicine.

## Medicinal plants

In the Middle Ages, observations concerning the medicinal properties of plants were assembled in publications called herbals. Perhaps the most celebrated example of an herbal is that by Nicolas Culpeper (1616-1654). The accuracy of some of the information he recorded is remarkable. Herbals widely recommended foxglove, *Digitalis purpurea*, for the treatment of dropsy (also called edema – fluid accumulation in body tissues caused by heart, kidney, or liver failure) long before William Withering published an account in 1785 of the action of the dried leaves of the foxglove plant on the weakened heart. It is now common knowledge that edema caused by heart failure can be treated with digitalis, which improves the efficiency of the heart.

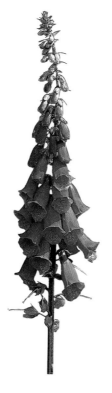

**Digitalis drugs**
*Digitalis from the leaves of the foxglove plant is used in the manufacture of drugs such as digoxin and digitoxin for heart conditions.*

## Explaining folk medicine

In some cases, science has been slow to provide a full explanation for successful treatments introduced many years ago. For example, although James Lind (1716-1794) knew as early as 1753 that scurvy (weakness of small blood vessels and poor healing of wounds caused by vitamin C deficiency) could be treated by eating citrus fruit, the vitamin responsible for the cure was not identified until the 20th century. Although Edward Jenner (1749-1823) introduced a vaccine against smallpox in 1796, scientists only recently have been able to understand how vaccination results in immunity.

### MERCURY DRUGS

From the earliest times, mercury was ingested in its metallic form (as quicksilver) and as various salts, especially mercurous chloride (calomel). Mercury salts are highly poisonous but, until the 20th century, they were the only known effective remedy for syphilis. Treatment with mercury had major toxic effects, including constant salivation, severe indigestion, tooth decay and tooth loss, loss of weight, weakness, emotional disturbances, and even death. It was not until the organic arsenical compound salvarsan was synthesized in 1907 that the use of mercury could be rendered a secondary treatment for syphilis.

## MORPHINE AND PAIN CONTROL

The pain-relieving and mood-altering properties of opium have been observed for thousands of years. Opium contains more than 20 natural alkaloids (organic substances found in plants that have medicinal uses), including codeine and morphine.

Morphine is chemically similar to the endorphins (substances in the body that relieve pain); this drug stops pain by occupying the same receptors on nerve cells as are occupied by the endorphins. This pain-relieving mechanism is unique to the opiate drugs. Although substitutes for morphine have been developed, most doctors agree that for severe pain morphine is unparalleled. Many doctors endorse the long-term use of morphine for severe pain; the relief of suffering is more significant than the risk of addiction.

**The opium poppy**
*Morphine is extracted from the juice of the unripe seed pod of the poppy* Papaver somniferum.

**Scientific analysis**
*Although doctors in earlier centuries identified many natural substances that had medicinal properties, it was not until the 19th and 20th centuries that chemists, using sophisticated laboratory equipment, were able to identify the active agents in those substances.*

## THE CHEMICAL REVOLUTION

During the 1800s, chemists began to investigate and extract the active ingredients of medicinal plants in a systematic way. Two methods were common. One was to extract the natural active agent in a pure form, which was then often crystallized or distilled, after which it could be weighed or measured. The other method was to find a synthetic substance that was equivalent to the natural drug and could be manufactured as a chemical. It became unnecessary to depend on the naturally occurring substance that in its earlier, cruder forms varied in potency and often required biological assay (laboratory analysis of components) to standardize the dose.

### Aspirin

Aspirin was one of the first great commercial successes in the pharmaceutical industry. Derived from salicin, a substance in the bark and leaves of some willow species, aspirin is acetylsalicylic acid, a chemical that was synthesized by Charles Gerhardt (1816-1856) in 1853 but was not fully appreciated until almost 50 years later. When a large pharmaceutical company began to look for a less irritating form of salicylic acid (a more basic derivative of salicin that was in widespread use as a painkiller and anti-inflammatory medication), Gerhardt's compound was reevaluated, given the trade name aspirin, and marketed around the world.

### The first antibacterial drugs

As recently as the 1930s, it was generally believed that bacteria could not be destroyed by drugs. In his research on dyes, Gerhard Domagk (1895-1964) experimented with a compound, known today as Prontosil, that had been synthesized in 1932. He found that Prontosil was effective in treating streptococcal bacterial infections in mice, while also being nontoxic. Domagk saved his daughter's life by treating her streptococcal infection and blood poisoning with Prontosil. It was later confirmed

### PENICILLIN

Penicillin is a substance that is produced by several molds. Penicillin was the first antibiotic used successfully to treat acute bacterial infections in humans. Allergy to penicillin is relatively common. Otherwise, penicillin is substantially nontoxic. Although some bacteria have become resistant, penicillin is effective against several common bacteria.

**Antibacterial and antibiotic drugs**
*Both antibacterial and antibiotic drugs are used to treat conditions caused by harmful bacteria, such as the streptococci (shown color-enhanced and magnified 4,000 times at right). All antibacterials were initially produced synthetically in the laboratory. All antibiotics were originally derived from molds and fungi but are now also made synthetically.*

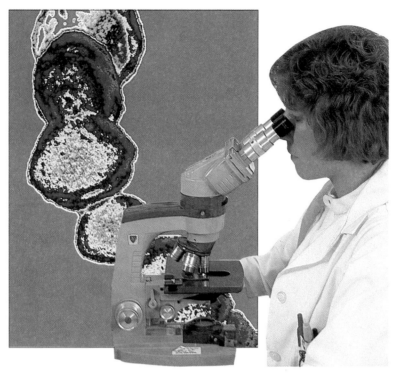

that Prontosil is converted in the body to sulfanilamide. Sulfonamide derivatives, developed from modifications of sulfanilamide, are now widely used to treat adult-onset diabetes. Sulfonamide research also led to the development of an important group of diuretic drugs, the thiazide drugs used to treat heart failure and high blood pressure.

The first anticancer drugs were developed in early 1940 by modifying mustard gas, a poison used in World War I. Chlorpromazine, a breakthrough in the treatment of severe emotional disorders, was developed in 1952 and was followed by the development of a number of antidepressant and tranquilizing drugs. Corticosteroids were introduced at about the same time for the treatment of autoimmune diseases (caused by a reaction of the body's immune system) and chronic respiratory diseases.

## PAUL EHRLICH'S "MAGIC BULLET"

The scientist Paul Ehrlich (1854-1915) had a dream that it was possible to find a substance – a "magic bullet" – that would seek out specific germs in the body and destroy them. He found that some arsenic compounds attached themselves to certain disease organisms by seeking out chemical groups called chemoreceptors in the organisms. Later, Ehrlich's compound 606 was found to be amazingly effective at seeking out and destroying the spirochetes (spiral-shaped bacteria) that cause syphilis. Named salvarsan, this compound was the "magic bullet" that Ehrlich had been so diligently seeking. It was used until treatment with penicillin became available after World War II.

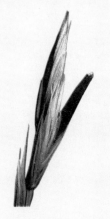

## THE IMMUNIZATION PROGRAM

In 1796, Edward Jenner developed a new medical technique that was to have worldwide consequences. In a series of experiments, he investigated the folk belief that contact with cows offered protection against smallpox. He confirmed that infection with a mild cowpox virus resulted in immunity to the much more dangerous smallpox virus. Since Jenner's discovery, immunization has been used against such diseases as diphtheria, pertussis (whooping cough), tuberculosis, and the rabies, measles, rubella, hepatitis B, poliomyelitis, mumps, and influenza viruses. Polio has now become very rare, but it remains a dangerous disease to those people who have not been vaccinated.

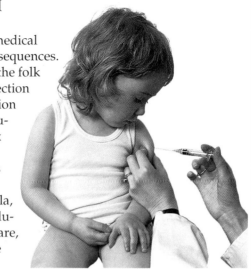

**The first beta blocker**
*Propranolol, the first beta blocker, slows the action of the heart and increases its efficiency, relieving high blood pressure, angina, and arrhythmias (forms of irregular heartbeat). It is also used to treat symptoms of anxiety and hyperthyroidism (overactivity of the thyroid gland) and to prevent migraine headache.*

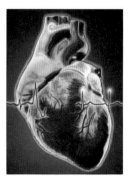

**Eradication of disease**
*It was confirmed in 1980 that smallpox has been eradicated worldwide by vaccination programs. Tuberculosis (TB), caused by the bacterium* Mycobacterium tuberculosis *(right, magnified 2,925 times), afflicts more than 20,000 people in the US each year. However, preventive measures, including antituberculous drugs and the BCG (bacillus Calmette-Guérin) vaccine are making inroads against TB.*

## TAILOR-MADE DRUGS

Many of the medications of the last few decades are tailor-made drugs, which are designed to perform a particular function in order to remedy a specific disease. Scientists have learned that, rather than hoping to develop a new medication by trial and error (as largely occurred in the past), they can analyze a medical disorder and design a drug that has precisely the needed beneficial effect on specific mechanisms of the body. Two examples are propranolol, arguably the first tailor-made drug, and cimetidine. Propranolol and cimetidine are selective

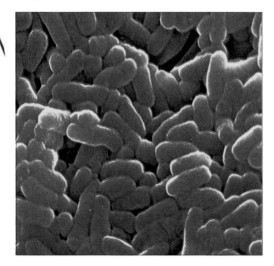

antagonists, which means they have an effect only on the cellular receptors they block.

### Propranolol

The drug propranolol acts as a blocker of a chemical agent called norepinephrine. Norepinephrine is a transmitter (messenger substance) that acts between nerves and muscles or between one set of nerves and another set of nerves. It stimulates changes in the body by acting on two types of receptors, which are found on the surfaces of certain cells throughout the body. When norepinephrine acts on alpha receptors in arteries, it causes the arteries to narrow, thus raising the blood pressure. However, when norepinephrine acts on beta receptors it causes the arteries to widen, lowering blood pressure. In addition, when norepinephrine acts on beta receptors in the heart, it increases the heart's rate and the force of its contraction.

Propranolol is chemically constructed to block the attachment of norepinephrine to the beta receptors. It does so by attaching to the beta receptors; thus it is called a beta blocker. Propranolol reduces the amount of work the heart needs to do, which is helpful in the treatment of cardiovascular diseases such as angina and high blood pressure.

## Cimetidine

When stimulated, some cells in the body release histamine, which reacts with two types of cellular receptors ($H_1$ and $H_2$ receptors). Histamine provokes an allergic reaction by interacting with the $H_1$ receptors. Histamine also interacts with $H_2$ receptors in the stomach, which causes release of gastric acid into the stomach. Cimetidine is an $H_2$ blocker – that is, it blocks the attachment of histamine onto these $H_2$ receptors. Cimetidine is used in the treatment of peptic ulcers, which usually occur in the lining of the stomach and duodenum (part of the small intestine), and occasionally occur in the esophagus. Rarely they are found farther down the small intestine in an appendixlike structure called Meckel's diverticulum. Cimetidine and other, more recently developed, $H_2$-blocker drugs reduce the release of gastric acid, allowing ulcers to heal.

**Cyclosporine**
*Cyclosporine is a drug derived from substances secreted by the fungus* Tolypocladium inflatum gams *(right). Cyclosporine has proved invaluable for organ transplant operations (below) because it inhibits the body's immune system and prevents it from rejecting the newly transplanted organ as a foreign body. Before cyclosporine was used, rejection of a transplanted organ was common.*

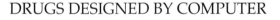

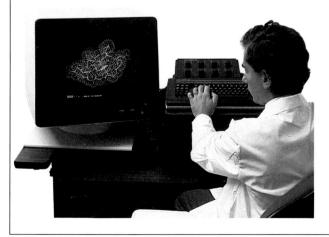

---

## DRUGS DESIGNED BY COMPUTER

In recent years, the development and production of tailor-made drugs has been made easier by the use of computers. Sophisticated analytical techniques such as X-ray crystallography allow researchers to visualize a receptor (see page 31) in three dimensions on a computer screen and to calculate the space into which a compound must fit in order to block the receptor. With this information, chemists can then modify the structure of new compounds to produce drugs that fit precisely into a particular receptor – the so-called tailor-made drugs.

A precise fit between a new compound and the receptor on a computer screen does not guarantee that a drug will be effective, but it provides a good starting point. The chemists who produce the compounds and the biologists who test the effects of these compounds develop a clear picture of the relationship between structure and activity of new compounds. The most promising compounds are selected to be tested on animals for toxic effects and then are used in human clinical trials. This procedure has yielded many of the new medications that have become available in recent years and is now an established means of developing new drugs.

# DRUGS MADE BY GENETIC ENGINEERING

All enzymes (substances that control the rate of chemical reactions in the body) and many hormones (messenger substances) are proteins. When the body does not produce enough of a particular protein, that protein can be administered in drug form to make up for the deficiency. For example, injections of insulin are given to diabetics, who do not have enough of this substance (produced by the pancreas). In the past, proteins such as insulin had to be extracted from animal tissue for medical use. Now many of these proteins can be made by genetic engineering, or recombinant DNA technology. DNA is the substance in cells that consists of strings of genes, with each gene providing the code for the production of a particular protein. Some genetically engineered drugs and their action on the body are listed below.

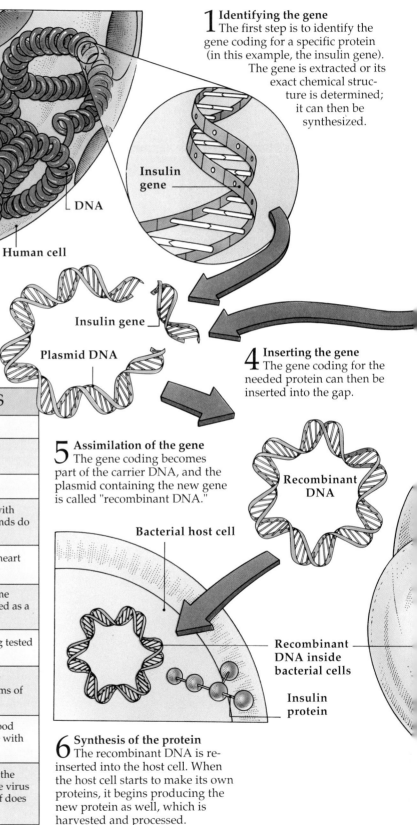

**1 Identifying the gene**
The first step is to identify the gene coding for a specific protein (in this example, the insulin gene). The gene is extracted or its exact chemical structure is determined; it can then be synthesized.

Insulin gene

DNA

Human cell

Insulin gene

Plasmid DNA

**4 Inserting the gene**
The gene coding for the needed protein can then be inserted into the gap.

**5 Assimilation of the gene**
The gene coding becomes part of the carrier DNA, and the plasmid containing the new gene is called "recombinant DNA."

Recombinant DNA

Bacterial host cell

Recombinant DNA inside bacterial cells

Insulin protein

**6 Synthesis of the protein**
The recombinant DNA is reinserted into the host cell. When the host cell starts to make its own proteins, it begins producing the new protein as well, which is harvested and processed.

## GENETICALLY ENGINEERED DRUGS

| DRUG | ACTION ON THE BODY |
|---|---|
| Human insulin | Controls blood sugar level; given to diabetics |
| Factor VIII | Clots blood; given to hemophiliacs |
| Growth hormone | Induces growth; given to children with stunted growth whose pituitary glands do not produce enough hormone |
| Tissue plasminogen activator (TPA) | Dissolves blood clots; used to treat heart attack victims |
| Interleukin-2 | Converts selected cells of the immune system into "attack" cells; being tested as a cancer treatment |
| Interferon | Inhibits production of viruses; being tested as a treatment for some cancers |
| Bone marrow white cell growth factor | Manipulates the immune system by stimulating growth in primitive forms of white cells |
| Erythropoietin | Stimulates the production of red blood cells; used to treat anemia in people with kidney disease |
| Hepatitis B vaccine | Contains only some components of the hepatitis virus type B (not the whole virus particle); therefore, the vaccine itself does not cause disease in the body |

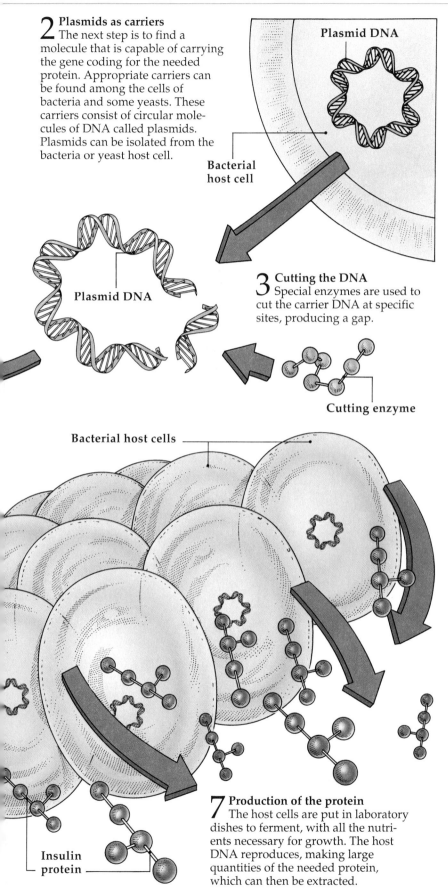

**2 Plasmids as carriers**
The next step is to find a molecule that is capable of carrying the gene coding for the needed protein. Appropriate carriers can be found among the cells of bacteria and some yeasts. These carriers consist of circular molecules of DNA called plasmids. Plasmids can be isolated from the bacteria or yeast host cell.

Plasmid DNA

Bacterial host cell

Plasmid DNA

**3 Cutting the DNA**
Special enzymes are used to cut the carrier DNA at specific sites, producing a gap.

Cutting enzyme

Bacterial host cells

**7 Production of the protein**
The host cells are put in laboratory dishes to ferment, with all the nutrients necessary for growth. The host DNA reproduces, making large quantities of the needed protein, which can then be extracted.

Insulin protein

# RESEARCH AND DEVELOPMENT

Many medications in current use are designed to treat symptoms, such as headache, rather than the physiological disorders that cause them. The pharmaceutical industry collectively is working to pinpoint basic problems in the body that cause symptoms in order to develop precisely targeted drugs that act on the underlying disorder.

Medical research is also attempting to identify the factors that control cellular function. Cancer, for example, involves the uncontrolled reproduction of cancer cells, so the genetic signals that cause cells (including cancer cells) to reproduce are now being investigated. Once scientists know more about these signals and the stimulation and inhibition of the growth of cells in general, they may be able to develop drugs that stop reproduction of cancer cells definitively and safely. Such a development would make obsolete all the current anticancer drugs, whose effects vary and which damage or kill healthy cells along with the cancer cells they are being used to treat.

## Future medications

The prospect for the future is that medications will be based increasingly on the body's own signals. For example, atrial natriuretic peptide is a natural substance produced by the heart that lowers blood pressure by causing blood vessels to widen. By finding out precisely how this substance works, scientists may be able to design a synthetic version. In the future many new drugs will be virtual clones of naturally occurring substances, manufactured by means of genetic engineering. Scientists theorize that, because such drugs are replicas of substances made by the human body, these drugs will be as effective as the natural substance and better tolerated by the body than are many of the synthetic compounds currently available.

# THE PHARMACEUTICAL INDUSTRY

The pharmaceutical industry has transformed the pattern of medical treatment over the last 50 years by introducing a succession of breakthroughs that include antibiotics, anticancer drugs, cardiovascular drugs, nonsteroidal anti-inflammatory drugs, and thrombolytic drugs (which dissolve blood clots).

## CHANGING PERCEPTIONS

The public perception of prescription drugs has changed over the years. The development of vaccines to prevent and antibiotics to treat life-threatening diseases once seemed to suggest that there would soon be a drug for every disorder. Uncritical acceptance of the idea of "a pill for every ill" led to some overprescribing and overuse of drugs such as antibiotics and tranquilizers. Doctors and consumer groups agreed that some drugs such as tranquilizers should be used more con-

servatively. In 1962 the world was shocked by the fetal deformities caused by the drug thalidomide (see ADVERSE DRUG EFFECTS on page 32). This tragedy led to a new awareness of the need for strict government controls over the testing and marketing of new drugs. The testing procedure has become long and expensive. But today, the consumer of a new drug can be assured that most if not all of the life-threatening characteristics (as well as the potential for fetal malformations and adverse effects on nursing infants) have been excluded.

## Alternatives to drugs

Attitudes about drug treatment changed in the 1980s. Doubts arose as to whether medication alone, rather than professional counseling, was the best approach for the treatment of conditions such as obesity and symptoms such as anxiety and unhappiness. Millions of Americans require drug therapy and drugs continue to be a cost-effective treatment for many problems. However, studies have shown that counseling or behavior modification along with supportive drug therapy provide the most effective means of dealing with addictions such as alcoholism or cigarette smoking.

**Drug dollars**
*More than $100 billion is spent on drugs every year, most of it in North America, Europe, and Japan. Prescription drugs account for about 80 percent of the total sales in these areas, although drugs available only by prescription in some countries may be available over-the-counter in others. The pharmaceutical industry invests about 15 percent of its sales income into research and development, a higher percentage than is common in other major industries.*

# HOW A NEW DRUG IS DEVELOPED

The development of a new drug often begins in a laboratory with the discovery of a new chemical entity. Researchers test the actions of the new chemical on animals and, if the results suggest that it may offer some advantages over existing drugs, they begin a program of long-term studies (clinical trials). According to Food and Drug Administration (FDA) regulations, the clinical trials are divided into three phases and are designed to establish the safety of a drug, its most appropriate form and dosage, its effectiveness, and its clinical value.

## Animal tests

Preliminary studies using animals provide a profile of how a new chemical entity affects all body systems. All potential new drugs must be tested on animals to determine toxic effects, including whether they could cause cancer or fetal abnormalities.

## Phase I trials

Phase I studies are usually carried out with fewer than 100 healthy people. These studies are designed to determine that the drug is safe and what its side effects might be. The studies also provide basic information about how a drug works in the body – such as how it is absorbed into the bloodstream, whether it undergoes chemical changes in the liver or kidney, how long it stays in the body, where it is stored, and how it is excreted.

## Phase II trials

Phase II studies test a new drug on several hundred patients who have the disorder it is intended to treat in order to evaluate the dosages needed. Carefully monitored studies show in detail how and why the drug works in the body and the side effects it causes. To be successful, the new drug must be effective and safe.

## FDA approval

During the course of a new drug's trials, the manufacturer and clinical investigators must provide interim reports to the FDA. Eventually the investigators file a new drug application with the agency. Approval of the application by the FDA is rendered on the basis of advice from committees of experts on drugs and disease. Once the drug is approved, it can be marketed throughout the US. Postmarketing surveillance may be required to ensure that unexpected drug reactions are detected, reported, and evaluated. Postmarketing research focuses on new indications for using the drug, problems of people with selected conditions who take the drug, and other quality-of-life issues.

## Phase III trials

Phase III studies extend the observations made in Phase II to a larger, more diverse group of patients (usually 2,000 to 3,000) who are treated in supervised studies. The studies confirm the clinical value of the new drug by comparing it with existing drugs and by tracking effects of the drug over time and providing statistics on adverse reactions.

NEW DRUG

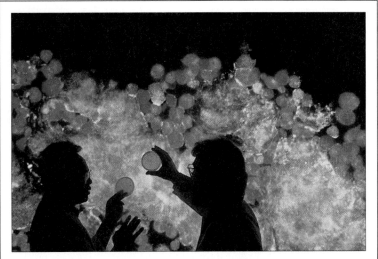

## "PARALLEL TRACK" DRUG TREATMENT

Although the testing of a new chemical entity normally takes between 6 and 10 years, people with AIDS and those with certain types of cancer have requested that experimental drugs that have been cleared for testing in volunteers be available not just to the patients in clinical trials, but (via a "parallel track") to all patients. This program was implemented in 1989 with the early introduction of zidovudine for treating AIDS. Researchers continue to study the human immunodeficiency virus (above) in search of a cure for AIDS.

## WHO INVENTS NEW DRUGS?

The roots of today's pharmaceutical industry can be traced to the development of the process for synthesizing aspirin in 1899. Important research on drugs (such as insulin and penicillin) has been and continues to be performed at colleges and universities. By the 1960s, however, the research and development departments of the pharmaceutical industry had become dominant.

With the worldwide introduction of drug-testing regulations and a dramatic rise in costs, developing new drugs has become expensive. Large, publicly owned drug companies have an advantage in financing research and development, but small drug companies (often called "boutiques") have also successfully developed new medications, particularly in areas involving genetic research. Academic research teams that

are developing innovative medications sometimes join forces with commercial drug companies.

## Advertising drugs

Once the Food and Drug Administration (FDA) has approved a new drug, the manufacturers usually begin a promotional campaign directed to doctors. The manufacturers who initiate these campaigns emphasize the informational aspect of acquainting doctors with a new drug, the high developmental costs (about $100 to $160 million for each new drug), and the brief period of patent protection remaining after the marketing approval. Once the patent expires, other manufacturers may produce generic versions of the same product. All claims that are made in advertisements are regulated by the FDA and must conform to the research results approved by the agency. Prescription drugs are now being advertised directly by name to the public; these advertisements must include a list of all possible adverse reactions that may be caused by the drug. Some drug advertisements do not give the name of the drug, but rather discuss a problem (such as baldness) and refer the consumer to a doctor for more information.

**Selling a new drug**
*Pharmaceutical company representatives introduce new medications to the medical profession. These visits to doctors serve both a promotional and educational function.*

# TAKING PART IN A CLINICAL TRIAL

The participation of patients in clinical trials is vital to the development of a new drug, yet many people have reservations about taking part. Their objections often center on the concurrent use of a placebo, or "dummy," version of the drug that is being tested in a clinical trial.

About 30 percent of patients report improvements in their symptoms when they take a drug on a trial basis, even if what they took is only a placebo (usually colored water or sugar tablets). This is known as the placebo response. The power of suggestion may be strong, but other factors involved may include the body's natural healing process, an incorrect diagnosis, or the use of other drugs by the patient. When a new drug is being tested, the first step is to demonstrate that it is superior to treatment with a placebo, ideally in a double-blind, randomized trial (see above right).

**Double-blind, randomized trials**

*In a controlled test, patients are randomly divided into two groups. One group takes the drug and the other takes a placebo that is identical in appearance. The drugs and placebos are assigned randomly by code; only when the code is broken at the end of the trial do the patients and investigators know which substance – the placebo or the drug – was being administered to a given individual.*

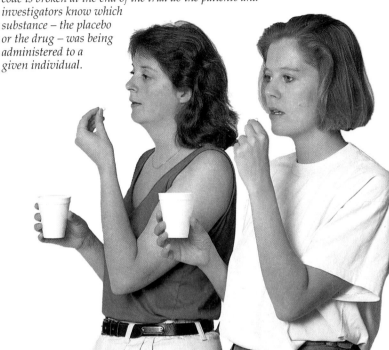

## ORPHAN DRUGS

Because of the high costs of developing new drugs, the pharmaceutical industry studies the potential sales of a new product before development begins. Most major drug companies do not invest in finding remedies for rare diseases because the number of potential consumers is too small for the research to be cost-effective. The drugs required for these rare disorders are called orphan drugs and the FDA helps finance the cost of developing these drugs. Changes in the tax laws have made it financially advantageous for a company to develop an effective orphan drug. Some orphan drugs have been used to treat other conditions than originally intended and therefore have been sold to a larger market.

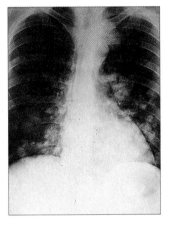

**Pentamidine for AIDS patients**
*This is a chest X-ray of an AIDS patient with pneumonia caused by the organism Pneumocystis carinii. Normally life-threatening, the infection can be treated successfully in many patients using an aerosol form of the orphan drug pentamidine.*

## The ethics of clinical trials

A major question about giving placebos to patients enrolled in clinical trials is whether giving placebos is ethical in the case of life-threatening conditions. There are clear guidelines for investigators. First, the investigator must believe that the new medication is likely to be effective but should have no conclusive evidence that it is effective. Second, placebos may be used as a control only when there is no established treatment for the condition against which the new drug can be compared. Third, patients must give their full and informed consent to participate in a placebo-controlled trial. Finally, in most large, placebo-controlled clinical trials, a panel of experts reviews the results every few months. If the medication being tested is found to achieve better results than the placebo, the trial may be discontinued to allow patients receiving the placebo to be switched to the medication being tested.

# CHAPTER TWO

# UNDERSTANDING DRUGS

INTRODUCTION

WHAT ARE DRUGS?

HOW DRUGS WORK

HOW DRUGS ARE
ADMINISTERED

A DRUG MAY BE defined as any substance introduced into the body to produce some alteration in the body's chemistry and in the functioning of one or more body organs. Some drugs, such as alcohol, nicotine, and caffeine, may be used to satisfy some need or compulsion of the user. A medication is any natural or synthetic substance intended to prevent, diagnose, treat, or cure a disease or other medical condition.

It is wise to consult your doctor about the selection and use of the more than 5,000 over-the-counter medications that are available today. Beneficial or dangerous interactions between different over-the-counter drugs, between different prescription medications, or between over-the-counter drugs and prescription medications should be considered. Symptoms that may not seem serious to you may require treatment with a prescription drug. Remember that drugs are not a "cure-all" for disease; sometimes their function is to help the body recover. One of the most astonishing aspects of today's medications is the ability of some drugs to do their work in the body at blood concentrations as low as one part per billion. These types of medications act at receptors, the specialized sites on the surface of a cell at which a chemical binds to produce a specific reaction.

Almost all medications can produce harmful as well as positive effects. When considering treatment with a drug, you and your doctor must carefully weigh the potential benefits against the possible risks. Furthermore, response to a drug can vary from person to person, depending on such factors as age, sex, and health status.

The first section of this chapter describes how drugs are categorized. We also explain the concepts of drug dependence and drug abuse, how you obtain medications, and the role of the pharmacist. The second section offers advice on how to obtain the medication you need at the best price. We explain clearly such terms as "generic substitution" and "bioequivalence." The third section reviews the principal ways in which drugs act on the body in terms of beneficial effects, adverse effects, and interactions with other drugs. The final section looks at the different ways in which drugs are administered, including new and future drug delivery systems. In addition, it examines the way in which our bodies process the drugs we take, from absorption (through the skin, various mucous membranes, or the small intestine) through excretion via the liver or the kidneys.

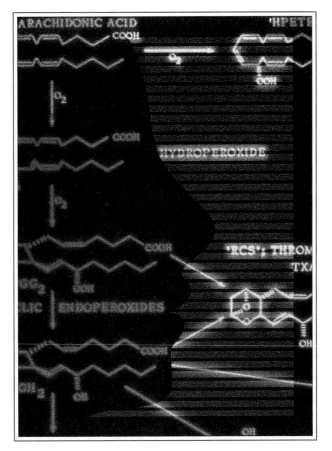

# WHAT ARE DRUGS?

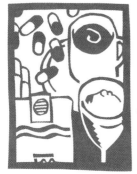

A T FIRST GLANCE the question "What are drugs?" might seem easy to answer – they are substances that your doctor prescribes for the treatment of disease or injury. However, drugs also include illegal agents such as LSD or heroin, as well as a variety of chemical products that you can buy from a drugstore or supermarket to relieve symptoms. Even ordinary table salt, sodium chloride, is sometimes used medicinally.

As discussed earlier in this chapter, "drugs" and "medications" have slightly different definitions, although the terms can often be used interchangeably. Many drugs are taken for medically approved purposes, usually to alter the course of a disease process or relieve a symptom. Narcotics and other drugs are used, sometimes without medical approval or justification, to change moods or emotions. Some foods contain chemicals that act as drugs. Some beverages contain drugs, examples being tea and coffee that contain the stimulant caffeine and alcoholic beverages.

## OBTAINING DRUGS

Until the 20th century, drugs were manufactured and sold freely, and many people bought and used traditional remedies without consulting a doctor. However, since the early 1900s, a series of food and drug laws have been passed in the US, placing drugs under the regulatory control of the Food and Drug Administration (FDA), which requires documentation that any new drug is both safe and effective. Drugs already in use when regulations come into force are assessed retrospectively, and those found to be unsafe or ineffective are ordered to be withdrawn from the market. Drugs are classified by the FDA into two broad groups – prescription and over-the-counter drugs. The FDA monitors both types of medications, although with different sets of regulations. Prescription drugs can be sold only by the order of a doctor in the form of a prescription. A patient takes the doctor's prescription to a pharmacist, who dispenses the medication. In some instances, doctors themselves dispense medications from their offices. Patient package inserts

**The role of the pharmacist**
*Pharmacists know the actions of drugs and their side effects. Many pharmacists keep computerized records of their customers' prescriptions. Thus, the pharmacist may alert you to the possibility of an interaction between drugs prescribed for you by different doctors.*

## WHICH SUBSTANCES ARE CONTROLLED?

The Controlled Substances Act of 1970 separates drugs that may be abused into five categories (called schedules) based on the use and biological effects of the drugs. Strict regulations for the use and supply of the drugs in each category are also established.

| | | Examples |
|---|---|---|
| Schedule 1 | Almost all the drugs in this category are illegal. All have a high potential for dependence and abuse, and it is illegal to have them in your possession. | Heroin, LSD, marijuana |
| Schedule 2 | These drugs are highly addictive but, despite that risk, they remain in medical use because no satisfactory nonaddictive alternative medication is available. Renewal of prescriptions is not allowed without a new prescription from your doctor. | Cocaine, amphetamines, morphine, some barbiturates |
| Schedule 3 | This category includes drugs that have some potential for abuse or dependence. Prescriptions can be renewed up to five times in 6 months if your doctor so authorizes. In some states, prescriptions phoned to the pharmacist by your doctor must be confirmed in writing. | Acetaminophen or aspirin with codeine, some appetite suppressants |
| Schedule 4 | These drugs are considered less likely to cause dependence or to be abused as much as the drugs in schedule 3, but the prescriptions are covered by the same regulations that govern schedule 3. | Diazepam, chloral hydrate, phenobarbital |
| Schedule 5 | These drugs are included in the regulations because they contain small amounts of narcotics. However, they are the least likely to be abused. | Some antidiarrheal medications and cough medicines |

### DRUGS OF ABUSE

Drug abuse is defined as any nonmedical use of drugs that causes physical, psychological, legal, economic, or social damage to the user or to people affected by the user's behavior. Abuse usually refers to illegal drugs but may also be applicable to drugs that are available legally, such as alcohol and nicotine, as well as some prescription medications. Addiction to drugs can also develop during the course of medical treatment, as occurs with some barbiturates. During the 1960s and 1970s many people became dependent on benzodiazepine tranquilizers. Because of this risk, doctors today are more cautious about prescribing any drugs that may cause dependence.

explaining the benefits and risks of the prescription drug are included with some medications. If you have any questions about your prescription medication, talk to your doctor or pharmacist.

Over-the-counter drugs are carefully evaluated by the FDA both for their effectiveness and for their safety for use by the public without the need for consulting a doctor. The FDA rules state that the labels on over-the-counter products must provide directions for safe use of the drug along with clear warnings about any possible side effects.

### Social attitudes

*Attitudes toward the nonmedicinal use of drugs vary from culture to culture. For example, consumption of alcohol is socially acceptable in some countries but illegal in others, while marijuana is illegal in most countries but acceptable in others. Attitudes also change over time, as evidenced by the growing antismoking movement against the public and private use of the drug nicotine.*

# THE DRUG CONTINUUM

All drugs may be considered in terms of their medicinal value and their potential for causing harm. Some drugs are effective medical treatments that have no apparent ill effects on the user, while others are not used as medication and may cause damage through abuse and addiction. These opposites are extremes, however, and other categories exist. Drugs cannot be easily categorized as "good" or "bad." Rather, they may be viewed as appearing on a continuum that reflects their medicinal value as well as their potential for causing harm.

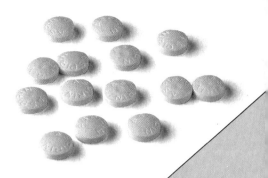

| ALWAYS USED MEDICALLY AND NEVER ABUSED | OFTEN USED MEDICALLY AND SOMETIMES ABUSED | SOMETIMES USED MEDICALLY AND FREQUENTLY ABUSED |
| --- | --- | --- |

### Antibiotics
*Used to treat infections caused by bacteria (below, magnified 9,000 times), antibiotics have no other effects that might lead to abuse (though they can be overused) and do not lead to dependence.*

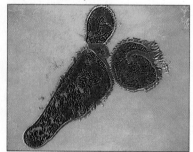

### Aluminum hydroxide
*This drug is widely used in antacids for the treatment of peptic ulcers and acid indigestion. The substance used alone may be constipating and is never abused.*

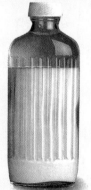

### Nonsteroidal anti-inflammatory drugs (NSAIDs)
*NSAIDs such as aspirin are painkillers and also reduce inflammation in joints and soft tissues. They have no other effects that might lead to abuse, but they are sometimes overused or used inappropriately.*

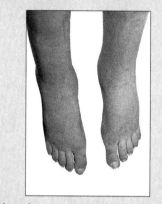

### Diuretics
*Diuretics are used to treat many conditions that can cause edema (above), including heart failure, kidney disorders, and cirrhosis of the liver. Because they help remove excess water from the body, diuretics are sometimes abused by jockeys and boxers to prevent weight gain and achieve rapid weight loss before a weigh-in.*

### Beta blockers
*Beta blockers are used primarily to treat heart disorders, but also to treat migraine and anxiety. Because these drugs reduce tremor and palpitations, beta blockers are occasionally abused by participants in activities that require a steady hand or voice.*

### Alcohol
*In medicine, alcohol is sometimes used as an antiseptic and a solvent. Consumption of alcoholic beverages may temporarily reduce anxiety, tension, and inhibitions. Alcohol becomes a drug of abuse when it is used to excess.*

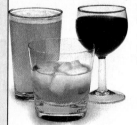

### Diazepam
*Diazepam, which may be the best known and most widely used benzodiazepine drug, is a tranquilizer mainly used to treat anxiety and insomnia. The drug is sometimes abused and is habit-forming.*

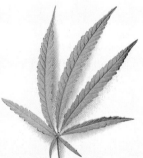

### Marijuana
*Marijuana comes from the plant Cannabis sativa (above); its active ingredient is called tetrahydrocannabinol (THC). In medicine, a synthetic derivative of THC is sometimes used to suppress the nausea and vomiting associated with cancer chemotherapy and radiation therapy. Marijuana is abused for its relaxing effects.*

### Caffeine

*In medicine, this stimulant is often combined with analgesic drugs to relieve pain, or with ergotamine to treat migraine headache. Used specifically in tablet form as a stimulant, it is often misused, especially by people attempting to reduce fatigue and drowsiness.*

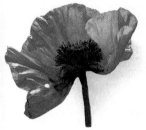

### Morphine

*Derived from the opium poppy, morphine is a potent painkiller used medically to relieve severe pain. Its euphoric properties can lead to abuse and an uncontrollable craving for the drug.*

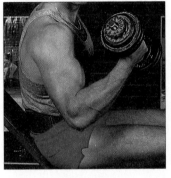

### Anabolic steroids

*Synthetic anabolic steroids increase muscle bulk. Even though their potential for serious adverse effects is well known, anabolic steroids are often abused by athletes such as football players, track stars, and weight lifters.*

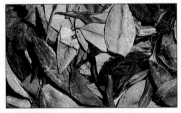

### Cocaine

*Extracted from the leaves of the coca plant, cocaine is used as a local anesthetic, primarily for minor surgical procedures. However, the drug is also widely abused in several forms as a stimulant.*

### Barbiturates

*Barbiturates are sedative drugs that are used medically as an anesthetic and to treat epilepsy and sleeplessness. Their use is strictly controlled, however, because there is a high risk of dependence.*

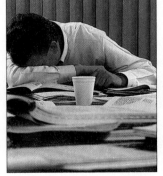

### Amphetamines

*These stimulant drugs were once commonly used to treat obesity because they suppress appetite. Many of the people who used amphetamines as appetite suppressants became addicted to these drugs. Amphetamines are now used medically only in the treatment of narcolepsy (abnormal sleepiness). Controversy surrounds the use of methylphenidate, a stimulant, in the treatment of attention disorders.*

### LSD

*LSD is a powerful hallucinogenic drug that was originally suggested for use in psychotherapy. However, the drug sometimes produces irreversible effects on the brain or psychotic paranoid reactions.*

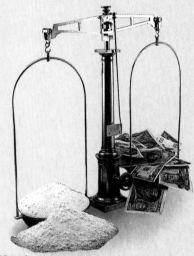

### Heroin

*Heroin is a narcotic synthesized from morphine. Heroin is the most potent, widely abused narcotic. Its use, after a level period of a few years, is once again increasing in the US.*

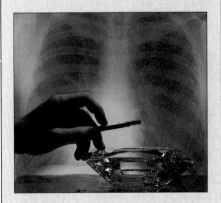

### Tobacco

*The drug nicotine in tobacco is highly addictive. In addition to having a calming effect, nicotine also decreases appetite or increases the body's metabolic rate. Any short-term desired effects of tobacco smoking are heavily outweighed by the damaging effects it has on many organs in the body.*

# DRUG LABELS AND COSTS

All drugs approved by the FDA for sale without a prescription must be packaged with a label that clearly explains the disorders for which the drug is recommended, precautions that should be followed, and possible adverse effects. The FDA approves the wording of these labels. In the event of any new information that requires a warning to consumers, it is mandatory that the label be modified.

In the case of prescription drugs, the FDA also approves the drug manufacturer's label (usually a package insert for doctors), which summarizes the results of research studies on the drug, warns about conditions for which it should not be prescribed, and lists adverse effects, interactions, and customary dosage ranges. The label is periodically revised and updated in light of new information obtained from clinical trials and reports.

The cost of a prescription drug can vary widely depending on the quantity prescribed and on pharmacy prices. Generally, the larger the quantity, the lower the unit price. Unless the doctor has marked the prescription "named drug only," the pharmacist may supply a generic alternative (see GENERIC AND BRAND NAMES, left). Some states permit even greater latitude in dealing with a prescription for a brand-name drug; "therapeutic substitution" allows the pharmacist to dispense a different drug than the one the doctor selected, primarily to lower drug costs to the patient.

## Generic substitution

The retail price of a generic drug is lower than the brand-name product. Your doctor does not always choose the less expensive alternative because, while the active ingredient may be the same, the two drugs are not necessarily identical in strength or in the form used to deliver the drug to the bloodstream (see GENERIC DRUGS AND BIOEQUIVALENCE on page 29). This can result in inadequate or excessive levels of the active drug reaching the bloodstream, thereby interfering with the desired therapeutic effect of the drug.

**Drug information for patients**
*The AMA recommends that for prescription drugs the label on the container should at least state the name of the drug, its strength, and how often you should take it. In 1982 the AMA began a drug information program and has now produced easy-to-read information sheets called patient package inserts for more than 100 commonly prescribed drugs. Each insert includes the action of the drug, its benefits, and any possible risks. Doctors can purchase the inserts to give to patients as supplements to any information that is discussed during the office visit.*

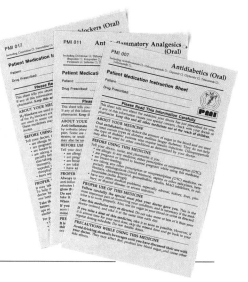

## GENERIC DRUGS AND BIOEQUIVALENCE

All generic drug manufacturers must prove to the FDA that the drugs they plan to sell are bioequivalent ("essentially similar" chemically in the body) to the original brand-name drug. The effect of a dose of drug given by mouth depends on how much of it is absorbed into the bloodstream and how quickly that absorption occurs. A variety of questions must be answered to ensure that the drugs are bioequivalent. The questions also apply to drugs that are injected.

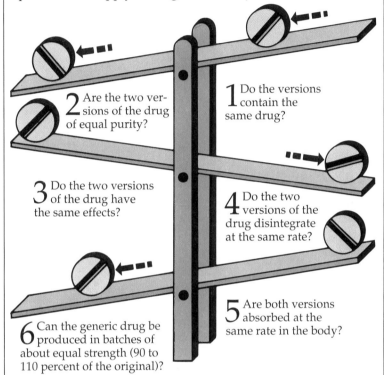

2 Are the two versions of the drug of equal purity?

1 Do the versions contain the same drug?

3 Do the two versions of the drug have the same effects?

4 Do the two versions of the drug disintegrate at the same rate?

5 Are both versions absorbed at the same rate in the body?

6 Can the generic drug be produced in batches of about equal strength (90 to 110 percent of the original)?

## Strict controls

In 1989, the FDA determined that some manufacturers of generic drugs were not following the specifications listed in their license applications. Extensive publicity highlighted examples of generic drugs that failed tests of bioequivalence (see box above). Also, in 1989, evidence of fraud was uncovered in applications for FDA approval of generic drugs. Some companies bribed FDA employees and substituted brand-name drugs for testing by the FDA. Dozens of generic drugs were removed from the market and the FDA began a program to inspect the generic drug industry. As a result, more doctors insist that pharmacists supply brand-name drugs.

## ASK YOUR DOCTOR
## PRESCRIPTION DRUGS

**Q** My doctor gave me a prescription for only a 2-month supply of my new oral contraceptive. Why can't she prescribe a year's supply of the pill and save me the cost of extra office visits?

**A** Doctors often prescribe only a limited amount of a drug at a time. This helps avoid waste if you need to change to another drug or if you lose your medication. Once you have adjusted to your new medication, your doctor may prescribe enough refills for 6 or 12 months.

**Q** Why is my new antibiotic so expensive? Don't the drug companies make huge profits?

**A** The major drug companies do make large profits but they maintain that some of the profit is reinvested in research. The development of a new drug may take 10 to 15 years and cost millions of dollars. In addition, there is no guarantee that production of a new drug will be profitable. Pharmaceutical companies are high-risk enterprises where failure is common but a successful product brings rich rewards.

**Q** I am soon moving to another country. My doctor prescribes thyroxine tablets for my underactive thyroid gland. How will I obtain my medication overseas?

**A** All developed countries have medical services that can provide you with any medication necessary to treat your condition. If you plan to move to a developing country make sure your medication is available there. If the drug is not available, ask your doctor how you can arrange to purchase it or if a different drug could be substituted.

# HOW DRUGS WORK

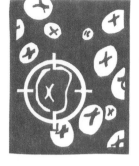

BECAUSE OF YEARS of research by doctors and scientists, we now know a great deal about the effects that drugs can have on the body. For example, we know that aspirin can relieve pain and that an antihistamine can help alleviate the symptoms of an allergy. However, we still have much more to learn about the mechanisms by which drugs produce these and other effects.

In the past 50 years, scientific knowledge has increased dramatically. Although the actions of some drugs have not yet been discovered, doctors today understand the manner in which drugs affect the body more completely than ever before. Most drugs act by subtly changing the activities of certain cells, tissues, or organs in the body. Some drugs act outside the cell, some act on receptors on the surface of the cell, and others act inside the cell, depressing or stimulating different physiological functions. The study of drugs is highly complex, because most drugs can have more than one action.

## DRUG ACTIONS AND DISEASE

To understand the many ways drugs can work in your body, consider the many purposes for which you may take drugs – from the relief of minor symptoms to the prevention and treatment of disease. Some drugs, such as antibiotics, destroy invading organisms. Drugs used to treat cancer (called cytotoxic drugs) work either by preventing reproduction of cancer cells or by killing the cancer cells directly. Biological drugs are

### THE PLACEBO EFFECT

In addition to the beneficial effect a drug provides through its action on the body, the effect of most drugs is enhanced by the patient's expectations that the drug will produce good results. This placebo effect ("placebo" is a Latin word meaning "I shall please") varies in intensity among individuals. The placebo effect may induce a desired effect or a variety of undesirable side effects.

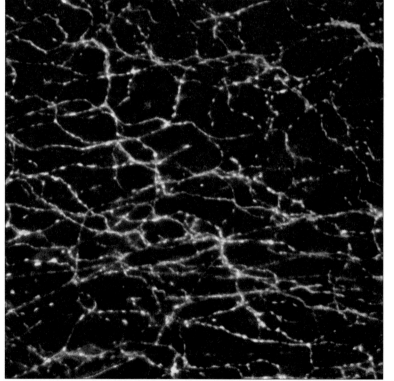

**Receptors**
*In this photograph (magnified 300 times), the fluorescent threads are nerve cell fibers, as revealed by a technique that shows the naturally occurring chemical norepinephrine (appearing to glow) coating the surfaces of the fibers. Norepinephrine attaches to receptors on the surface of the nerve cells and helps transmit their signals. One cell can have several different types of receptors on its surface. Each receptor has a link with a specific type of chemical. For example, histamine receptors respond only to histamine in the body. Drugs can be designed to bind to specific receptors to trigger or block their signals.*

derived from human tissue and are used to supplement or replace substances missing in the body. For example, factor VIII, made from human plasma, provides a clotting substance that reduces the bleeding tendency of hemophiliacs.

Other drugs change the course of a disease. For example, lipid-lowering drugs reduce the level of fatty substances such as cholesterol in the blood. Although these drugs work in different ways, they generally prevent the production of cholesterol in the liver or interfere with its reabsorption into the bloodstream from the intestine.

## Replacement of absent chemicals

To function, our bodies need adequate levels of certain chemicals, such as vitamins and minerals. A balanced diet usually supplies these, but deficiencies can occur during pregnancy or because of disease, problems with intestinal absorption of nutrients, or poor eating habits. The function of some drugs is to replace absent chemicals. For example, vitamin $B_{12}$ is given to patients who have pernicious anemia, a condition caused by the body's failure to absorb this vitamin. Other deficiency diseases occur because of lack of hormones, substances produced in glands that regulate the rate of chemical reactions in the body. For example, insulin-dependent diabetes mellitus, caused by inadequate production of the hormone insulin by the pancreas, is treated with injections of insulin.

## Interference with chemical processes

Many drugs act on receptors, which are found on the surface of cells throughout the body. Chemicals that occur naturally in the body, such as neurotransmitters (substances that transmit signals between nerves or between nerves and muscles), bind to receptors and trigger a response in the cell. Drugs can be given to increase or decrease the response.

## DRUGS AND RECEPTORS

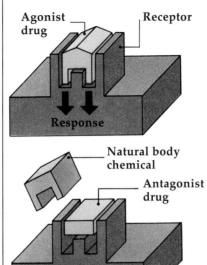

**Agonist drugs**
*Drugs that initiate the same response as a natural body chemical when they bind to a receptor are known as "mimics" or agonists. The action of such drugs is to enhance or restore a cell's normal activity.*

**Antagonist drugs**
*Some drugs stop a natural body chemical from reaching a receptor by occupying the receptor themselves, without causing any response. These drugs are called "blockers" or antagonists. Their action is to prevent or decrease cellular activity.*

**Partial agonist or partial antagonist drugs**
*Some drugs combine with a receptor to partially block or stimulate the action of natural body chemicals. These drugs, known as partial antagonists or partial agonists, are used to regulate a cell's activity.*

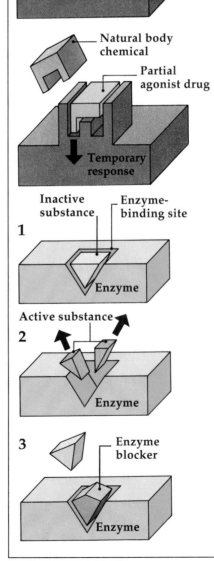

**Enzyme blockers**
*Enzymes, the group of proteins that regulates chemical processes in the body, have binding sites that can be used in drug treatment. Normally, when certain substances in the body combine with an enzyme-binding site, the substances are modified and become active (see 1 and 2). Some drugs are designed to block these sites and stop the activation of these substances (see 3).*

# ADVERSE DRUG EFFECTS

Almost all drugs have effects beyond their intended therapeutic actions. This is because most drugs have more than one action in the body and because of the unpredictability of each patient's response to a drug. There are two broad kinds of additional effects – side effects and adverse reactions.

## Side effects

The side effects of a drug are unwanted effects that can be predicted. They include any frequently experienced or infrequent but expected reactions. For example, an antihistamine such as diphenhydramine dries up a runny nose caused by hay fever but may also be expected to cause undesired effects such as drowsiness and clumsiness.

Sometimes a so-called "side effect" becomes a therapeutic effect. For example, narcotics cause constipation, so small doses of narcotics are sometimes prescribed to stop diarrhea.

Many side effects are temporary and may gradually disappear as the body becomes accustomed to the drug. If unpleasant side effects persist, your doctor may change the dosage or prescribe a different drug that has similar actions.

## Adverse reactions

An adverse drug reaction is an unexpected, unpredictable, and infrequent response that is potentially harmful and

## DRUG DISASTERS

Probably the most notorious drug disaster involved thalidomide, a sedative. Although thalidomide was never approved for use in the US, it was used in other countries to treat morning sickness and other symptoms in thousands of pregnant women. When more than 5,000 babies were born with limb deformities to women who had taken the drug while pregnant, thalidomide was quickly withdrawn from distribution. All new drugs are now rigorously screened for possible adverse effects. However, because drug testing cannot be performed on pregnant women, there is still a chance of a new drug harming a fetus.

Apparently valuable drugs have been withdrawn because they are found to have serious, unpredictable toxic effects. Public overreaction to the possible adverse effects of a drug can lead to a drug being banned. Another drug used to treat morning sickness was withdrawn in response to claims that babies had been born deformed because the mother had taken the drug during pregnancy. However, it has never been clearly proved that this drug was responsible for the deformities.

**The aftermath of thalidomide**
*The thalidomide disaster, which left thousands of babies throughout the world with limb deformities, starkly illuminated and brought to public consciousness the potential problems of taking drugs while pregnant. Today, most women do not take any drug during pregnancy without approval by their doctor.*

## THE THERAPEUTIC RANGE

The intended effects of any drug tend to increase as dosage is increased, but adverse effects increase as well. For example, the painkilling effects of acetaminophen increase with the dose but, above a certain dose, acetaminophen can cause serious liver damage. The goal of drug treatment is to achieve a concentration of medication in the body that lies between the minimum level that will produce a therapeutic effect and the maximum level above which toxic effects are more likely to occur. The difference between these levels is known as the therapeutic range of a drug.

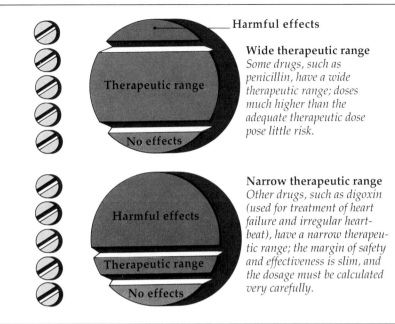

Harmful effects

**Wide therapeutic range**
*Some drugs, such as penicillin, have a wide therapeutic range; doses much higher than the adequate therapeutic dose pose little risk.*

**Narrow therapeutic range**
*Other drugs, such as digoxin (used for treatment of heart failure and irregular heartbeat), have a narrow therapeutic range; the margin of safety and effectiveness is slim, and the dosage must be calculated very carefully.*

not related to the usual effects of a drug. An adverse reaction can occur because of the amount of a drug that is taken, because a drug acts as a poison in the body, or because the patient is allergic to a drug. Common allergic reactions include a rash, painful joints, facial swelling, wheezing, or jaundice. Some people are genetically prone to experience adverse reactions to certain drugs. In most cases, however, the cause of an adverse reaction is unknown.

You should report adverse reactions to your doctor. He or she may change the dosage, or may tell you to stop taking the drug and start you on a different medication. On rare occasions, anaphylactic shock may occur; this life-threatening allergic reaction to a drug occurs when an extreme sensitivity has resulted from previous exposure to that drug.

## Risks versus benefits

Because an element of risk is associated with taking any drug, the most important consideration for you and your doctor is whether the benefits of a treatment outweigh the risks. This assessment depends on the likelihood or severity of the adverse effects of a drug, on whether effective alternative drugs are available, and on the severity of the disease being treated. For example, cancer treatments cause unpleasant side effects (such as hair loss, sores in the mouth, and severe vomiting) and dangerous side effects (such as suppression of bone marrow production). However, people endure these side effects because the disease itself is life-threatening.

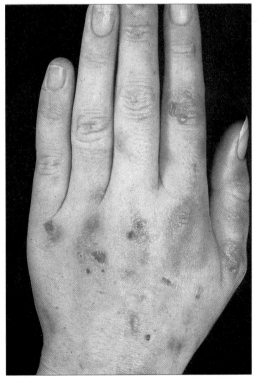

**Porphyria**
*The porphyrias are a group of uncommon inherited disorders. Use of some drugs, such as barbiturates, oral contraceptives, and tetracyclines, can cause acute attacks of porphyria in people with this genetic disorder. These attacks are characterized by symptoms such as abdominal pain, nervous system disturbances, and increased sensitivity of the skin to sunlight, which can lead to a rash and blistering (left).*

# COMMON SIDE EFFECTS OF DRUGS

It is not unusual for drugs to cause side effects. One recent study found that more than 40 percent of all patients experience some kind of unwanted reaction to the prescription drug they are taking. However, most side effects are not serious and are short-lived. Certain side effects are more commonly caused by specific drugs or groups of drugs. While some side effects are very common, others rarely occur.

### Drowsiness
Any drug that has a depressant effect on the brain can cause drowsiness. Examples include antidepressant drugs, tranquilizers, antihistamines, sleeping pills, narcotic painkillers such as codeine and morphine, antianxiety drugs, and anticonvulsant drugs.

### Osteoporosis
Osteoporosis, or bone thinning, can be caused by long-term use of corticosteroid drugs. A fracture (arrow) from a fall is a typical sign.

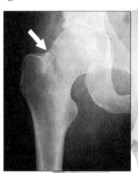

### Hives
Hives, or urticaria, is characterized by itchy wheals (raised white patches of skin surrounded by red inflamed skin) on the limbs and trunk. The condition is most commonly caused by an allergic reaction to drugs.

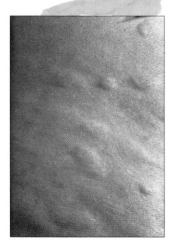

### Diarrhea
Many drugs can cause diarrhea. Classic examples are antibiotics and anti-cancer drugs, which can affect the lining of the intestines. Diarrhea is one of the most commonly experienced side effects of drug treatment.

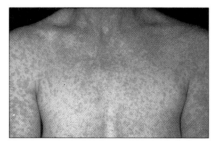

### Dizziness
Many drugs can cause dizziness. Some drugs, such as quinine, streptomycin, and aspirin, can affect the part of the inner ear that controls balance.

### Headache
Headache is a side effect associated with many drugs. Nitroglycerin, which is used to widen blood vessels in the heart, also widens blood vessels in the brain, causing a headache.

### Alopecia
Alopecia (loss of body hair, usually noticeable only on the scalp) is a common side effect of treatment with anticancer drugs.

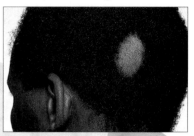

### Nausea and vomiting
Nausea and vomiting can be caused by a wide range of drugs. Opiates, anti-inflammatory drugs, antibiotics, anticancer drugs, and hormones can all cause nausea and vomiting.

### Rash
Any drug can cause a rash. This reaction may suggest an allergy to the drug (see ADVERSE DRUG EFFECTS on page 32). Anti-infective drugs, such as penicillin, ampicillin, and the sulfonamides, are often associated with a rash. A rash occurs in about 10 percent of people taking the drug captopril, which is used to treat high blood pressure and heart failure.

**Skin thinning**
Thinning of the skin is a common side effect of prolonged use of topical corticosteroids for rashes. The degree of thinning depends on the corticosteroid used, the strength of the preparation, and the duration of use. The skin can become so thin and fragile

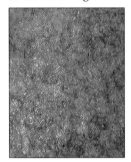

that small blood vessels can be seen just under the surface. A strong corticosteroid preparation can cause some skin thinning after only 2 weeks; a milder form used sparingly and infrequently is unlikely to produce thinning.

**Pruritus**
Pruritus, or itchy skin, may be associated with rash caused by an allergic reaction to a drug. Pruritus is also a common side effect of narcotic painkillers such as codeine.

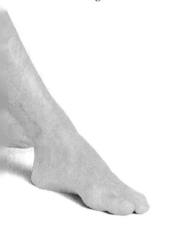

# UNUSUAL SIDE EFFECTS

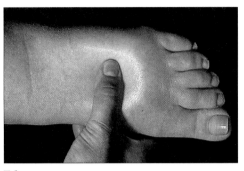

**Edema**
Edema is swelling of body tissues caused by retention of fluids. It occurs as an unusual side effect in people with heart failure who are taking beta blockers or some types of anti-inflammatory drugs.

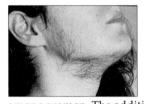

**Hirsutism**
Hirsutism is excessive growth of body and facial hair. It can occur in both sexes but is more common among women. The additional hair conforms to a male pattern of distribution (for example, on the face). Hirsutism can be a side effect of corticosteroid drugs, the anticonvulsant drug phenytoin, and the antihypertensive drug minoxidil.

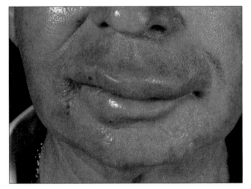

**Angioedema**
Angioedema is sudden swelling of the lips, face, neck, and sometimes the throat. It is accompanied by difficulty breathing, speaking, and swallowing. A common cause of angioedema is a food allergy. Angioedema may also result from an allergic reaction to a drug, insect sting, animal, or pollen or from emotional stress, exposure to cold, or an unknown cause.

**Gynecomastia**
Gynecomastia is abnormal breast development in men. It can be caused by drugs that mimic the actions of female sex hormones. However, it can also result from other treatments such as the antiulcer drug cimetidine, the diuretic spironolactone, or the drug digitalis, which is used to treat heart failure or irregular heartbeat.

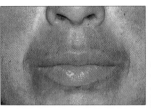

**Chloasma**
Chloasma (also called melasma) is a condition in which brown pigmentation of the skin appears on the face. Chloasma can occur in persons with chronic liver disease and in women taking oral contraceptives that contain estrogen. The condition is aggravated by exposure to sunlight. There is no treatment, but the pigmentation usually fades after women stop taking the estrogen-containing oral contraceptives.

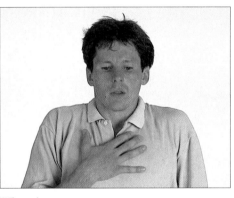

**Wheezing**
Wheezing, or difficulty breathing, is caused by narrowing of the bronchioles (small airways) in the lungs. Aspirin can cause wheezing in people who are allergic to the drug. Some beta blockers have a direct effect on the lungs, causing wheezing in people who have respiratory disorders.

**Dyskinesia**
Dyskinesias are disorders of muscle movement that can be caused by medications from several drug groups. Most notable of these are antipsychotic drugs. For example, haloperidol can cause tremor, a shuffling walk, and other symptoms similar to those of Parkinson's disease.

# DRUG INTERACTIONS

Some medications can interact with certain foods or with alcohol and other drugs to produce abnormal effects – either an increase or a decrease in the normal effects. These interactions can occur with prescription drugs, with over-the-counter medications, or with combinations of both. Always read the warning labels on over-the-counter drugs and discuss with your doctor any possible interactions of your prescription medications.

The most obvious type of drug interaction occurs when two drugs are prescribed to produce the same therapeutic effect. Your doctor may prescribe two drugs to increase their effectiveness, for example, in treatment with antibiotics.

However, drug interactions can produce unwanted or even harmful effects. Taking two drugs that have similar actions can cause death. For example, both alcohol and some sedative hypnotic drugs depress the activity of the central nervous system. Taking them together can cause breathing to cease. The main types of interactions are listed below.

## Inactivation

Some drugs, when taken at the same time, can inactivate, or neutralize, each other. This inactivation reduces the amount of active drug available for use in the body.

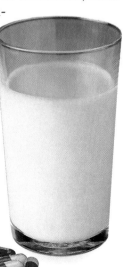

**Impaired tetracycline absorption**
*Drinking a half pint of milk within 1 hour before or 2 hours after taking an average dose of the antibiotic tetracycline will prevent the absorption of the drug almost completely.*

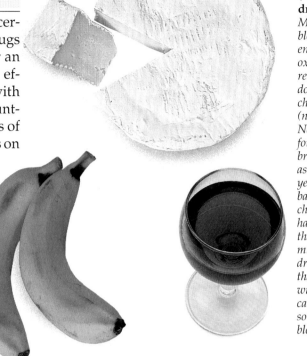

## Altered absorption

The rate of absorption of a drug can be altered in several different ways. Some drugs, such as alcohol, can change the rate at which the stomach empties its contents into the small intestine. This in turn can alter the rate of absorption of other drugs being taken.

Sometimes two drugs bind together in the stomach to form a substance that cannot be readily absorbed. The antibiotic tetracycline binds with iron, milk, and antacids in this way; therefore, tetracycline must be taken at least 1 hour before or 2 hours after consuming these substances or foods containing them. Some drugs can also modify the availability of other drugs by altering the bacteria found in the intestines. Antibiotics have this action and cause a decrease in the absorption of oral contraceptives.

## Metabolic effects

Many drugs are broken down, or metabolized, by enzymes in the liver. If two drugs that are metabolized in this way are taken together, they may compete for

**Monoamine oxidase (MAO) inhibitor drugs**
*MAO inhibitor drugs block the action of the enzyme monoamine oxidase, which is responsible for breaking down excitatory chemicals (neurotransmitters). Neurotransmitters are found naturally in the brain. Some foods such as cheese, red wine, yeast extracts, beer, and bananas contain a chemical (tyramine) that has an action similar to that of the neurotransmitters. MAO inhibitor drugs taken with foods that contain tyramine or with certain drugs can cause a severe and sometimes fatal rise in blood pressure.*

**Reduced absorption in the intestine**
*Absorption of a drug can be reduced if the drug combines with a food molecule or another drug in the intestine.*

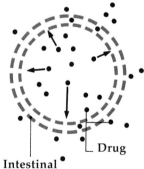

Drug

Intestinal wall

**Food molecule or another drug**

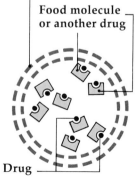

Drug

## PROTEIN BINDING

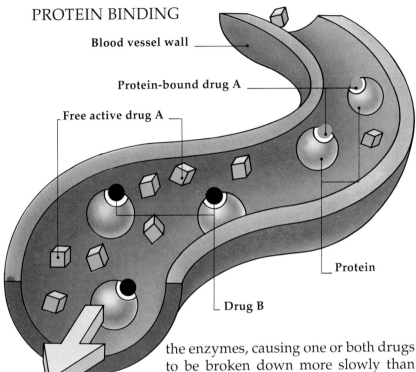

Blood vessel wall

Protein-bound drug A

Free active drug A

Protein

Drug B

**How protein binding is reduced**
*A portion of most drugs becomes bound to a protein in the blood, making that portion of the drug inactive. If one such drug (drug A) is taken and then another (drug B) is taken, drug B can displace some of drug A from the protein so that more of drug A is free to be active. For example, a portion of the anticoagulant warfarin is bound to protein but can be readily displaced by many commonly used anti-inflammatory drugs. This is potentially very dangerous because the amount of unbound (active) warfarin in the blood must be carefully regulated to prevent abnormal bleeding.*

the enzymes, causing one or both drugs to be broken down more slowly than usual. Some drugs can affect the production of enzymes in the liver, which interferes with the rate at which other drugs are activated or inactivated.

Another type of metabolic interaction can occur when a drug works by blocking an enzyme reaction elsewhere in the body. The monoamine oxidase inhibitor drugs, which are used to treat depression, are enzyme inhibitors and can cause serious or fatal reactions when taken with certain foods or other medications such as meperidine, a narcotic.

## Reduced excretion

The kidney's ability to excrete a drug (such as penicillin) can be blocked by another drug, causing the blocked drug to stay in the body for a longer time.

## Receptor effects

If two drugs that act at the same receptor sites are taken together, the effects of the drugs can be enhanced or one drug can block the other's action. For example, naloxone, the drug given to reverse the effects of a narcotics overdose, blocks the receptor sites used by narcotics and prevents the narcotics from working.

## ASK YOUR DOCTOR SIDE EFFECTS AND INTERACTIONS

**Q** My doctor has prescribed the antibiotic metronidazole for an infection I have. Can I drink alcohol when I'm taking this drug?

**A** No. Drinking alcohol while you are taking metronidazole can cause dangerous reactions. When combined with alcohol, metronidazole has effects that are similar to those of disulfiram, the drug given to alcoholics to help prevent them from drinking. These effects include flushing, an increased heart rate, severe headache, dizziness, nausea, and vomiting.

**Q** I take iron tablets every day for my anemia. I bought some nonprescription medicine for indigestion today but the label on the bottle says that I should not take it with iron tablets. Why not?

**A** Many indigestion remedies contain salts that react with iron to form insoluble substances. These substances cannot be absorbed from the intestines so your iron tablets are ineffective if you take an antacid at the same time.

**Q** Can I take vitamin and mineral supplements while I undergo kidney dialysis?

**A** You should avoid taking vitamin and mineral supplements or any medications unless you have consulted your doctor. People with kidney disease have higher-than-normal levels of vitamin A and some minerals and do not readily excrete certain substances. These substances thus can reach toxic levels in the bloodstream.

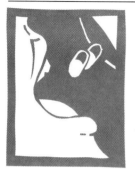

# HOW DRUGS ARE ADMINISTERED

D RUGS CAN BE GIVEN in different forms, including tablets, drops, creams, lotions, ointments, suppositories, or injectable liquids, and in different ways. The route chosen depends on factors such as the severity of the illness, the part of the body being treated, and the properties of the drug being administered.

In the past, most drugs were taken by mouth or given by injection. In recent years, however, other types of administration have been increasingly used.

## ROUTES OF ADMINISTRATION

Some of the most important routes of administration are discussed here.

## Oral administration

The majority of drugs are still taken by mouth because it is often the most acceptable, convenient, and cost-effective way to use a drug. However, drugs taken by mouth must be absorbed from the digestive tract and processed by the liver before they reach the bloodstream. Thus, oral preparations are not generally used when a rapid effect is needed. One exception is sublingual tablets, which are placed under the tongue. The drug is absorbed through the lining of the mouth and passes directly into the circulation.

## Topical application

Topical preparations – the most common forms being ointments, creams, lotions, or drops – are used to treat such disorders as inflammation or infection of the skin, ears, and eyes. Topical drugs are applied directly to the affected area.

More and more people are taking drugs in suppository form. The advantage of taking a medication in suppository form is that irritation of the stomach can be avoided. Suppositories can be used to treat irritation and infection of the vagina or rectum. Rectal suppositories are also used for administering drugs that are destroyed by the stomach's acid or digestive enzymes or if vomiting is likely to occur and thus prevent absorption of the drug into the bloodstream.

## Inhalation

Substances in sprays, aerosols, powders, or gaseous forms are readily absorbed in the lungs and nasal passages. Gases used to produce general anesthesia and drugs used to treat conditions such as asthma and hay fever are often given by inhalation through the nose and mouth.

**Injections**
*There are four common types of injection (see below). Drugs can also be injected into body cavities and into the spinal canal. Injections are given to produce a rapid effect, the intravenous route being the fastest.. Sometimes depot injections are given into a muscle. With a depot injection, the drug is injected in a relatively insoluble form and is released slowly into the body.*

**Intradermal**
Into the skin

**Intravenous**
Into a vein

**Intramuscular**
Into a muscle

**Subcutaneous**
Under the skin

# NOVEL METHODS OF DRUG DELIVERY

Several new methods of administering drugs have been developed in recent years (see below). These new methods provide drug dosages that are delivered more evenly and more accurately.

## TARGETING DRUGS

Targeting where a drug will go in the body is particularly useful in the treatment of hormonal disorders and cancer, conditions for which it is important to deliver drugs to specific sites. A variety of carriers that are related to substances produced naturally in the body have been developed. These drug carriers include monoclonal antibodies (artificially produced antibodies that attach to receptors on tumor cells), a patient's own blood cells, and liposomes (artificial structures similar to cell membranes that enclose the drug between their layers). It may also be possible to combine metal particles with a drug that can then be injected and directed to specific sites using external magnets.

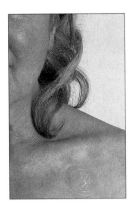

### SLOW RELEASE

Many of the new methods are designed to deliver a drug by slow release, by delayed release, or in regulated doses. These systems of drug administration have several advantages over conventional drug formulations. They are more convenient (one dose can supply the drug continuously over several hours or even days) and they can reduce the risk of adverse reactions and overdose because the dose entering the bloodstream is better controlled.

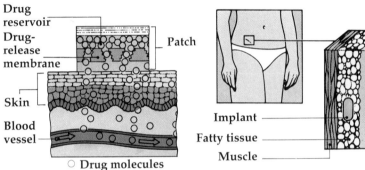

Drug reservoir
Drug-release membrane
Patch
Skin
Blood vessel
○ Drug molecules
Implant
Fatty tissue
Muscle

**Skin patches**
*Adhesive drug-containing patches (shown above in cross section) adhere to the skin. The drug passes through the skin slowly and is absorbed into the bloodstream. An antiangina drug, hormone replacement therapy, a local anesthetic, and a drug for motion sickness are available in skin patch form.*

**Implants**
*Pellets containing a drug can be surgically implanted under the skin. Implanted pellets are used to deliver a drug (usually a hormone) over long periods of time.*

**Monoclonal antibodies**
*Anticancer drugs are highly toxic to healthy cells. Such drugs can be attached to monoclonal antibodies. These antibodies are copies (made in a laboratory) of molecules naturally produced by the body's immune system. The monoclonal antibodies are designed to attach to the receptors of specific cancer cells but not to healthy cells.*

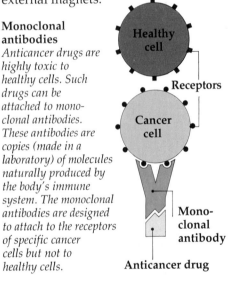

Healthy cell
Receptors
Cancer cell
Monoclonal antibody
Anticancer drug

**The eye system**
*There is now a slow-release system for treatments of the eye that can deliver a drug over a full week. The device, consisting of two membranes enclosing a drug, is inserted into the eye like a contact lens.*

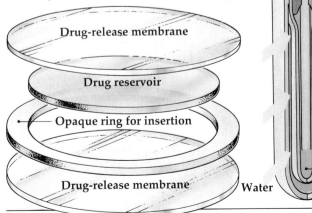

Drug-release membrane
Drug reservoir
Opaque ring for insertion
Drug-release membrane

Modulator

**The minipump**
*The minipump is implanted under the skin; as water from surrounding tissues moves in through the minipump's outer membrane, the drug solution is forced out through a modulator, delivering the drug (or hormone) over a period of 1 to 4 weeks.*

Outer membrane
Drug solution
Water   Water

**Slow-release tablets and capsules**
*Technological developments have resulted in a number of sophisticated slow-release systems. In slow-release capsules, the drug is enclosed in tiny coated balls. The physical and chemical characteristics of the coatings determine how quickly the drug is released.*

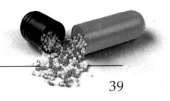

# DRUG FORMULATIONS

Drugs can be given in many forms. Most drugs are specially formulated so that they are easy and convenient to take to ensure that people have little difficulty taking their medication. Sometimes formulations contain inactive ingredients (those with no therapeutic effect), such as stabilizers or flavorings, as well as the drug. Some formulations contain dyes that may cause allergic reactions. Here are some of the most common formulations.

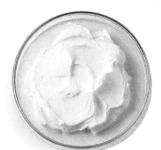

## TABLETS

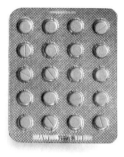

**Tablets** contain a fixed amount of powdered drug compressed or molded by machine into a solid form. Some inactive ingredients are usually added (see WHAT'S IN A TABLET? on page 41).

## CAPSULES

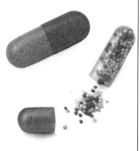

**Capsules** are made of a gelatin shell, with the drug in powdered form inside. The drug is usually mixed with an inactive filler. Sometimes the drug is formulated into tiny slow-release balls (see NOVEL METHODS OF DRUG DELIVERY on page 39).

## LIQUIDS

**Liquids** are a common form for some medications. The drug is combined with inactive ingredients, such as preservatives, dyes, flavoring agents, or stabilizers.

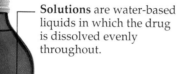

**Solutions** are water-based liquids in which the drug is dissolved evenly throughout.

**Elixirs** are sweetened, aromatic solutions of a drug; they often contain a large amount of alcohol, sugar, and flavoring.

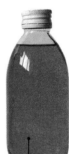

**Emulsions** are mixtures of two liquids that do not mix naturally (such as oil and water), with the drug dispersed throughout both liquids. An emulsifying agent – used to stabilize the suspension of one liquid in the other – is often included.

**Suspensions** are water-based liquids containing an undissolved drug. Suspensions must be well mixed to distribute the drug.

**Mixtures** are liquids containing several drugs that are dissolved or diffused in water or another solvent.

## TOPICAL PREPARATIONS

There are several different preparations for application to the skin or to other surfaces of the body. Most preparations include preservatives to minimize bacterial growth.

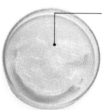

**Ointments** are semi-solid preparations based on substances such as petroleum jelly. Ointments can be used to deliver a drug or to protect dry skin.

**Pastes** are similar to, but firmer than, ointments and contain a high proportion of powder. They are useful in the treatment of skin problems such as leg ulcers or to protect healing skin.

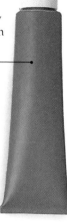

**Creams** are emulsions of water in oil (aqueous cream) or oil in water (oily cream). In addition to being used as a vehicle to "carry" a drug, creams are also used to soothe or moisten the skin.

**Lotions** are solutions or suspensions of a drug used to bathe and cool the skin.

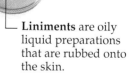

**Liniments** are oily liquid preparations that are rubbed onto the skin.

**Shake lotions** cool by evaporation, leaving an inert powder behind. An example is calamine lotion.

## INHALERS

**Inhalers** are used to deliver a drug via the nasal passages or by inhalation through the mouth. Aerosol inhalers contain solid or liquid drug particles under pressure. When released, the drug is suspended in a fine mist. Other types include dry-powder inhalers and nasal sprays that contain the drug in solution.

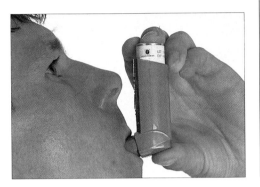

## EAR AND EYE DROPS

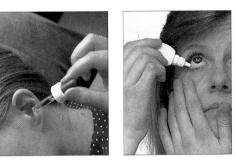

**Drops** are sterile solutions or suspensions of a drug that are introduced into the eye or the ear by dropper.

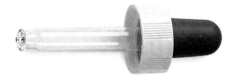

## SUPPOSITORIES

**Suppositories** are medicated bullet-shaped solids that dissolve after insertion into the rectum or vagina.

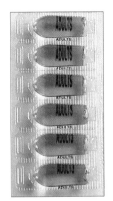

## WHAT'S IN A TABLET?

The active drug is only part of a tablet. Other ingredients are included to hold the ingredients together, to make the tablet easier to swallow, and to ensure the drug is released in the correct part of the digestive system to produce the desired effect.

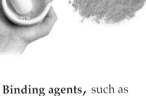

**Binding agents,** such as acacia, gelatin, glucose, or sucrose, to hold ingredients together.

**Bulking agents or diluents,** such as sucrose, lactose, or sodium chloride, to give bulk to a tablet.

**Granulating agents** to make particle size uniform.

**Drug**

**Disintegrating agents,** such as starch, cocoa butter, or sodium bicarbonate, to help the tablet break up and release the drug in the intestines.

**Coatings** such as sugar to conceal taste or a special coating to delay disintegration in the stomach and absorption by the body.

**Lubricants,** such as magnesium stearate or purified talc, to make a tablet easier to swallow.

# DRUG DOSAGE AND METABOLISM

When a drug enters the body, it goes through several stages before and after it exerts its effect. The study of the processes a drug moves through in the body is called pharmacokinetics. The first stage is absorption into the bloodstream; the second is distribution throughout the body; the third is metabolism, or utilization and then breakdown; and the fourth is elimination from the body.

## Absorption

The time it takes for a drug to work after you take it depends on its absorption characteristics – the rate at which the drug passes from the intestines into the bloodstream and the amount of the drug that passes into the bloodstream. If a drug is injected directly into the bloodstream, it bypasses the absorption stage and is said to have been completely absorbed. However, when a drug is taken by mouth, absorption depends on the form in which the drug is taken, how efficiently the intestine can process the drug, and whether other drugs or food are present. Absorption rates vary a great deal from person to person. Some drugs, such as certain resins used in the treatment of high cholesterol, are insoluble and cannot be absorbed into the bloodstream. Such cholesterol-reducing drugs combine with cholesterol-carrying bile salts in the intestine and are excreted.

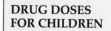

## DRUG DOSES FOR CHILDREN

Because children have a smaller body mass than adults, smaller drug doses are given. For some drugs, the dosage for a child is calculated by taking the child's weight as a percentage of a standard adult's weight and reducing the dosage by the same proportion. As an alternative, body surface area may be used to calculate a child's dosage.

## HOW A DRUG PASSES THROUGH THE BODY

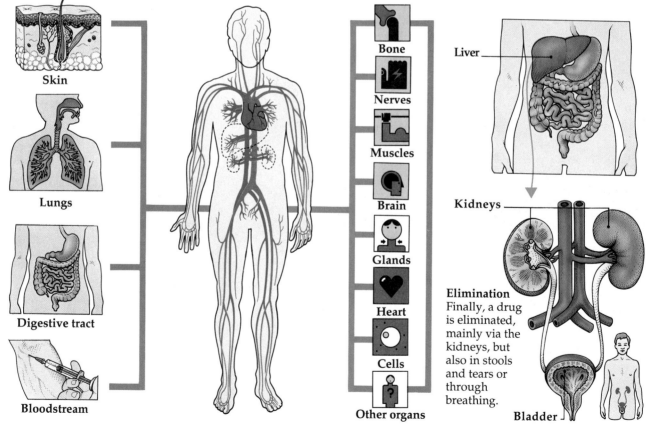

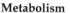

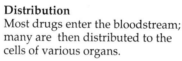

**Absorption**
The site at which a drug enters the body affects its rate of absorption.

Skin

Lungs

Digestive tract

Bloodstream

**Distribution**
Most drugs enter the bloodstream; many are then distributed to the cells of various organs.

Bone

Nerves

Muscles

Brain

Glands

Heart

Cells

Other organs

**Metabolism**
A drug is partially broken down, usually in the liver, before or after distribution.

Liver

Kidneys

**Elimination**
Finally, a drug is eliminated, mainly via the kidneys, but also in stools and tears or through breathing.

Bladder

## Distribution

Once a drug has been absorbed into the bloodstream, the drug is distributed to the rest of the body. Some drugs pass through the entire body, moving out of the blood into the tissue spaces, across the protective chemical "fence" around the brain called the blood-brain barrier, and even – in pregnant women – across the placenta into the fetus. Having entered the body's tissues, some drugs may enter body cells. Your doctor considers the distribution properties of a drug when prescribing your medication. For example, the older antihistamine drugs cross the blood-brain barrier to cause unwanted drowsiness. Newer antihistamines have been developed that do not pass into the brain, so they can be used to treat allergy symptoms without also causing drowsiness.

## Metabolism

Drug metabolism is the breakdown of a drug within the body to another chemical. This conversion usually occurs in the liver and often results in inactivation of the drug. The liver is a vital part of the body's natural defense mechanism that works to rid the body of a foreign substance. Many drugs must be metabolized before they can be eliminated from the body. Occasionally, however, a drug is given in an inactive form as a pro-drug (a precursor of a drug) and is converted to its active form after absorption by the liver. This process can be useful with drugs such as dopamine that cannot be absorbed from the gastrointestinal tract in their active form or that are harmful to the stomach.

## Elimination

Most drugs and their breakdown products are excreted in the urine. Small amounts of a drug may be excreted in breast milk, saliva, sweat, tears, or feces or via the lungs. Drugs excreted in feces are those that are never absorbed and those eliminated by the liver.

### THE "FIRST-PASS" EFFECT

Most drugs taken by mouth are absorbed through the wall of the small intestine into the bloodstream. Once the drug enters the bloodstream, it passes via the portal vein to the liver before reaching the rest of the body through the general circulation. Many drugs are broken down in the liver so that only a part of the amount absorbed reaches the rest of the body. This is called the "first-pass" effect. A drug such as nitroglycerin, if it is swallowed, may be broken down so much by this first-pass effect that it would be virtually inactive. This is why other formulations for various drugs have been developed, such as tablets that dissolve under the tongue, skin patches, suppositories, and implants (see NOVEL METHODS OF DRUG DELIVERY on page 39 and DRUG FORMULATIONS on page 40). The newer methods of delivery allow the drug to be absorbed directly into the general circulation via the skin, the lining of the mouth, or the lining of the rectum, rather than to pass first through the liver.

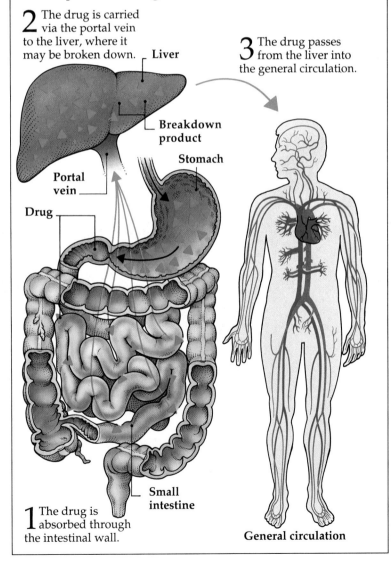

2 The drug is carried via the portal vein to the liver, where it may be broken down.

**Liver**

3 The drug passes from the liver into the general circulation.

**Breakdown product**

**Stomach**

**Portal vein**

**Drug**

1 The drug is absorbed through the intestinal wall.

**Small intestine**

**General circulation**

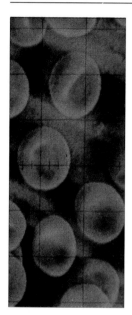

**An inherited disorder**
*G6PD deficiency is an inherited disorder that affects the chemistry of red blood cells. This deficiency makes these blood cells vulnerable to damage caused by some medications such as sulfa drugs (antibacterials) and antimalarial drugs. It is most common among blacks, affecting about 15 percent of the black male population in the US.*

# INDIVIDUAL DRUG RESPONSES

In addition to the drug interactions and the side effects and adverse reactions that may occur, several other factors may influence the overall effects that a drug has on your body.

## Personal factors

Your age, weight, and health and any nutritional problems you may have can change the manner in which a drug is broken down and used by your body. Kidney disease can change drug absorption, distribution, metabolism, and elimination. Liver, lung, and heart disease can all reduce the rate at which some drugs are broken down and eliminated. Gastrointestinal problems may affect drug absorption, and both pregnancy and obesity may impair drug metabolism, distribution, and elimination.

## Genetic and racial factors

Genetic and racial factors can also influence the way in which a drug is broken down and used by the body. People of Far Eastern ancestry are more susceptible to the effects of alcohol because they have a genetic deficiency of the enzyme that metabolizes alcohol. Blacks seem to be more resistant to the actions of beta-blocker drugs used to treat high blood pressure and generally need higher doses of these drugs or a different medication.

## Psychological factors

Scientists believe that psychological factors may play a part in drug response. Some people think a drug given by injection is more powerful than the same drug given orally. Their response to a drug may be influenced by the placebo effect (see THE PLACEBO EFFECT on page 30).

## Other factors

The time at which you take a drug can be important because biological rhythms in the body can affect the activity of some drugs such as aspirin and corticosteroids. However, apparently similar people sometimes respond differently to a drug; this phenomenon is called idiopathic (unexplained) variation. There are major differences in how the body uses drugs that cannot be explained by age, race, or environment. Therefore, while a standard drug dosage is used to start treatment, drug dosages are then tailored to the response of each individual. Your doctor will ask about your symptoms, examine you for changing signs of illness, and measure the levels of the drug in your blood.

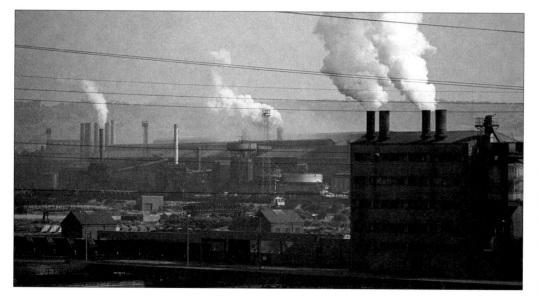

**Environmental factors**
*Even environmental factors such as air pollution can influence drug response, as can exposure to glues, solvents, and other chemicals. Some pollutants stimulate certain enzymes to break down drugs (for example, the painkiller pentazocine) faster.*

# CASE HISTORY
## DECREASING DRUG EFFECTIVENESS

ERNEST HAS BEEN experiencing chest pains during exertion. About 6 months ago he went to see his doctor, who sent him for an exercise stress test. The doctor diagnosed Ernest's chest pains as angina and prescribed nitroglycerin tablets, to be taken as soon as he felt the pain and as often as necessary. About a month ago, Ernest noticed that, although the attacks were not occurring more frequently, one tablet seemed to relieve his ...ncerned about his angina ...on, Ernest made an ...ment with his doctor.

**...RSONAL DETAILS**
...ne Ernest Jones
...e 55
...upation Carpenter
...ily Father died of a heart ...ck at 55. Mother has high ...d pressure, diabetes, and ...ina.

**...E DIAGNOSIS**
...results of the second stress test ...w no major changes since the ...inal test. The doctor explains to

Ernest that his problem is a result of DRUG TOLERANCE. Ernest's doctor tells him that the drug tolerance has developed because his body has become less sensitive to the actions of the nitroglycerin. When drug tolerance occurs, an increased dosage of the drug is necessary to produce the original, prompt, full effect.

Ernest's doctor tells him that tolerance to nitrate drugs usually wears off once use of the drug is stopped. One option would be to replace Ernest's nitroglycerin with another type of drug that produces the same effect, such as the calcium channel blocker nifedipine. Alternatively, Ernest's doctor could prescribe another nitrate, isosorbide dinitrate, the effects of which last longer than some of the other nitrates.

**THE OUTCOME**
The doctor prescribes isosorbide dinitrate because nitrates have been effective for Ernest. His doctor tells him that the calcium channel blocker drug nifedipine may be added to Ernest's treatment in the future if his condition worsens.

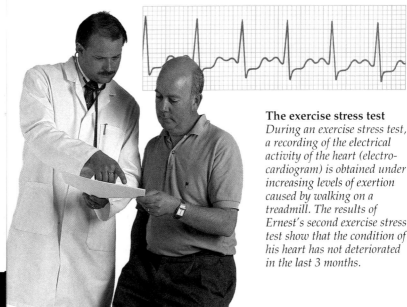

**The exercise stress test**
*During an exercise stress test, a recording of the electrical activity of the heart (electrocardiogram) is obtained under increasing levels of exertion caused by walking on a treadmill. The results of Ernest's second exercise stress test show that the condition of his heart has not deteriorated in the last 3 months.*

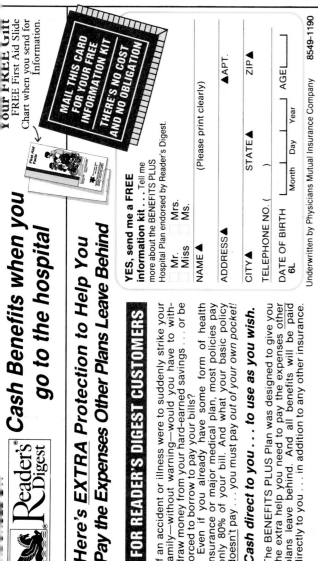

# CHAPTER THREE

# USING DRUGS WISELY

WHETHER THEY ARE prescribed by your doctor, purchased over-the-counter, or consumed in the form of alcohol, drugs are all around us. However, the fact that drugs are so familiar should not lead us to forget that all drugs are powerful substances that cause changes in the body, some of which can be harmful or even fatal in certain circumstances. This chapter discusses the importance of using all drugs with care, both to receive maximum benefit and to protect yourself from any possible harm.

The first section explains why there is much more to a course of drug treatment than simply purchasing the drug from your pharmacist. For the best results, you should talk to your doctor about your medication – what time of day it should be taken, the correct dosage, the prescribed frequency of doses, and possible side effects. It is vital that you

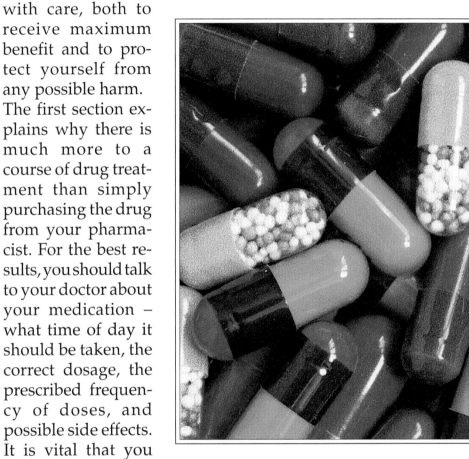

communicate openly and clearly with your doctor; your medical history may have an important bearing on the drug that he or she prescribes. Prompt reporting of adverse reactions and unexpected side effects helps your doctor to make adjustments in your treatment, such as a change in medication. Although all drugs in the US are manufactured to rigorous safety standards, many medications have recognized side effects,

and you must be prepared for them. The second section outlines the side effects that can be expected to occur when you take certain drugs and describes how you and your doctor can work together to keep any adverse reactions to a minimum. We discuss the effect that one drug might have on another. We list a variety of drugs that interact with other drugs to increase or decrease their effect or to result in yet another drug action. Medication must be stored correctly to prevent loss of potency. The third section describes storage techniques for drugs and how to safely dispose of any leftover or outdated medications.

Any woman who is planning a pregnancy must be very careful about every drug she takes. The fourth section contains important information for the mother-to-be. Most drugs pass from the woman to the fetus via the placenta or to the infant via the mother's breast milk. A doctor should approve all medications that a woman takes during pregnancy or while breast-feeding to prevent harm to the fetus or infant. Drugs of abuse are a threat to child and adult alike. The fifth section lists the drugs that carry a risk of physical and/or psychological dependence. The last section offers tips on assembling a medical kit for the individual or family about to take a trip.

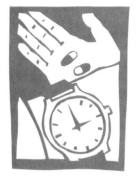

# FOLLOWING YOUR PRESCRIPTION

TAKING THE DRUG YOUR DOCTOR prescribes in the manner suggested is called compliance. Reasons for noncompliance include failure to understand instructions and a fear of possible side effects. If you do not take your medication as instructed, the drug's effectiveness may be decreased, your medical condition may worsen, or unpleasant or harmful effects may occur.

To receive maximum benefit from your medication and to reduce the chance of experiencing an adverse reaction, you must talk to your doctor to learn how to use your medication correctly.

## EXCHANGING INFORMATION

Make sure your doctor tells you the brand name and generic name of the drug being prescribed and what symptom or disorder the drug is being prescribed to treat. For other information you should know about your medication, see WHAT SHOULD I ASK MY DOCTOR? on page 52. Your doctor may ask you questions about your medical history. Tell him or her about any previous unpleasant side effects you have had when taking a drug. Also, be sure you tell your doctor about allergies that you have; allergies can affect the way a drug works. Do not take any nonprescription remedies when you are taking prescription drugs unless you have discussed with your doctor the possible interactions of these remedies (see ADVERSE DRUG INTERACTIONS on page 58).

### WARNING

A single extra dose of most types of drugs is unlikely to cause any adverse effects. In some cases, the effect of the drug may intensify temporarily. However, exceeding the recommended dose can be dangerous with some types of drugs such as anticonvulsants. If an overdose has been taken, or a child has accidentally taken a drug, call a poison control center, an emergency room, or your doctor immediately. If you are instructed to induce vomiting, you may be advised to use syrup of ipecac. To avoid choking and inhalation of vomit, make sure the person leans far forward before vomiting begins. Do not induce vomiting in a person who is drowsy or unconscious.

**Avoid mixing drugs**
*If you are taking any nonprescription medications, make sure you tell your doctor. Nonprescription medications may affect the way a prescription drug works.*

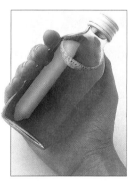

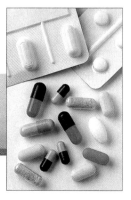

## Missing a dose

If you miss one dose of a drug, the amount of drug in your body is temporarily reduced; the importance of this reduction is in part dependent on the illness or disorder being treated by the medication and the actions of the medication you are taking. Call your doctor for instructions about taking the missed dose. For most medications, as long as the time when you take your medication varies by only a few hours, there is usually no harm done. However, missing just one dose of some drugs can have serious consequences (for example, insulin treatment for diabetes). For some drugs you are directed to take a missed dose as soon as you remember; for others, you can wait for the next scheduled dose.

**Risk of pregnancy**
*Any woman who misses a dose of a progestin-only contraceptive pill has an increased risk of pregnancy if she does not use additional methods of contraception for the next 14 days, even if she takes the pill as soon as she remembers.*

## USING MEDICATIONS SAFELY

### WHAT YOU SHOULD DO

 Take the recommended dose and follow the timing schedule closely. If the drug is making you sick, call your doctor.

 Always take the full treatment course of your medication even if you start to feel better or your symptoms disappear.

 Consult your doctor if you think your medication is not working, but remember that it may take a few days for the drug to have a noticeable beneficial effect.

 If the medication you are taking is a drug in the form of a liquid suspension, you must shake the medication thoroughly before taking each dose. This will ensure that the ingredients are uniformly distributed; otherwise your dosage will vary with how evenly the drug is distributed in the liquid.

 If your medication is a tablet or capsule, drink some water before taking the medication to help moisten your esophagus. Swallow the tablet or capsule with plenty of water and don't take it while lying down. These measures reduce the chance of the tablet or capsule getting stuck in your esophagus and causing a chemical burn.

### WHAT YOU SHOULD NOT DO

 Never take more than the recommended dose unless your doctor tells you to. A larger dose won't make the drug work any better or quicker and may cause adverse reactions.

 With rare exceptions, don't stop taking a drug without checking with your doctor, even if you notice side effects. Use of some drugs must be stopped gradually with tapered doses to prevent withdrawal symptoms or a recurrence of the condition.

 To avoid taking an accidental overdose, do not take any medication in the dark, and do not keep medications by your bed. It is easy for someone half-asleep to take an extra dose mistakenly or even take the wrong drug.

 Do not break up a capsule to make it easier to swallow. Doing so could have an effect on the way in which the drug is absorbed. Some tablets can and should be broken to vary the dosage but always ask your doctor first.

 Don't take a drug that was prescribed for someone else, even if you think you have the same symptoms. The drug may be inappropriate for your symptoms or could even cause a dangerous adverse reaction.

# AIDS TO COMPLIANCE

Many people want to comply with their prescribed drug treatment but may not receive clear, accurate, and complete instructions or cannot remember these instructions. There are several methods to help you follow your doctor's instructions. If you need to take different drugs at different times of the day, you can prepare a chart and check off each dose as you take it. This reduces your risk of taking the same dose twice or missing a dose. Other people may benefit from medication organizers. These containers are designed to help the person remember to take the medication or to help someone who has several different medical conditions and thus is taking several drugs.

**Medication organizers**
*For people taking medications, containers are available that consist of a series of small compartments into which a full day's or week's supply of pills and tablets is placed. Each compartment can then be labeled with the day and/or the time of day that the drug should be taken.*

**Measuring liquids**
*Always use a measuring spoon, measuring cup, or dropper to measure the correct dose; a household teaspoon cannot provide an accurate dose.*

**Special packaging**
*Blind people can ask their pharmacist for special labels or bottles of different shapes for their drugs, enabling them to differentiate one medication from another.*

## Pill cutters
*For some medications, the correct dose is less than a whole tablet. Special cutting devices can be used to divide pills into the appropriate amounts.*

## Pill crushers
*People who are not able to swallow whole tablets can buy pill crushers to pulverize their tablets.*

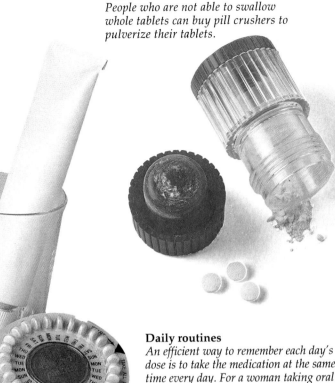

## Easy-open lids and caps
*For people with arthritis, specially designed lids and caps are available to make containers easier to open.*

## Labeled blister packs
*Some packages, such as those for oral contraceptives, are marked with the days of the week so that you can tell whether you have taken your dose each day.*

## Daily routines
*An efficient way to remember each day's dose is to take the medication at the same time every day. For a woman taking oral contraceptives, the easiest time may be first thing in the morning, with the pill package kept in the bathroom (near a toothbrush, for example).*

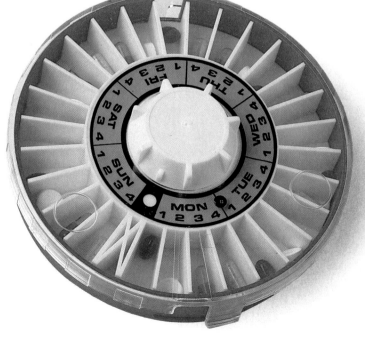

## Pill dials
*Containers are available with a dial that moves forward to release one pill at a time, helping to ensure that the correct dosage is taken each day.*

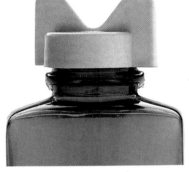

## Warning labels
*Warning labels may be placed on your medication. These labels provide a variety of information and are usually brightly colored and illustrated with simple symbols. If you have any questions about a warning label, ask your pharmacist or doctor.*

# WHAT SHOULD I ASK MY DOCTOR?

Lack of information is one of the most common reasons for failing to take a drug properly. Other reasons include forgetfulness, fear of taking drugs, the cost of the drug, and side effects of and adverse reactions to a drug. Whenever your doctor writes a prescription for you, there are several things you should know. Some questions can be answered by reading the medication's label and package insert. However, feel free to ask your doctor any questions you have about your new medication.

| | QUESTION | WHY YOU NEED TO ASK |
|---|---|---|
| | How soon will the drug start working? | If you do not know when you may start to feel the effects of the drug, you may think that the medication is not working and may be tempted to increase the dosage or stop taking the drug. This can be dangerous. |
| | How should I take the drug? | This is important to know because different forms of drugs work differently. For example, you need to dissolve some types of tablets in your mouth rather than swallow them. If you do not take the medication correctly, it may not be effective, or it may even have an adverse effect. |
| | Do I have to wake up at night to take my medication? | Timing of doses influences the effectiveness of your medication. In most cases, "once daily" can be at any time, but should be at about the same hour each day. "Twice daily" means approximately every 12 hours. If "four times a day" is specified, ask your doctor if you should wake up during the night to take your medicine. |
| | Can I take all three of my medications at the same time? | If you are taking several different drugs, ask your doctor if you can take them at the same time, or if they must be taken several hours apart. Some drugs interfere with the absorption of others. |
| | Should I take the drug after eating? | Food and liquids can make some medications less effective by reducing the amount of drug that is absorbed into the bloodstream; for these medications, you must take the drug at least 1 hour before eating. Other drugs must be taken with or after a meal to reduce the risk of stomach irritation. |
| | When I am taking the drug, do I need to avoid any other medications or foods? | Some drugs and other substances can have adverse interactions if taken simultaneously (see page 58). For example, fruit juices reduce the effectiveness of some antibiotics by breaking them down in the stomach. You should avoid drinking alcohol while taking most drugs. |
| | Do I need to take the full course of treatment? | If you are taking an antibiotic, the infection may return and the bacteria may become resistant if you stop taking the drug before you are supposed to. However, for other drugs it may be acceptable to discontinue treatment as soon as you feel better. Always ask your doctor before you stop taking any drug in advance of the end of the scheduled treatment course. |
| | Are there likely to be any side effects and what should I do if there are? | Any drug, even aspirin, can cause an adverse reaction in some people. Ask your doctor about expected side effects and possible adverse reactions that can be caused by your medication. If your medication makes you feel dizzy or drowsy, do not drive, operate machinery, or climb ladders. You should report any unexpected side effects to your doctor. |
| | Can I use the drug safely over a prolonged period of time? | With some drugs there is a possibility of complications with long-term use. For example, some antibiotics, especially when taken for prolonged periods, may result in overgrowth of yeast in the mouth, vagina, or bowel or in infection of the gastrointestinal tract. |

# CASE HISTORY
## AN INCOMPLETE COURSE OF ANTIBIOTICS

CAROL FELT THE URGE to urinate every 10 minutes, and she felt a burning pain each time she urinated. Rather than make an appointment with her doctor, Carol decided to take some antibiotics that she had left over from a recent urinary tract infection. Her urinary symptoms cleared up. However, a few days later, Carol awoke with shaking chills, a fever, and a severe pain on the right side of her back. She decided to call her doctor.

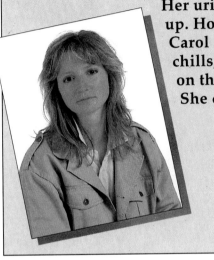

**PERSONAL DETAILS**
**Name** Carol Brown
**Age** 27
**Occupation** Stage technician
**Family** Carol's mother suffers from stress incontinence.

### MEDICAL BACKGROUND
Carol has had two urinary tract infections during the last 12 months. Aside from these infections, she has had no other medical problems.

### THE CONSULTATION
Carol tells her doctor that, since she called to make her appointment, she has started to feel nauseated and has vomited twice. She tells him that she had taken leftover antibiotics from her previous urinary tract infection. While examining her, the doctor finds an area over the right side of her back that Carol indicates is tender. Her temperature is very high (102°F). Carol is asked to provide a specimen of urine for urinalysis and culture for bacteria and other microorganisms.

### THE DIAGNOSIS
The pain and tenderness in Carol's back and her high fever, along with Carol's history of urinary tract infections, suggest a diagnosis of acute PYELONEPHRITIS – inflammation of a kidney due to a bacterial infection. This infection has spread into her right kidney because of an incomplete course of antibiotic treatment of the previous infection.

### THE TREATMENT
The doctor prescribes a new course of antibiotic treatment for Carol and instructs her to take all the medication, even though her symptoms may disappear in a few days. The doctor administers the first dose of antibiotics by injection. He advises Carol to drink large amounts of water and to take aspirin or acetaminophen every 4 hours as needed to control her fever and ease pain. Within 24 hours, Carol's temperature returns to normal and the right side of her back feels much less tender.

### THE OUTLOOK
The laboratory analysis of Carol's urine sample shows a few red and numerous white blood cells and a trace of protein. This is what doctors call a "nonspecific finding," which means that it supports the doctor's diagnosis but does not confirm it. Carol's doctor discusses with her the necessity of taking a full course of antibiotics and offers advice on how to help prevent a recurrence of the infections. He tells her to drink plenty of water, urinate often, and wipe herself properly after a bowel movement (women should always wipe from front to back). Carol's doctor also informs her that pyelonephritis can be very serious if not treated promptly; he tells her that she may now be more susceptible to recurrent infections and that she should call him immediately if she experiences a recurrence of any symptoms. Carol's doctor asks her to return in a month to have the urinalysis and the urine culture repeated to make certain that the current infection has been cured. Carol assures her doctor that she will take all the medication and will make the follow-up appointment.

**The spread of bacteria**
*Carol's incomplete course of antibiotics was inadequate to kill all the bacteria causing her infection. Although her symptoms had subsided, the surviving bacteria continued to multiply and the infection spread into her right kidney.*

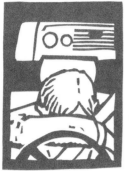

# DEALING WITH SIDE EFFECTS

W HEN YOUR DOCTOR prescribes a new drug, ask him or her which side effects to watch for and what to do if they occur. Not all side effects develop within the first few days of taking a new drug. During long-term treatment, some side effects can occur months, or even years, after use of the drug was started. Occasionally, side effects appear after treatment has ended.

**Dizziness or drowsiness**
*Always discuss the possible side effects of your medication with your doctor. Some side effects may be safely ignored while others may be a warning of a dangerous reaction that requires you to stop taking the drug immediately. If a drug causes dizziness or drowsiness, do not drive, operate machinery, or work on an elevated site.*

Many drugs have predictable side effects. Some side effects represent "too much" of the intended effect and are relatively harmless (for example, a tranquilizer may make you sleepy). Other side effects may be more serious, such as hives or a rash (caused by an allergy) or poisoning of the liver or kidneys. If you experience any new or unusual symptoms during treatment, do not stop taking the drug (the result of this action may be worse than the side effects). Report

the problem to your doctor immediately. Reporting unusual symptoms is especially important if you are taking a drug that has been on the market for only a short time; your symptoms may represent previously unknown side effects.

## PREVENTING SIDE EFFECTS

As scientists have learned more about the ways in which drugs work, it has become possible to predict many of the more common side effects and to reduce the risk and severity of an unwanted reaction during treatment. Before starting a new drug, tell your doctor about any allergic or unusual response you

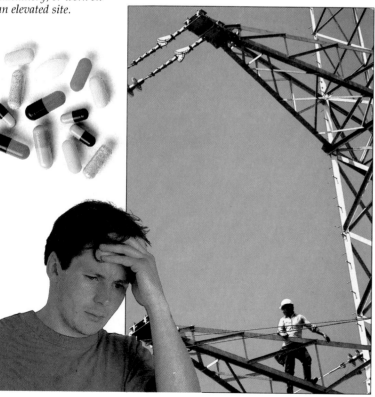

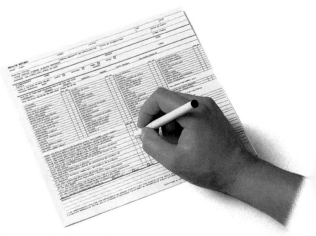

**Your medical records**
*Your doctor asks questions about your medical history and habits to ensure that the safest and most effective drug is chosen for your treatment.*

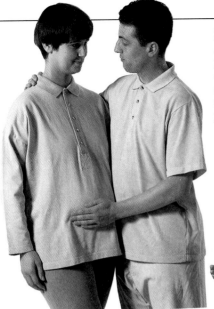

**Drugs and pregnancy**
*If you are breast-feeding, pregnant, or planning to conceive, tell your doctor. Some drugs can have a harmful effect on your fetus or infant (see pages 64 to 66).*

**Sensitivity to sunlight**
*During treatment with drugs that cause increased sensitivity to sunlight, such as phenothiazines (used to suppress vomiting or to treat mental illness) or tetracyclines (antibiotic drugs), restrict the time you spend in the sun and use a sunscreen on any exposed areas of skin. If you are taking these drugs, excessive exposure to the sun can lead to a severe sunburn.*

have had to drugs you have taken in the past. This ensures that you will not be given the same product or any chemically similar substance. You should keep a record of all drugs (including vaccines) to which anyone in your family has experienced an adverse reaction. Remember, too, that some drug preparations can be inappropriate for people on special diets or people who have certain medical disorders. For example, a diabetic may need a sugar-free formulation of a particular product. In addition, if you are allergic to certain food additives or preservatives, do not take a medication that contains that substance as an ingredient.

## SPECIAL PRECAUTIONS

Follow all precautions your doctor has told you to observe while taking a drug (see captions above). Do not exceed the recommended dosage of a drug unless an increase has been discussed with and approved by your doctor. Ask your doctor about any likely interaction between and among prescription drugs or nonprescription drugs you may be taking. Also ask your doctor about possible interactions that your medication may have with food or alcohol. Interactions may reduce the effectiveness of the treatment and also cause serious adverse reactions (see page 58).

## COMMON SIDE EFFECTS

Predictable side effects are reactions to a drug that can be expected to occur because of the way the drug works on different body tissues. Side effects are inevitable for most types of drugs. Some of the common side effects for several different drug groups are listed below.

| DRUG GROUP | COMMON SIDE EFFECTS |
|---|---|
| Angiotensin-converting enzyme (ACE) inhibitors | Dizziness, dry mouth, vomiting, cough, rash |
| Antibiotics | Diarrhea, thrush (a fungal infection, often in the vagina), rash |
| Anticholinergic drugs | Blurred vision, dry mouth, retention of urine |
| Antidepressants | Drowsiness, dry mouth, blurred vision, constipation |
| Antihistamines | Dizziness, drowsiness, clumsiness |
| Barbiturates | Dizziness, drowsiness, clumsiness |
| Benzodiazepines | Dizziness, drowsiness |
| Beta blockers | Wheezing, cold hands and feet, impotence |
| Cytotoxic anticancer drugs | Hair loss, diarrhea, vomiting, sores in the mouth |
| Narcotic analgesics | Constipation, nausea, vomiting, drowsiness |
| Nonsteroidal anti-inflammatory drugs (NSAIDs) | Indigestion, nausea, diarrhea, black bowel movements |
| Thiazide diuretics | Sensitivity to light, impotence |
| Vasodilators | Dizziness, fainting, ankle swelling |

## HAVING YOUR TREATMENT MONITORED

If you are taking a drug regularly for longer than a couple of weeks, or you are prescribed a drug that you have not previously taken, your doctor may want you to return for periodic checkups to monitor your drug treatment.

### Monitoring for effectiveness

First, your doctor will want to assess your response to the drug you are taking. For example, if you are undergoing treatment with antihypertensive drugs, your blood pressure will be measured at each appointment to ensure that it is under control. If the blood pressure readings remain abnormally high, you may need a higher dose of the drug, an additional medication, or a different type of drug treatment. The effectiveness of many drugs is evaluated in terms of both how well your symptoms respond and how much

**Specific tests**
*If you are taking antibacterial drugs to treat a serious infection, such as pneumonia, your doctor will perform a physical examination and take a chest X-ray to monitor your recovery. An inadequate response to drug treatment requires reevaluation of the diagnosis or a change to other antibacterial drugs.*

the results of one or several specific tests change. For diabetes, the success of drug treatment is primarily reflected in how well the blood sugar level is controlled. There may also be a demonstrable effect on your symptoms, such as a decrease in thirst and excessive urination. Your doctor may recommend that you measure your urine and blood sugar levels at home, in addition to undergoing medical supervision, to provide the most effective control of your diabetes.

### Monitoring for side effects

Another important reason for monitoring drug therapy is to find out if you are experiencing any adverse effects. Some drugs may cause complications that do not produce obvious symptoms at first,

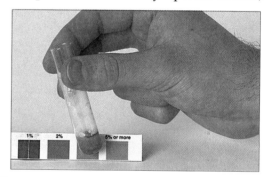

**Self testing**
*In addition to regular appointments with their doctors, people who have diabetes are usually asked to participate in their own care by keeping a record of their condition and treatment. This can be done by measuring the level of sugar in the urine and/or the blood on a day-to-day basis using a special testing kit.*

so inform your doctor at each appointment whether you have any new symptoms. Examples of such drugs include gold compounds and penicillamine, used in the treatment of rheumatoid arthritis; propylthiouracil, used to treat overactivity of the thyroid gland; and carbamazepine, which is an anticonvulsant used in the treatment of seizures.

Both gold compounds and penicillamine may cause kidney damage and affect blood cell production by the bone marrow; therefore, blood counts and urinalyses are done frequently during treatment. Propylthiouracil can impair the body's immune system by reducing the production of white blood cells by the bone marrow, so blood counts are performed regularly. In addition, a sore throat or mouth ulcer may indicate a serious drop in the white blood cell count. Because carbamazepine can damage the liver and bone marrow, blood tests are recommended periodically. If these tests uncover an abnormality that has been caused by the drug, a different anticonvulsant drug is substituted. In most cases,

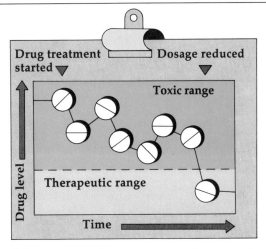

this reverses the process and prevents serious or permanent damage.

The blood levels of other drugs, such as theophylline, digoxin, and phenytoin, are periodically monitored by your doctor. Most people respond best to these drugs when the drug concentrations in the blood and other body fluids are within a specific range (called the therapeutic range). When levels are above this range, the person is more vulnerable to toxic effects of the drug; when the levels fall below the range the person is less likely to be responding optimally to the drug.

**Blood tests**
*If your doctor is uncertain about the most effective dosage of a drug for your condition, a blood test may be taken shortly after you start your treatment to measure the level of drug that is actually reaching your bloodstream. The dosage may then be increased or decreased, depending on whether the level is below or above the amount required to produce the best therapeutic effect. This form of monitoring is usually needed for only a few drugs. In most cases the drug dosage is calculated on the basis of previous studies in which the drug was used by many other patients; subsequently the dosage may be adjusted according to your response to the drug.*

**Charting drug effectiveness**
*The treatment of asthma with bronchodilators is evaluated in part by measuring the patient's ability to exhale forcibly after a deep inhalation. The dosage of drugs used in the treatment of arthritis is sometimes adjusted as a result of measuring the patient's grip strength or the time the patient needs to walk a measured distance. Eye drops for glaucoma are regulated by measuring the pressure of the fluid inside the eye (see right).*

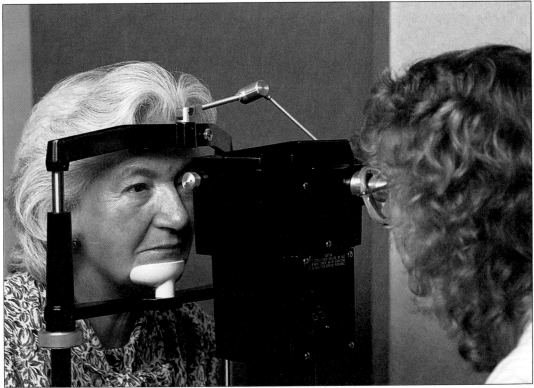

## ADVERSE DRUG INTERACTIONS

Before you take a new drug, your doctor will want to make sure that the drug will not interact negatively with any medication you are already taking or other substances you might consume. Because small amounts of a drug may remain in your body for several weeks after you have stopped taking the drug, tell your doctor about all medications you have taken in the past several months.

### Nonprescription drugs

Interactions can occur not only between prescription drugs but also between a prescription drug and another substance. Seemingly harmless over-the-counter remedies, including laxatives, antacids, painkillers, and vitamins, can interfere with a normal response to a drug. Alcohol, nicotine, caffeine, and some foods can also interact with medications to produce unwanted, harmful, or life-threatening reactions. Ask your doctor or pharmacist for a list of substances to avoid while you are taking a particular drug. Before purchasing an over-the-counter medication, ask your doctor or pharmacist about potential interaction with your current prescription drug. Many pharmacies have computerized records of each customer's prescription drugs. The pharmacist is thus able to check your prescription medications for potential interactions with any over-the-counter drug you plan to use.

### Mention your medication

If you are seeing more than one doctor, always keep each doctor informed about any drugs that the others have prescribed for you. If you are taking medication that is known to have a life-threatening interaction with other drugs or if you know you have an allergic reaction to a drug, you should wear or carry some form of drug alert in case you need emergency treatment for an illness or injury.

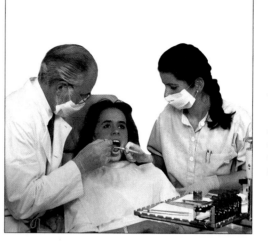

**Drugs before surgery**
*If you are having any kind of surgery, including dental procedures, tell the surgeon, anesthesiologist, or dentist which medications you have been taking. Some drugs increase the risk of abnormal bleeding or interact with anesthetic drugs.*

## COMMON DRUG INTERACTIONS

Several drugs are known to interact with specific substances and cause potentially serious consequences.

| SUBSTANCES | INTERACTIVE SUBSTANCES | CONSEQUENCES |
|---|---|---|
| Hypoglycemic drugs used to lower the blood sugar level of diabetics | Alcohol or sulfonamide antibacterial drugs | Further lowering of blood sugar level and risk of hypoglycemia |
| Depressants of the central nervous system (e.g., sleeping pills, narcotic analgesics, antihistamines, and alcohol) | Any of the central nervous system depressants listed at left | Dangerous oversedation and respiratory failure |
| Anticoagulants | Aspirin, nonsteroidal anti-inflammatory drugs, alcohol, or antibiotics | Increased anticoagulant effect and risk of abnormal bleeding |
| Certain types of tetracycline antibiotics | Iron supplements, milk, or antacids | Reduced effectiveness of antibiotics if taken within 1 hour before or 2 hours after the antibiotics |
| Oral contraceptives | Barbiturates or some types of antibiotics | Reduced effectiveness of contraceptive and increased risk of pregnancy |
| Monoamine oxidase inhibitor antidepressants | Meperidine, decongestants, amphetamines, cheese, bananas, red wine, beer, yeast extract, or chocolate | Dangerous rise in blood pressure and risk of seizures or brain hemorrhage |

# CASE HISTORY
## SELF-MEDICATION FOR FLU SYMPTOMS

MARTHA HAD A SORE THROAT with a fever for several days. Aches and pains then developed all over her body. When the glands in her neck became swollen, Martha thought she had the flu. She began taking a variety of nonprescription medications from the medicine cabinet. However, she started to feel worse instead of better. After Martha complained of a splitting headache and became very weak and drowsy, her mother called for an ambulance.

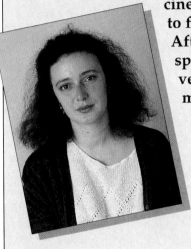

**PERSONAL DETAILS**
**Name** Martha Andrews
**Age** 19
**Occupation** College student
**Family** Parents are in good health.

## MEDICAL BACKGROUND
Martha had an appendectomy at age 11 and an operation to remove her tonsils at age 14. Other than these operations, she has seen a doctor only for school checkups.

## IN THE EMERGENCY ROOM
Martha has lapsed into unconsciousness upon arrival at the hospital, but her breathing is normal and her heartbeat and pulse rate are stable. A doctor in the emergency room checks Martha's neurological functions; Martha does not respond when the doctor talks to her, but she has normal reflex reactions to painful stimuli. Martha's mother tells the doctor the names of the flu medications that Martha has been taking. Martha has also been taking two tablets of acetaminophen every 4 hours for her muscle and joint pain and, just recently, for her headache. Blood samples are taken to establish the level of acetaminophen in Martha's body and to check the function of her liver, which could be damaged by excessive amounts of acetaminophen.

## THE DIAGNOSIS
The doctor concludes that Martha lost consciousness as the result of an OVERDOSE OF ACETAMINOPHEN caused by taking several medications simultaneously, all of which contained acetaminophen. The doctor explains to Martha's mother that taking several multiple-ingredient medications at the same time can accidentally lead to drug overdose if the medications contain the same ingredient.

## THE TREATMENT
The results of the blood tests confirm a dangerously toxic level of acetaminophen, but Martha's liver function is normal. Her stomach is pumped to remove any acetaminophen that was taken over the last few hours that has not yet passed beyond her stomach. An intravenous infusion of the drug acetylcysteine is started. Acetylcysteine reduces the production of toxic substances that occurs during the breakdown of acetaminophen. Martha is kept at the hospital for observation.

## THE RECOVERY PERIOD
Martha slowly regains consciousness over the next 24 hours. Blood tests show a steady decrease in the level of acetaminophen but, on the second day in the hospital, the blood tests also indicate that her liver function is deteriorating. After 4 days her liver function improves and soon she is ready to leave the hospital. Martha's doctor tells her that she was very lucky because liver failure caused by an overdose of acetaminophen can be fatal if not treated within a few hours of the overdose.

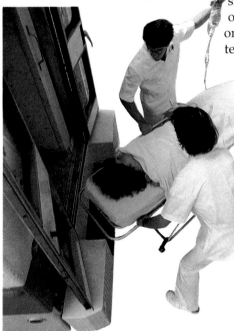

**A disturbing discovery**
*Looking in on her daughter, Martha's mother was frightened to find that Martha seemed very weak and drowsy and complained of a severe headache. She immediately called an ambulance.*

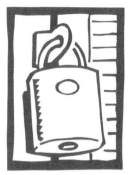

# DRUG STORAGE AND DISPOSAL

IN YOUR HOME you probably have a variety of remedies for common problems such as headaches, indigestion, diarrhea, and ñasal congestion. Also, someone in your family may be taking a prescription drug, either on a regular basis or to treat a short-term illness. It is important to know how to store the drugs in your home safely and how to dispose of any medications that have passed their expiration date or are no longer needed.

**Drugs and children**
*All medications should be kept out of the reach of children. Children easily mistake drugs for candy; accidental poisoning or death can result.*

All drugs should be stored in an easily remembered place, but always out of the reach of children. Purses and briefcases are among the worst places to "hide" drugs from children. If you are worried that you will forget to take a dose, write yourself a note or leave an empty medicine container out as a reminder. Medication organizers that have a series of small compartments can be filled once a week or daily and carried with you.

## STORING YOUR MEDICATIONS

It is important that a drug be stored under conditions that ensure its effectiveness; if improperly stored the drug can become inactive or toxic. If you have any questions, ask your pharmacist or doctor. Illustrated here are a few tips on proper storage.

**Close lids and caps**
*Keep the lid of the medicine container tightly closed to keep the medication fresh and to prevent spilling if the drug is a liquid. Childproof caps are required by law for many types of medications that are taken orally.*

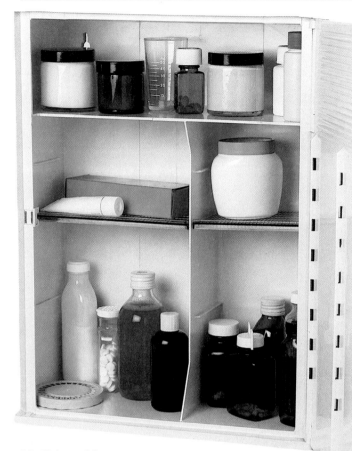

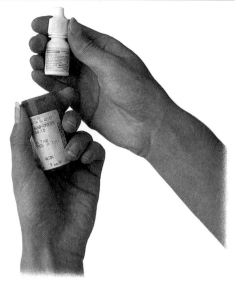

## Appropriate containers
*Drugs should always be stored in their original containers so that you can review the label for directions for use. Your pharmacist may place eye drops (shown above) in a container large enough to hold the instruction label.*

## Medicine cabinet
*The best place to store drugs is in a wall cabinet that is out of the reach of children. Most drugs should be kept at room temperature in a dark, dry place. Some drugs should not be kept in the bathroom because a warm, humid atmosphere may cause them to lose their effectiveness.*

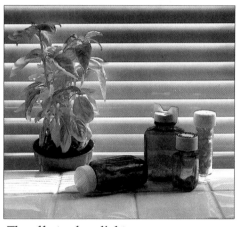

## The effects of sunlight
*Drugs should be kept away from direct sunlight, even when they are in a darkened container. Sunlight can cause a drug to deteriorate, resulting in a loss of effectiveness.*

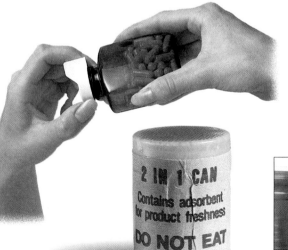

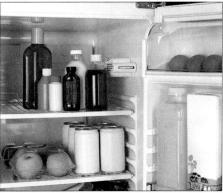

## Refrigerated drugs
*Some drugs need to be stored in the refrigerator, but you should never let them freeze.*

## Desiccants
*If a medication is particularly susceptible to the effect of moisture, your pharmacist may place a drying material (desiccant) inside the container to absorb any moisture. Don't swallow it by mistake.*

## DRUG DISPOSAL

As a rule, you should have used up your entire prescription after you have completed the treatment period recommended by your doctor. However, you may have a small amount of your prescription drug left over. Dispose of all leftover drugs. Flushing them down the toilet is a safe and convenient way to ensure that children will not find the drugs and mistake them for candy. Safely disposing of leftover drugs also prevents other family members from taking them, perhaps because they think that they have the same symptoms as you. The medication could be inappropriate or even harmful to others (see USING MEDICATIONS SAFELY on page 49).

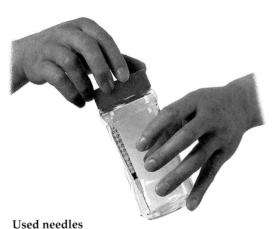

**Used needles**
*If you inject yourself with a drug, such as insulin for diabetes, ask your doctor or pharmacist for suggestions on how to safely dispose of your used needles and syringes.*

## WHEN TO DISPOSE OF DRUGS

The following signs should prompt you to throw away drugs:

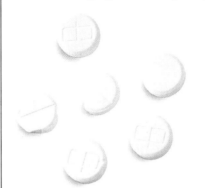

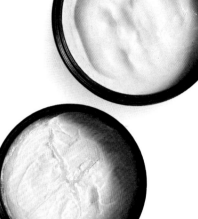

◆ Tablets or capsules are more than 2 years old or are chipped, cracked, powdery, or discolored.

◆ An ointment or cream is hardened, discolored, or separated.

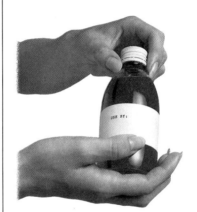

◆ The expiration date has passed.

◆ Do not refrigerate your medication unless instructed to do so by your pharmacist.

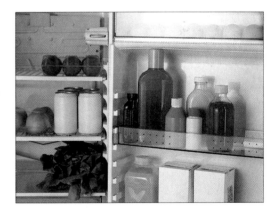

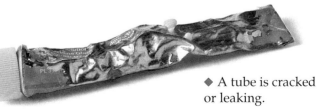

◆ A tube is cracked or leaking.

◆ Capsules are softened, cracked, or stuck together.

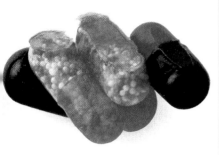

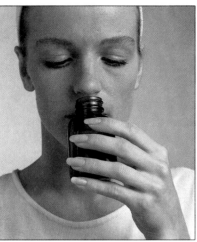

◆ The odor of a medication has changed (for example, aspirin tablets begin to smell of vinegar).

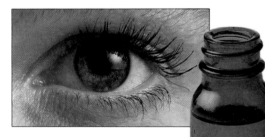

◆ A bottle of eye drops has been opened for more than 28 days (there is a risk of contamination).

◆ A liquid is thickened or discolored.

## ASK YOUR DOCTOR
## DRUG STORAGE AND DISPOSAL

**Q** I take nitroglycerin tablets for my angina, but my doctor says that I must dispose of any leftover tablets every few weeks and get a fresh supply. Isn't that a waste?

**A** No. Nitroglycerin is a relatively unstable compound and begins to break down as soon as the sealed container is opened and the drug is exposed to the moisture in the air. After several weeks the drug is much less effective. Keep the bottle tightly closed and recap it as quickly as possible after taking out a tablet. Do not store the tablets in a pillbox, which may not be airtight, and do not expose the drug to sunlight.

**Q** I recently bought some aspirin but found that the expiration date on the bottle was 2 months ago. Should I use them?

**A** No. Any medication that has passed its expiration date should not be used. You should return the aspirin to the store and ask for a refund or a new bottle.

**Q** My grandmother died recently. When I was sorting through her things, I found that her medicine cabinet was full of old prescription drugs and other medications. What should I do with them?

**A** Dispose of all the medications. Some medications may have become ineffective or dangerous if they have been stored for a long time. Never throw them in the garbage. Flush them down the toilet. Do not try to donate the leftover medications to your hospital pharmacy for the benefit of indigent patients. Hospital pharmacies are not permitted to accept the drugs.

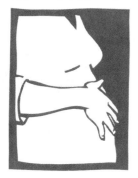

# DRUGS, PREGNANCY, AND BREAST-FEEDING

SOME DRUGS CAN BE harmful to pregnant women, developing fetuses, or breast-fed babies. A small amount of virtually any drug taken by a pregnant woman passes to the fetus via the placenta; drugs can also be passed from a woman to her infant via breast milk. A pregnant or breast-feeding woman should check with her doctor before taking any drugs, including alcohol. Use of illegal drugs during pregnancy can have devastating consequences.

Although drugs no longer enter the market without rigorous testing, it is rarely possible for doctors to know whether a certain drug is completely safe for every pregnant woman or breast-fed infant. Therefore, the safest course of action is to avoid taking any drug during pregnancy or when breast-feeding, unless your doctor believes there are compelling medical reasons for doing so.

## THE THREE TRIMESTERS

The 9-month duration of pregnancy is divided into three stages of 3 months each, known as trimesters. Whether a medication is likely to have an adverse effect on a developing fetus is determined by the trimester in which the drug is taken, its potential to produce abnormalities in the fetus, and the quantity of medication taken. Some medications are considered to be safe to take during one trimester but not during another.

**First trimester**
A drug taken during the first trimester may disrupt the early development of the embryo's major organs. The result may be birth defects or, in some cases, miscarriage.

**Second trimester**
Some drugs taken between the fourth and sixth months of pregnancy, the second trimester, may slow the rate of growth of the fetus and cause the infant to have a low birth weight.

## DRUGS AND PREGNANCY

Drug treatment during pregnancy is prescribed only if the potential benefits of treatment outweigh any risk to the mother and fetus. It is common to continue taking long-term medication for conditions such as diabetes, hypertension, or epilepsy. However, sometimes a drug that poses a risk may be replaced with one that is safer for the fetus. A woman taking long-term medication should notify her doctor if she is planning to become pregnant. It may be necessary to change the medication before conception occurs.

**Third trimester**
Possible adverse effects of drugs taken during the last trimester include breathing difficulties in the baby and bleeding abnormalities in the mother and baby.

## Crossing the placenta

The placenta acts as a filter between mother and fetus, allowing small molecules of oxygen and nutrients through, while keeping out larger particles such as blood cells. Most drugs taken during pregnancy pass easily from the mother's bloodstream through the placenta into the bloodstream of the developing fetus. Most drugs are found in the same blood concentrations in the mother and the fetus. However, because the fetal circulatory system contains a much smaller volume of blood compared to the mother's circulatory system, some drugs may be found in relatively high concentrations in the fetus.

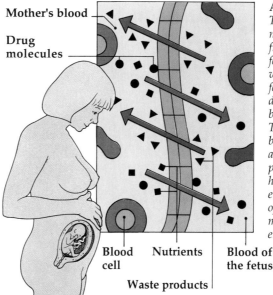

Mother's blood

Drug molecules

Blood cell

Nutrients

Blood of the fetus

Waste products

**A two-way filter**
*The placenta allows nourishment to pass from the mother to the fetus and allows the waste products of the fetus such as carbon dioxide and urea to pass back to the mother. There is no exchange of blood between mother and fetus. Although the placenta prevents most harmful substances from entering the circulation of the fetus, most drug molecules are small enough to pass through.*

---

## WHICH DRUGS COULD HARM THE FETUS?

An estimated 2 to 3 percent of birth defects are caused by the use of some form of drug or chemical. The drugs featured below are widely available and yet are known to be harmful to the fetus when taken during pregnancy.

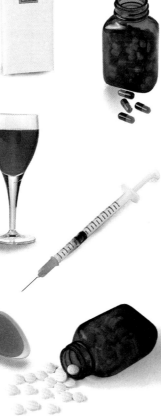

### Tobacco
Smoking tobacco during pregnancy increases the mother's risk of premature labor and abnormal bleeding before birth. The babies of women who smoke during pregnancy tend to have a lower birth weight and are more susceptible to illness. Inhaled carbon monoxide reduces the level of oxygen carried to the placenta. Nicotine restricts the supply of oxygen and nutrients to the fetus.

### Alcohol
Heavy consumption of alcohol during pregnancy significantly increases the risk of the baby being born with fetal alcohol syndrome (characterized by developmental problems and mental retardation). Consumption of even small amounts of alcohol may increase the risk of birth defects, miscarriage, and stillbirth. It is best to abstain completely from alcohol during pregnancy.

### Cough medications
Some cough preparations contain iodine compounds, which may cause enlarged and underactive thyroid glands in newborn babies, leading to growth problems. Talk to your doctor before taking any cough medication.

### Prescription drugs
If you are taking any prescription drug and you are planning to become pregnant, talk to your doctor about it now. Some prescription drugs, such as anticonvulsants, oral contraceptives, isotretinoin, warfarin, and lithium, can cause serious deformities in the developing fetus.

### Vaccines
If there is a possibility that you are pregnant, talk to your doctor before getting any vaccination. Some vaccines, such as the polio vaccine and the measles, mumps, and rubella vaccine, are best avoided during pregnancy because of risk to the fetus.

### Aspirin and NSAIDs
Taken in the later stages of pregnancy, aspirin and other NSAIDs (nonsteroidal anti-inflammatory drugs), such as ibuprofen, can cause excessive bleeding in both the mother and baby at the time of birth by interfering with the normal coagulation of blood. Aspirin can cause high blood pressure in the newborn. High doses of aspirin may increase the average length of pregnancy and prolong the duration of labor.

## DRUGS AND BREAST-FEEDING

When a woman is breast-feeding, small amounts of any drug she is taking may pass from her bloodstream into her breast milk. The amount of the drug that reaches the breast milk is determined by several factors, including the dosage the woman takes, how small the drug molecules are, and whether the drug molecules dissolve in fat. A fat-soluble drug passes into breast milk in greater concentrations than one that is soluble in water.

### Effects on the baby

Most drugs that pass into breast milk usually do so in concentrations that are too low to have any effect, adverse or otherwise, on the breast-fed baby. How-ever, a breast-feeding woman who must continue drug treatment for a long-term medical problem should ensure that her baby's condition is closely monitored for any possible adverse effect. In some cases, a drug that is safer for the infant may be substituted or, if this is not possible, the doctor may recommend bottle-feeding.

Antibiotics, antibacterials, and sedatives are among the drugs known to have unwanted effects on a breast-fed baby. Exposure to an antibiotic or antibacterial in breast milk may sensitize an infant so that he or she will be allergic to that drug if it is prescribed for the infant at a later date. Sedatives may make a baby drowsy, affect the baby's coordination, and cause feeding problems. Other drugs, such as diuretics, may reduce a baby's intake of nutrients by decreasing the amount of breast milk produced.

### HOW DRUGS PASS INTO BREAST MILK

The milk-producing glands in the breast are surrounded by a network of tiny blood vessels. Nutrients such as glucose (sugar) pass from these blood vessels into the breast milk, and antibodies in the mother's bloodstream pass into breast milk to help protect a baby against infection. Any substance made up of small molecules that is carried in the bloodstream is quickly absorbed through the thin walls lining the milk glands. Drug molecules pass easily into breast milk, so the baby receives small doses of any drug taken by the mother. Some drugs can cause unwanted effects on the baby.

**Protecting your child**
*Drug molecules pass easily from a mother's bloodstream into her breast milk. Newborn babies are particularly vulnerable to harm caused by certain drugs passed on in this way. Your doctor may recommend bottle-feeding if you must take medication.*

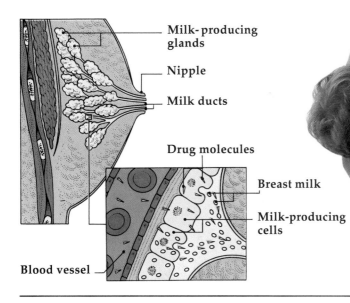

Milk-producing glands

Nipple

Milk ducts

Drug molecules

Breast milk

Milk-producing cells

Blood vessel

# CASE HISTORY
# ACNE TREATMENT AND PREGNANCY

WENDY HAS HAD ACNE **for several years. During one severe outbreak her doctor prescribed isotretinoin tablets. This therapy was effective and she has not taken any more tablets for a year. Two months ago, Wendy's acne became much worse again. At the same time Wendy began to suspect that she was pregnant. Although she still had some isotretinoin tablets, her doctor had warned her that the drug should never be taken during pregnancy. Wendy made an appointment to see him.**

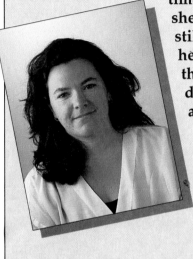

**PERSONAL DETAILS**
**Name** Wendy Malkovich
**Age** 24
**Occupation** Secretary
**Family** Wendy's parents are both healthy.

### MEDICAL BACKGROUND
Wendy had most of the illnesses that commonly occur during childhood, but she has never had any serious medical problems. Wendy does not have any allergies or skin disorders other than acne.

### THE CONSULTATION
Wendy's doctor examines her. He notes that her acne is particularly bad but finds that she is otherwise healthy. A blood test confirms that she is pregnant. Her doctor is relieved to learn that she remembered his instructions about isotretinoin and that she did not take any of the tablets left over from the previous treatment, because the drug is known to cause severe abnormalities in the organs of the developing fetus.

### THE DIAGNOSIS
Wendy's doctor tells her that her ACNE FLARE-UP and her pregnancy are probably linked and that the acne is likely to improve once her baby is born. Having established that Wendy has not taken any isotretinoin for a year before becoming pregnant, her doctor tells her that the use of any drug must be reevaluated when pregnancy is being planned or occurs. He explains that, although her acne is physically and emotionally disturbing to her, drug treatment for her acne during her pregnancy poses too great a risk to the developing fetus compared to the cosmetic benefit that would be achieved. To help her control the acne during her pregnancy without endangering the fetus, her doctor recommends an antibacterial skin lotion containing benzoyl peroxide, which can be purchased without a prescription. Wendy's doctor tells her to apply the lotion twice a day after washing her face. He reminds Wendy to tell her obstetrician about her treatment for acne and to check with her obstetrician before taking any other drugs, including over-the-counter medications, during her pregnancy.

### THE OUTCOME
Wendy's pregnancy progresses normally. Her acne stays under control with regular use of the antibacterial lotion. Seven months after her first appointment, Wendy gives birth to a healthy baby girl. Within a few weeks, her acne improves without any further drug treatment.

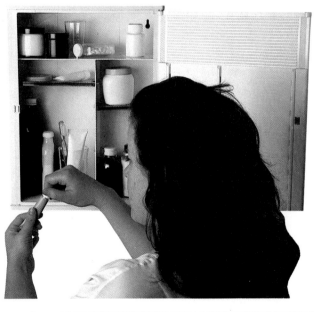

**Awareness of side effects**
*Drugs such as isotretinoin that are safe to use under most circumstances can endanger the development of the embryo and fetus in the early months of pregnancy. Women using isotretinoin should use two methods of birth control until several months after they stop taking the drug and should discuss the situation with their doctor.*

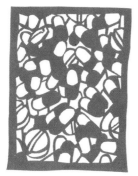

# SUBSTANCE ABUSE AND DRUG DEPENDENCE

DEPENDENCE on a drug develops from a compulsive desire to experience the enjoyable effects of a drug or a need to prevent the unpleasant withdrawal reactions that occur when use is discontinued (or both). In addition to the recognized problem of dependence on illegal drugs in the US, millions of Americans are dependent on legal drugs such as alcohol and nicotine; others are dependent on prescription drugs such as tranquilizers.

**Drug tolerance**
*Many of the drugs that cause dependence also increase tolerance. This means that a progressively larger amount is necessary to achieve the desired effect. A smoker tends to increase the number of cigarettes he or she smokes unless the habit is deliberately curtailed. Likewise, heavy drinkers can tolerate levels of alcohol in their blood that would cause severe intoxication in other people. Doctors review the dosage of some prescription drugs from time to time to detect increasing tolerance to a drug.*

The terms abuse, addiction, and dependence are often confused. Abuse connotes the improper use of a drug for pleasure or psychological reasons. Addiction means an intense, habitual craving with physical and psychological dependence and withdrawal reactions if use of the substance is stopped.

## TYPES OF DRUG DEPENDENCE

Drug dependence may be psychological, physical, or both. A person is psychologically dependent if he or she experiences craving or emotional distress when not taking the drug. Physical dependence develops when the body adapts to the presence of a drug. Higher doses of the drug may be required to achieve the desired effect. If use of the drug is stopped, severe physical signs and emotional distress can occur.

Not all substances that cause psychological dependence result in physical dependence. However, drugs that produce physical dependence are associated with psychological dependence because of the drug user's desire to prevent the unpleasant reactions that develop when he or she stops taking the drug and because of the rapid relief and pleasure obtained by taking the drug. Another factor in drug dependence is drug tolerance (see DECREASING DRUG EFFECTIVENESS on page 45).

### How do dependence and addiction develop?
Drug dependence and addiction occur as the result of regular or excessive use of a drug. Only a few groups of drugs can produce either psychological or physical dependence; most of these are substances that are capable of altering an individual's mood or behavior.

The factors that may influence whether a person will become dependent on or addicted to a drug include availability of that drug in the community; social and economic factors such as poverty, unemployment, and a disrupted family life;

## HOW THE BODY ADAPTS TO A DRUG AS TOLERANCE DEVELOPS

When the presence of a drug is maintained in the body by means of a habit such as smoking or by taking medication for a prolonged period of time, the cells of the body adapt to the substance. For many drugs that cause dependence, the processes of adaptation are not fully understood, but one well-established model is that of morphine dependence and the effect it has on pain receptors in the body.

| PAIN IS STOPPED FOR SHORT PERIODS | PAIN IS STOPPED FOR LONGER PERIODS | PAIN SIGNALS ARE TRANS-MITTED DIRECTLY FROM BRAIN WITHOUT BUFFER |
|---|---|---|
| **Normal perception of pain**<br>A painful stimulus such as heat applied to some part of the body causes signals to be sent to pain receptors (also called opiate or endorphin receptors) in the cerebral cortex of the brain. These receptors interpret the signals and transmit another set of signals that the body experiences as pain. Pain receptors in the brain are later blocked by naturally occurring chemicals (endorphins) and the pain briefly diminishes. | **Morphine dependence**<br>Morphine molecules affect the same pain receptors in the brain that are normally acted on by endorphins. Thus morphine decreases the sensation of pain for a prolonged period. Morphine also suppresses the body's production of endorphins. The suppressed production of endorphins that normally act as buffers between the pain receptors in the brain and pain sensation in the body can cause dependence on morphine to provide relief from pain. | **Morphine withdrawal**<br>In the absence of endorphins or morphine to act as a buffer, pain signals are freely transmitted. Withdrawal from morphine produces a severe reaction in the portion of the nervous system that controls involuntary activities. Reactions include diarrhea, nausea, vomiting, excessive salivation, yawning, sweating, runny nose, goose flesh ("going cold turkey"), painful cramps, and listlessness. |

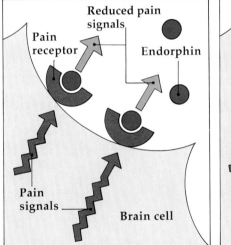

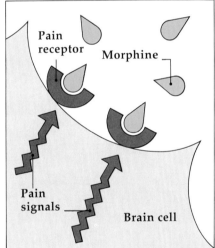

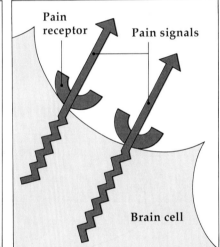

and pressure from friends and associates. Inherited genetic factors are also believed to play a part in causing addiction to alcohol.

## WITHDRAWAL FROM DRUGS

Therapy with most types of drugs can usually be stopped without causing symptoms of withdrawal. However, an unpleasant reaction may develop in anyone who tries to stop taking a drug that causes physical dependence and has been taken for a long time. Each type of drug has its own characteristic pattern of withdrawal symptoms (see SYMPTOMS AND TREATMENT OF DRUG WITHDRAWAL on page 70). For example, use of a corticosteroid drug can cause physical dependence because the drug suppresses the natural production of corticosteroid hormones by the adrenal glands. Corticosteroids can also cause psychological dependence because they may produce a heightened sense of well-being and feelings of euphoria. Symptoms of withdrawal from long-term use of tranquilizers or sleeping pills may include shaking, wakefulness, or convulsions.

# SYMPTOMS AND TREATMENT OF DRUG WITHDRAWAL

| DRUG | | SYMPTOMS OF WITHDRAWAL | TREATMENT OF WITHDRAWAL |
|---|---|---|---|
| Benzodi-azepines | | Recurrence of anxiety symptoms up to 2 weeks after last dose of the drug. | A medically supervised gradual reduction in dosage over several weeks is recommended if benzodiazepines have been taken for longer than 2 weeks. |
| Cortico-steroids | | Sudden withdrawal can result in collapse of the circulatory system and death if the person is subjected to severe stress. | A phased reduction in dosage is recommended. Normal functioning of the adrenal glands may not return for 6 months to a year after use of the drug has been stopped. |
| Barbiturates | | Sleeplessness, twitching, nightmares, and convulsions. Symptoms may appear within 24 hours of the last dose of the drug. Coma occurs in some cases. | A medically supervised gradual reduction in dosage over several weeks is recommended. |
| Amphet-amines | | Severe tiredness, dizziness, increased appetite, and a need to sleep for long periods. | A medically supervised withdrawal program is strongly recommended for heavy users of amphetamines. |
| Alcohol | | Trembling, sweating, nausea, anxiety, abdominal cramps, and vomiting. Symptoms normally start within 8 hours of consuming the last drink and may last up to 7 days. In severe cases, withdrawal can cause confusion, delirium tremens (hallucinations), seizures, and death. | Tranquilizers may be prescribed to reduce withdrawal symptoms; use of tranquilizers should be medically supervised to prevent development of dependence. Professional counseling can help reduce psychological dependence on alcohol. |
| Nicotine | | Intense craving for nicotine, irritability, difficulty concentrating, headaches, and restlessness. Symptoms develop gradually over 48 hours after stopping smoking and can persist for many weeks. | Nicotine chewing gum is available by prescription. However, millions of people have quit smoking through sheer determination and by using the behavior modification techniques taught at stop-smoking clinics. |
| Caffeine | | Fatigue, headache, drowsiness, and irritability commonly occur in people who drink excessive amounts of coffee, tea, or cola. Symptoms may begin within hours of consuming the last caffeinated drink. | Consumption of caffeinated beverages is gradually reduced. Psychological dependence can be alleviated by using decaffeinated brands of coffee, tea, or cola. |
| Marijuana | | Chronic users of marijuana report tremor, nausea, vomiting, diarrhea, sweating, irritability, and difficulty sleeping. | The quantity of marijuana smoked can be gradually reduced or completely eliminated. Professional counseling can help reduce psychological dependence. |
| Cocaine | | Users of excessive amounts of cocaine suffer severe depression and physical symptoms such as tremor and sweating. | A medically supervised withdrawal program that includes behavior modification is strongly recommended for heavy users of cocaine. |
| Heroin and morphine | | At first, restlessness, sweating, yawning, watery eyes, and a runny nose, accompanied by an overwhelming desire to obtain more of the drug. Later, diarrhea, vomiting, abdominal cramps, dilated pupils, tremor, irritability, weakness, depression, and goose flesh. Symptoms start between 8 and 12 hours after the last dose of the drug. | Medically supervised programs are available in special centers and hospitals. These programs usually recommend a gradual reduction in dose. However, abruptly imposed abstinence is the treatment of choice in some centers. In some cases, drug therapy (such as the narcotic methadone) may be used to relieve the withdrawal symptoms. |

# CASE HISTORY
# TRANQUILIZER DEPENDENCE

MARSHA HAS HAD a difficult time emotionally since her husband's death 6 months ago. Her doctor prescribed a benzodiazepine tranquilizer to help her cope with her loss. She continued taking the tranquilizer until a friend cautioned her about the risk of addiction. Marsha abruptly stopped taking the pills. Before long she had become increasingly tense and anxious and was experiencing a variety of disturbing physical symptoms. She called her doctor to make an appointment.

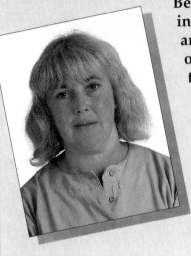

### PERSONAL DETAILS
**Name** Marsha Simmons
**Age** 49
**Occupation** Free-lance editor
**Family** Mother is healthy. Father had a nervous breakdown 5 years ago and is taking an antidepressant drug.

## MEDICAL BACKGROUND
Marsha visited her doctor 2 weeks after her husband's death because she had lost her appetite and was feeling very nervous and depressed. The doctor prescribed a benzodiazepine tranquilizer. She continued to take the tranquilizer during the 6 months after the death of her husband despite the fact that her anxiety and depression had eased.

## THE CONSULTATION
Marsha explains that she has been having nightmares and has awakened in the early morning hours with a feeling of tightness across her chest, sweating profusely, shaking uncontrollably, and unable to catch her breath. Marsha's doctor explains to her that she has developed a physical dependence on the tranquilizer she has been taking and that she is also experiencing symptoms of hyperventilation caused by anxiety.

## THE DIAGNOSIS
Marsha is experiencing a moderately severe WITHDRAWAL REACTION. The chemical equilibrium in her body changed while she was taking the tranquilizer. When she stopped taking it, the chemical balance in her body became unstable, resulting in her distressing symptoms.

The doctor tells her that the best way to withdraw from the drug is slowly, under his supervision.

## THE TREATMENT
The doctor prescribes a different type of benzodiazepine for Marsha to stabilize the chemical balance in her body and relieve her withdrawal symptoms. Marsha begins a program of controlled withdrawal with a daily dose equivalent to the dose of the tranquilizer she had been taking. Every 2 to 3 weeks (after Marsha discusses her physical and emotional health with her doctor), the dosage is reduced by a small amount.

To help relieve her anxieties and withdraw successfully from the drug, Marsha also does daily relaxation exercises and abstains from caffeine-containing beverages, which, when consumed in excess, can increase anxiety in some people.

## THE OUTLOOK
After 1 month, the daily dose of the tranquilizer has been reduced by half and Marsha has experienced no ill effects. She continues to experience progressively milder symptoms, occurring less frequently, that she has come to recognize as anxiety. The dosage will continue to be reduced gradually until she is no longer taking the drug.

**Benzodiazepine tranquilizers**
*Marsha's severe withdrawal symptoms were caused by a chemical imbalance that was created when she stopped taking the tranquilizer. Long-term therapy with benzodiazepine tranquilizers requires a medically supervised, gradual withdrawal program.*

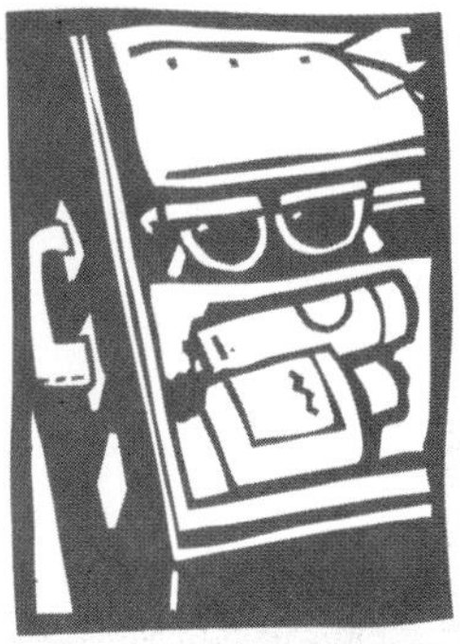

# DRUGS AND TRAVEL

THE ITEMS YOU NEED TO INCLUDE in your medical travel kit depend on the country you visit and how far from medical care you will be, as well as on your individual needs. Few travelers need all the items shown, but every item could be useful. Some of the drugs listed are available only by prescription.

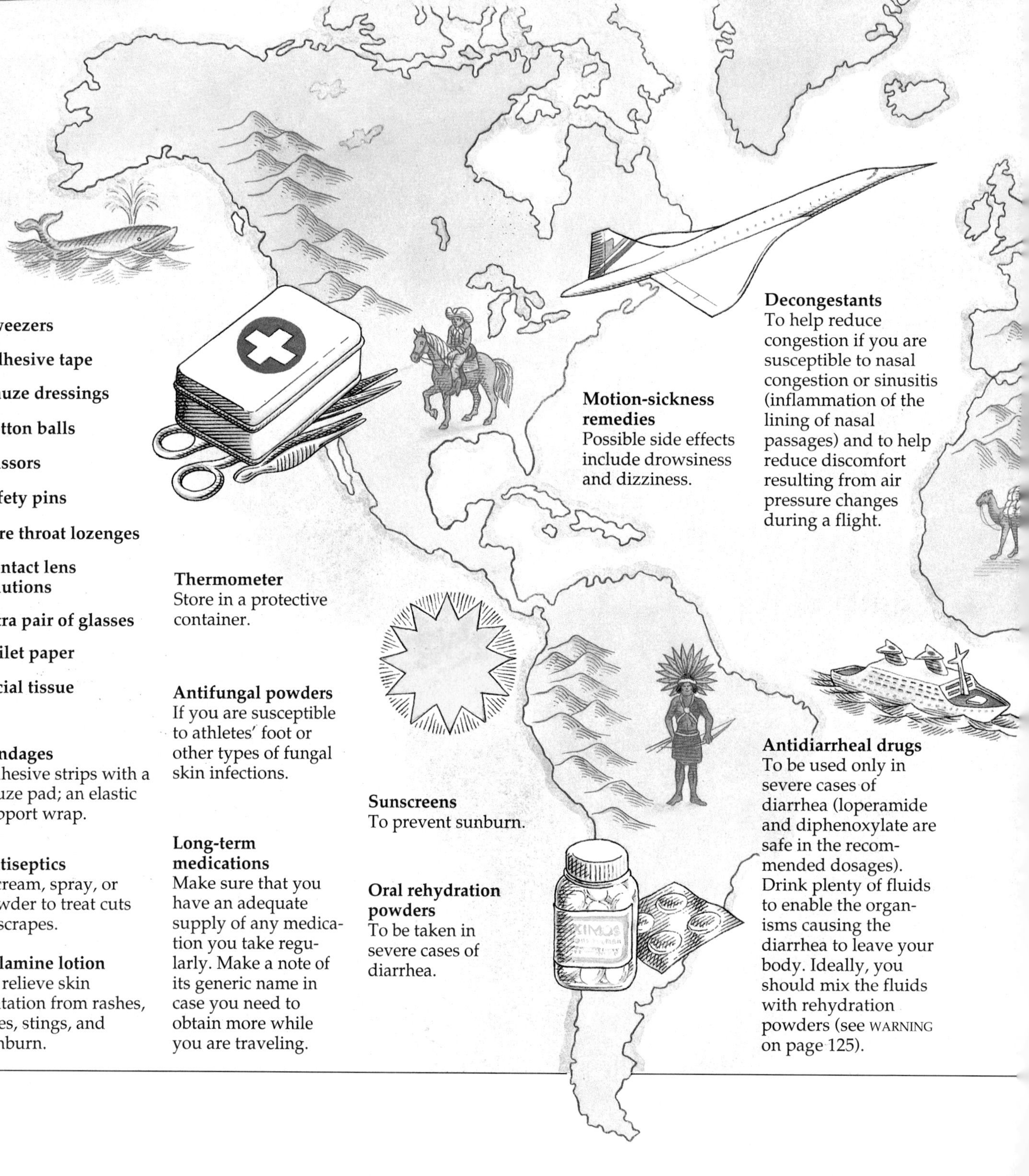

Tweezers

Adhesive tape

Gauze dressings

Cotton balls

Scissors

Safety pins

Sore throat lozenges

Contact lens solutions

Extra pair of glasses

Toilet paper

Facial tissue

**Bandages**
Adhesive strips with a gauze pad; an elastic support wrap.

**Antiseptics**
A cream, spray, or powder to treat cuts or scrapes.

**Calamine lotion**
To relieve skin irritation from rashes, bites, stings, and sunburn.

**Thermometer**
Store in a protective container.

**Antifungal powders**
If you are susceptible to athletes' foot or other types of fungal skin infections.

**Long-term medications**
Make sure that you have an adequate supply of any medication you take regularly. Make a note of its generic name in case you need to obtain more while you are traveling.

**Sunscreens**
To prevent sunburn.

**Oral rehydration powders**
To be taken in severe cases of diarrhea.

**Motion-sickness remedies**
Possible side effects include drowsiness and dizziness.

**Decongestants**
To help reduce congestion if you are susceptible to nasal congestion or sinusitis (inflammation of the lining of nasal passages) and to help reduce discomfort resulting from air pressure changes during a flight.

**Antidiarrheal drugs**
To be used only in severe cases of diarrhea (loperamide and diphenoxylate are safe in the recommended dosages). Drink plenty of fluids to enable the organisms causing the diarrhea to leave your body. Ideally, you should mix the fluids with rehydration powders (see WARNING on page 125).

## Antibiotics
In case a skin, sinus, or throat infection develops; also for bacterial infections such as cystitis or bronchitis.

## Antibiotic eye ointments or drops
To treat eye irritation.

## Antihistamine tablets
To relieve skin irritation from insect bites or stings and allergic reactions.

## Insect repellents
Slow-burning coils that release an insecticidal smoke are an effective repellent. You can also take repellent to apply to exposed parts of your body.

## Antacid tablets
Indigestion may be caused by eating unfamiliar foods, overeating, or drinking too much alcohol. Antacids should be taken in moderation, as stomach acids help protect against intestinal infection.

## Painkillers (analgesics)
Aspirin and acetaminophen reduce pain caused by headaches, toothaches, sunburn, or minor injuries. They also help to reduce a fever. Acetaminophen is recommended for children and teenagers.

## Laxatives
Constipation may be caused by dehydration, jet lag, a change in diet, or stifling the urge to defecate (sometimes because of a reluctance to use unhygienic toilets). Laxatives should always be used sparingly.

## Water sterilization tablets

## Needles and syringes
If you have a medical condition (such as diabetes) that requires self-administered injections, it is wise to carry your own injecting equipment along with a letter from your doctor stating your medical condition.

## Antimalarial tablets
Essential before going to a country where transmission of malaria is likely to occur. Check with your doctor about the exact type of antimalarial medication to take. The organisms that transmit malaria in the area you are visiting may be resistant to some forms of antimalarial drugs. Ask your doctor whether you should also take a course of a curative drug after you leave the malaria zone.

## Epinephrine
Available in a spray if you are susceptible to serious allergic reactions to insect stings.

73

# CHAPTER FOUR

# TYPES OF DRUGS

A SPECTACULAR RISE in the number of medications available for a growing range of physical and mental disorders has occurred during the 20th century. Development of many of these new drugs has resulted from our increased understanding of the ways in which natural substances work in the body. The pharmaceutical industry has synthesized some of these substances made in the body for use as drugs; many other drugs have been developed to mimic, or to interfere with, the action of the body's natural substances.

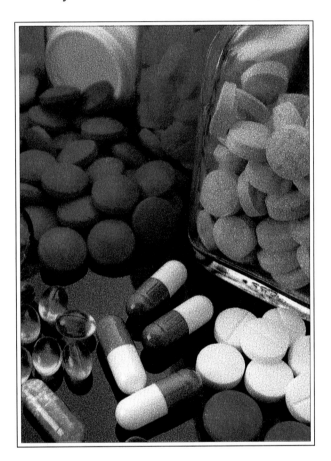

People who are taking prescription drugs sometimes have only a limited understanding of how these drugs produce their desired effects. This chapter explains the actions of the major drug groups on the body. Each subsection explains a major drug category and includes a description of the disorders treated with the drugs and the effects that the drugs have on the disorders. You may not find your medication mentioned here; a comprehensive listing of the generic names of commonly prescribed drugs can be found in the DRUG GLOSSARY (see page 134).

Although every drug undergoes exhaustive testing for effectiveness and safety before it is approved for use, most drugs can cause side effects. Some of these side effects are common and others are rare. We list some of these possible side effects, together with appropriate warnings to people who may be at risk if they take the drugs.

Some of the subsections concern groups of drugs that have the same end result but achieve that result in different ways. For example, several drugs are used to lower blood pressure. Some drugs do so by acting on the heart, some act on muscles in blood vessel walls, some act on the nerve endings in these muscles, and some act in the brain – the end result being a widening of the blood vessels and a lowering of blood pressure. In other subsections, there may be only one drug that is used to treat a specific disease. For example, regular injections of insulin are the only known treatment for insulin-dependent diabetes. This chapter deals only with those conditions for which drug therapy is the treatment of choice.

It is unrealistic to believe that a pill exists for every ill. And it is important to remember that people with certain medical conditions (heart disease, for example) receive the maximum benefit from their medications by also making changes in their diets and life-styles. In some cases, such as certain forms of cancer, surgery may be the most effective means of treatment available.

# DRUGS AND THE CENTRAL NERVOUS SYSTEM

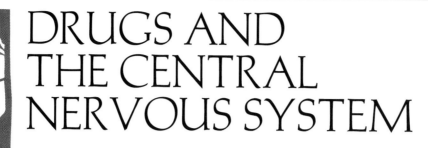

THE NERVOUS SYSTEM can be divided into two main parts – the central nervous system, which is made up of the brain and spinal cord, and the peripheral nervous system, which consists of a vast network of motor and sensory nerves connecting the central nervous system to the rest of the body.

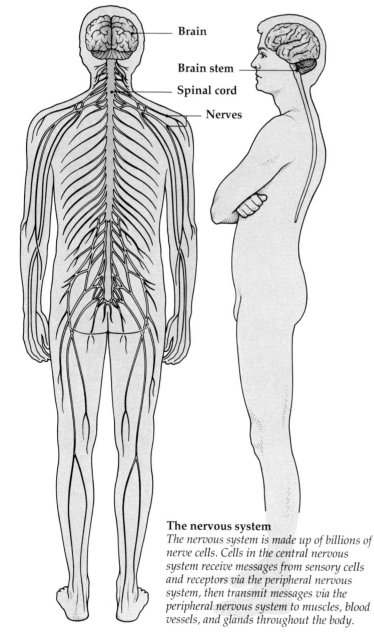

Brain

Brain stem

Spinal cord

Nerves

**The nervous system**
*The nervous system is made up of billions of nerve cells. Cells in the central nervous system receive messages from sensory cells and receptors via the peripheral nervous system, then transmit messages via the peripheral nervous system to muscles, blood vessels, and glands throughout the body.*

The brain is like a computer that receives messages from every part of the body, interprets these messages, and then sends back instructions. The brain is also the center for emotion, mood, personality, thought, and reasoning. Disorders of the central nervous system can result in conditions as diverse as epilepsy, Parkinson's disease, depression, anxiety, schizophrenia, or sleep disturbance.

Several groups of drugs have been developed to act on the central nervous system. Most of these drugs work by modifying the way in which signals are transmitted to, from, and within the brain. Some of these drugs are called agonists; they stimulate receptors in the brain. Others are antagonists; they depress brain cell activity. (See DRUGS AND RECEPTORS on page 31.)

## ANTIANXIETY DRUGS

Anxiety is the feeling of fear without any apparent cause or an overreaction to a stressful life event. Antianxiety drugs, sometimes called minor tranquilizers or sedatives, are used to alleviate these feelings of fear. These drugs can be effective for short-term treatment of the symptoms of anxiety; however, they can cause an increase in the symptoms when treatment is stopped. Antianxiety drugs do not treat the underlying causes of the feelings of fear; professional counseling or psychotherapy offers the best long-term solution. There are several classes of antianxiety drugs, among them benzodiazepines and beta blockers.

## How they affect you

Benzodiazepines depress activity in the part of the brain that controls emotion. They reduce anxiety and promote relaxation (see SLEEP-INDUCING DRUGS on page 81).

A beta blocker is often prescribed when anxiety causes physical symptoms such as chest pains or bowel disturbances. These symptoms result from overactivity of the part of the nervous system that releases the neurotransmitter norepinephrine. Beta blockers block the action of norepinephrine.

## ANTIPSYCHOTIC DRUGS

Antipsychotic drugs (sometimes called major tranquilizers or neuroleptics) are used in the treatment of psychoses (mental disorders) such as schizophre-nia, paranoid psychosis, and manic-depressive illness. These drugs are sometimes prescribed in very small doses for anxiety and agitation, dizziness, nausea, and vomiting. Antipsychotic drugs are prescribed to modify psychotic behavior; they do not cure the underlying cause of the behavior. Several types of drugs are available; the main class is the phenothiazines, which include chlorpromazine, one of the oldest and most widely used antipsychotics, and prochlorperazine. Other antipsychotic drugs are the butyrophenones, the thioxanthenes, and lithium.

## How they affect you

Antipsychotic drugs frequently cause side effects. Muscular rigidity and tremor and jerking movements of the mouth, tongue, face, hands, and feet may occur. Other adverse effects include a fall in blood pressure upon standing, weight gain, dry mouth, blurred vision, constipation, and difficulty passing urine.

### WARNING

Lithium is the drug of choice to treat manic-depressive illness. It controls the intensity of the mood swings that characterize this condition. Lithium can be harmful if the level of the drug in the blood rises too much, so concentrations in the blood are checked regularly. Symptoms of lithium poisoning may include blurred vision, twitching, vomiting, and diarrhea. Lithium may also cause kidney damage.

## HOW NERVE SIGNALS ARE TRANSMITTED

Signals travel through the nervous system by electrical and chemical means along nerve cell pathways. A pathway is made up of two or more nerve cells (neurons) connected in a line. Nerve cells have long projections called axons. Signals are carried by electrical impulses from one end of a nerve cell to the other via its axon. For the signals to cross the gap (called a synapse) between two nerve cells, chemical neurotransmitters must be released from the ends of an axon; the messages cross over the synapse and attach themselves to receptors on the neighboring nerve cell. An electrical impulse is then generated through that nerve cell to the next synapse, and so the impulse is passed along. Once the neurotransmitters have carried their message across the synapse, they are either taken back into the cell that released them for later reuse, or they are converted to inactive substances.

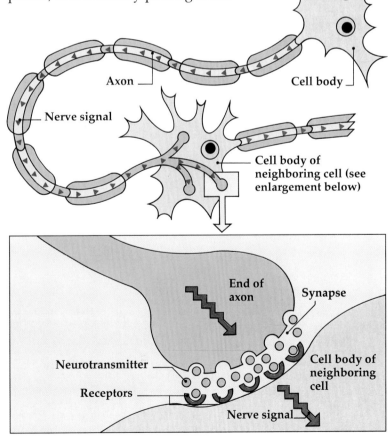

Axon — Cell body

Nerve signal

Cell body of neighboring cell (see enlargement below)

End of axon — Synapse

Neurotransmitter

Receptors

Cell body of neighboring cell

Nerve signal

# HOW DRUGS AFFECT THE BRAIN

Medications that act on the brain are thought to do so by affecting the way nerve signals are transmitted. However, each type of medication acts by a different mechanism. A variety of chemical substances in the brain serve as neurotransmitters. The most important of these neurotransmitters are serotonin, dopamine, and norepinephrine, as well as acetylcholine and gamma-aminobutyric acid (GABA). Some drugs block the action of these neurotransmitters, some mimic their actions, and others affect the way they are used by the brain.

### Antipsychotic drugs

*The activity of the brain is partially controlled by the action of dopamine, a stimulatory neurotransmitter. In psychotic illnesses, the brain cells are thought to release too much dopamine, which causes overstimulation. Antipsychotic drugs block the stimulatory actions of dopamine.*

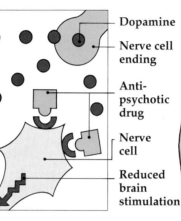

Dopamine

Nerve cell ending

Antipsychotic drug

Nerve cell

Reduced brain stimulation

### The vomiting reflex

*Nausea and vomiting occur when the vomiting center in the brain stem is stimulated. This stimulation may be caused by signals sent from the place in the brain that reacts to harmful chemicals (chemoreceptor trigger zone), from the balancing mechanism in the ear, or from the lining of the digestive tract.*

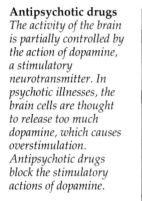

Brain

Nerve signals

Digestive tract

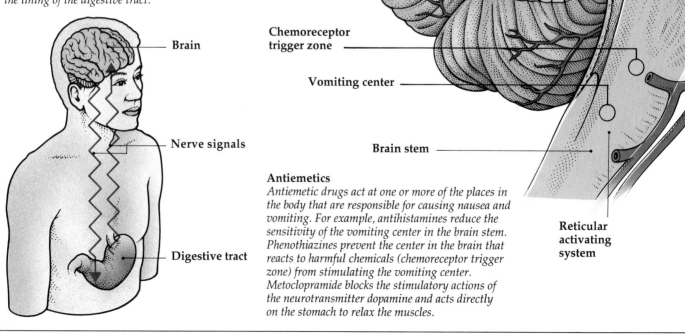

Chemoreceptor trigger zone

Vomiting center

Brain stem

Reticular activating system

### Antiemetics

*Antiemetic drugs act at one or more of the places in the body that are responsible for causing nausea and vomiting. For example, antihistamines reduce the sensitivity of the vomiting center in the brain stem. Phenothiazines prevent the center in the brain that reacts to harmful chemicals (chemoreceptor trigger zone) from stimulating the vomiting center. Metoclopramide blocks the stimulatory actions of the neurotransmitter dopamine and acts directly on the stomach to relax the muscles.*

### Stimulant drugs

*Stimulant drugs act on the reticular activating system (which regulates the level of mental activity) to increase the number of signals (purple arrows) being sent from this part of the brain to areas in the surface of the brain that control the body's functions.*

### Antidepressant drugs

*Depression is associated with reduced levels of the neurotransmitters norepinephrine and serotonin in the brain, leading to decreased brain stimulation. These neurotransmitters are constantly released and reabsorbed by brain cells, and then broken down by an enzyme called monoamine oxidase (MAO). Antidepressants either raise the levels of these neurotransmitters or prevent their inactivation in the brain.*

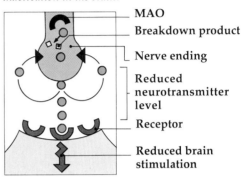

- MAO
- Breakdown product
- Nerve ending
- Reduced neurotransmitter level
- Receptor
- Reduced brain stimulation

### MAO inhibitors

*MAO inhibitor drugs increase the levels of neurotransmitters by blocking the enzyme (monoamine oxidase) that metabolizes them.*

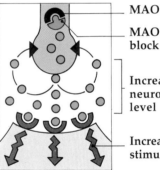

- MAO
- MAO inhibitors block enzyme
- Increased neurotransmitter level
- Increased brain stimulation

### The tricyclics and serotonin reuptake inhibitors

*Tricyclic drugs increase the levels of both serotonin and norepinephrine by blocking the reabsorption of these neurotransmitters into the nerve cell ending. Serotonin reuptake inhibitors specifically block the reabsorption of serotonin. This specific action is thought to decrease the incidence of many of the undesirable side effects caused by the tricyclics.*

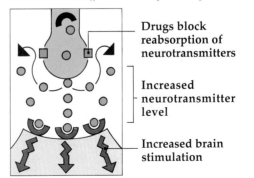

- Drugs block reabsorption of neurotransmitters
- Increased neurotransmitter level
- Increased brain stimulation

**Benzodiazepines decrease signals to centers of the brain that control conscious body movement**

- GABA
- Nerve cell
- Benzodiazepine
- GABA receptor
- Reduced brain activity
- Benzodiazepine receptor

### Benzodiazepines

*Benzodiazepines depress the reticular activating system, which regulates the level of activity in the brain. Benzodiazepines enhance the action of the inhibitory neurotransmitter gamma-aminobutyric acid (GABA) by fitting into receptors alongside GABA receptors. This decreases brain stimulation and has a calming and relaxing effect, making these drugs useful in the treatment of insomnia, anxiety, epilepsy, and muscle spasms. The duration of use of benzodiazepines should be limited because of the risk of addiction.*

# CASE HISTORY
## PROBLEMS WITH EPILEPSY TREATMENT

S EVERAL YEARS AGO **George experienced a seizure and was diagnosed as having epilepsy. His neurologist prescribed the anticonvulsant drugs phenobarbital and phenytoin. This treatment was successful until 2 months ago, when George had another seizure. He was rushed to the emergency room, where the seizure was controlled with an injection of diazepam. An increased dosage of his medications has prevented further seizures. However, George is now experiencing other symptoms; he arranges to see his neurologist.**

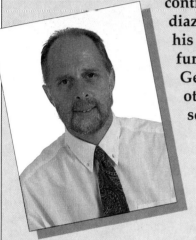

### PERSONAL DETAILS
**Name** George Atkins
**Age** 27
**Occupation** Chemical engineer
**Family** Father has epilepsy. Mother is well.

### MEDICAL BACKGROUND
Aside from his epilepsy (caused by abnormal electrical activity in the brain), George has been in good health. His epilepsy has been effectively controlled with anticonvulsant drugs. At the time of his last seizure, the levels of phenobarbital and phenytoin in George's blood were checked and were found to be low. At that time, his neurologist increased the dosage of both phenobarbital and phenytoin in order to prevent more seizures.

### THE CONSULTATION
George explains to his neurologist that he has now begun to have frequent headaches and to feel drowsy (sometimes so drowsy that he is unable to stay awake during the day), lethargic, and unsteady on his feet. His neurologist examines George and reviews the change in the dosages of George's medications that were made after his last seizure.

### THE DIAGNOSIS
The neurologist informs George that the symptoms he is now experiencing are SIDE EFFECTS FROM ANTICONVULSANT DRUG THERAPY. The neurologist changes the therapy to a combination of two newer drugs – carbamazepine and valproic acid. These drugs decrease the excess electrical activity in the brain, but should not produce the side effects that George is experiencing from the increased dosages of the combination of phenobarbital and phenytoin. The neurologist also impresses upon George the importance of taking his drugs regularly as prescribed to prevent further seizures.

### THE OUTCOME
A month after starting the new drug combination, George's symptoms have disappeared and he has had no serious adverse effects. George reports that he feels more alert and productive at work. To monitor the effect of the new drug treatment on George's brain activity, his neurologist performs an electroencephalogram. Levels of the two drugs in George's blood are monitored regularly to ensure that the amount of medication in his blood remains high enough to control his epilepsy.

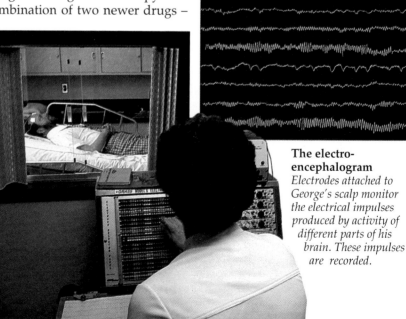

**The electroencephalogram**
*Electrodes attached to George's scalp monitor the electrical impulses produced by activity of different parts of his brain. These impulses are recorded.*

80

## HOW SLEEP-INDUCING DRUGS AFFECT SLEEPING PATTERNS

Normal sleep can be divided into three types – light sleep (nonrapid eye movement, or non-REM), dream sleep (REM), and deep sleep (non-REM). The length of time spent in each type of sleep varies with age and can be altered by sleep-inducing drugs and by the body's response to withdrawal of the drug after use for a prolonged period.

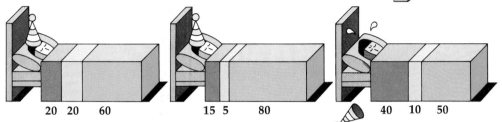

Dream sleep

Deep sleep

Light sleep

| 20 | 20 | 60 | | 15 | 5 | 80 | | 40 | 10 | 50 |

**Percentage of total sleep time**

**Normal sleep** In young adults, normal sleep is predominantly light sleep, with about equal proportions of dream and deep sleep.

**Drug-induced sleep** Sleep induced by drugs is predominantly light sleep, with much less deep sleep and a little less dream sleep.

**Sleep after drug withdrawal** After withdrawal from sleep-inducing drugs, there is an increase in dream sleep, accompanied by nightmares.

> **WARNING**
>
> Sleep-inducing drugs (hypnotics) may cause dizziness, daytime drowsiness, impaired coordination, and forgetfulness, which can interfere with the ability to drive or operate machinery. Alcohol should never be used when taking a hypnotic because alcohol also depresses brain function; alcohol and hypnotics used in combination can produce a dangerous level of sedation, or even coma.

> **A NEW TREATMENT FOR EPILEPSY**
>
> A new anticonvulsant drug – not yet available in the US – has been developed to treat epilepsy. Scientists believe that some neurotransmitters are involved in initiating and spreading the electrical signals that cause seizures, while the neurotransmitter gamma-aminobutyric acid (GABA) is responsible for switching off these signals. This investigational anticonvulsant drug irreversibly inhibits the enzyme that breaks down GABA. This increases GABA concentrations in the brain and thus reduces the risk of seizures.

## SLEEP-INDUCING DRUGS

Sleep-inducing drugs (also known as hypnotics) are prescribed to induce sleep in people who have persistent insomnia that is affecting their general health and sense of well-being. However, because sleep-inducing drugs can cause physical and psychological dependence, they should be used only for very short-term treatment of insomnia.

### How they affect you

Most sleep-inducing drugs promote sleep by depressing the part of the brain that controls wakefulness. Benzodiazepines are the most commonly prescribed group of sleep-inducing drugs, which includes flurazepam, triazolam, and temazepam. These drugs are also used in lower doses to treat anxiety. People who take benzodiazepines for more than about 2 weeks can become psychologically and physically dependent upon them (see DRUG DEPENDENCE on page 68).

Barbiturates are rarely used to treat insomnia because of the risk of abuse and because they are addictive; an overdose can be fatal. The sedative chloral hydrate and antihistamines such as promethazine are commonly used drugs that are particularly useful in the treatment of insomnia in children and in the elderly.

## ANTIDEPRESSANT DRUGS

Antidepressant drugs are used to treat severe depression that has lasted for longer than a few days and has caused symptoms such as a feeling of despair, loss of appetite, decreased sexual desire, early-morning awakening, low self-esteem, headache, and suicidal thoughts.

### How they affect you

All antidepressant drugs increase the availability of stimulating neurotransmitters in the brain. There are two main groups of antidepressant drugs – the tricyclics and the monoamine oxidase (MAO) inhibitors. Other drugs used as antidepressants include the tetracyclics, heterocyclics, serotonin reuptake inhibitors, and lithium.

The tricyclics include imipramine, amitriptyline, and desipramine. Some tricyclics have a mainly sedative effect and are used to treat concurrent anxiety and depression. Others have a more stimulating effect and are used to treat feelings of tiredness or drowsiness. Common side effects of tricyclics include dry mouth, blurred vision, constipation, dizziness, insomnia or drowsiness, weakness, fatigue, palpitations, seizures, sweating, and shaky hands.

The MAO inhibitors are particularly effective in the treatment of anxiety and phobias as well as depression. These inhibitors have side effects similar to those caused by tricyclics and can cause dangerous side effects when interacting with some foods and other drugs (see DRUG INTERACTIONS on page 36). The serotonin reuptake inhibitor fluoxetine is the first in a new class of more specific antidepressants; side effects include brief headaches, nausea, drowsiness, loss of appetite, rhinitis (inflammation of the lining of the nose), and anxiety.

# ANTIEMETIC DRUGS

Antiemetic drugs are used to suppress nausea and vomiting. The most commonly used antiemetic drugs are metoclopramide, antihistamines (such as meclizine and promethazine), and the phenothiazines (such as prochlorperazine and promazine).

## How they affect you

Antihistamines are used in the treatment of motion sickness; you should not take these drugs for longer than 2 days without consulting your doctor. Metoclopramide and the phenothiazines are the drugs that are currently being used to treat nausea caused by anticancer drugs and radiation therapy. Antiemetics are not recommended for use during pregnancy unless symptoms are severe. All antiemetics may cause drowsiness.

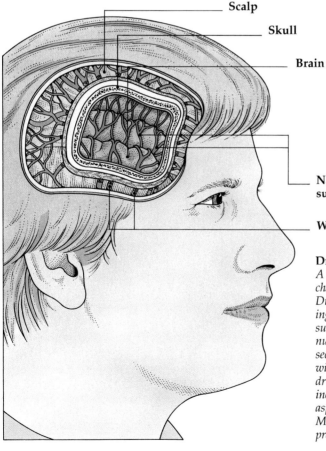

Scalp
Skull
Brain

Narrowed blood vessels surrounding the brain

Widened blood vessels in scalp

**Preventing migraine**
Migraine is prevented with drugs that block the narrowing of blood vessels surrounding the brain.

**Relieving migraine**
Ergotamine causes blood vessels to narrow, returning the widened blood vessels in the scalp to their normal size.

**Drugs for migraine**
*A migraine is a severe headache caused by changes in the blood vessels in the brain. During the first stage, vessels surrounding the brain narrow, causing symptoms such as flashing lights before the eyes and numbness in the arms and legs. In the second stage, blood vessels in the scalp widen, leading to a severe headache. The drugs often used to relieve migraine pain include ergotamine and the analgesics aspirin and acetaminophen with codeine. Methysergide or propranolol may be prescribed to prevent migraine pain.*

**STIMULANT DRUGS**

Stimulant drugs (for example, the amphetamines) are not widely used today because they are addictive. The amphetamine derivative methylphenidate hydrochloride is used in the treatment of attention-deficit disorders in children, although its use is controversial because of its addictive potential. In addition, stimulants can reduce appetite and the ability to concentrate; cause palpitations, tremor, sleeplessness, and anxiety; and precipitate drug-induced severe mental disorders.

## DRUGS FOR PARKINSON'S DISEASE

Parkinson's disease is caused by an imbalance of dopamine and acetylcholine – the neurotransmitters that are responsible for the transmission of nerve signals from the brain to coordinate muscle movement. In Parkinson's disease, the cells in the brain that produce dopamine degenerate. This causes an insufficient level of dopamine, so acetylcholine is overactive.

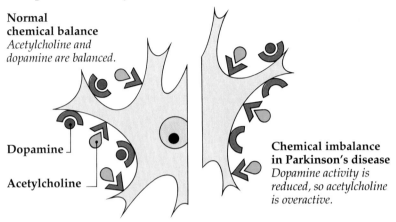

**Normal chemical balance**
*Acetylcholine and dopamine are balanced.*

**Dopamine**

**Acetylcholine**

**Chemical imbalance in Parkinson's disease**
*Dopamine activity is reduced, so acetylcholine is overactive.*

The balance between the two neurotransmitters can be restored either by taking a drug that blocks the action of acetylcholine (an anticholinergic drug), such as benztropine and orphenadrine, or by giving a dopamine-boosting drug. Dopamine activity cannot be increased by giving dopamine directly because dopamine is metabolized in the digestive tract; also, dopamine cannot cross from the blood into the brain. Therefore, the substance from which dopamine is formed, levodopa, is prescribed. Levodopa is converted to dopamine in the brain.

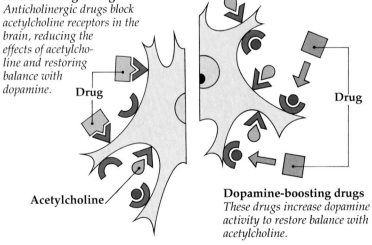

**Anticholinergic drugs**
*Anticholinergic drugs block acetylcholine receptors in the brain, reducing the effects of acetylcholine and restoring balance with dopamine.*

**Drug**

**Drug**

**Acetylcholine**

**Dopamine-boosting drugs**
*These drugs increase dopamine activity to restore balance with acetylcholine.*

Dopamine levels can also be increased by treatment with deprenyl, which reduces the breakdown of dopamine, or by amantadine, which increases dopamine levels by stimulating dopamine release. Bromocriptine is also used to treat Parkinson's disease. This drug has characteristics that are very similar to those of dopamine and mimics its action in the brain.

## ASK YOUR DOCTOR
## ANTIANXIETY AND SLEEPING DRUGS

**Q** Sometimes I wake up in the middle of the night, even after I have taken a sleeping pill. Is it all right to take another pill?

**A** No. You should never exceed the recommended dose of any medication, including sleeping pills. If you are waking up during the night, you may need a sleeping pill that has a longer duration of action. Talk to your doctor about the possible causes of your insomnia and ask him or her to review your medication.

**Q** About how many hours before I go to bed should I take my sleeping pills?

**A** Sleeping pills begin to be absorbed about 30 minutes after they are taken. Most people usually fall asleep within an hour of taking a sleeping pill. You should try to be in bed within about half an hour after taking them.

**Q** I have been taking chlordiazepoxide for 20 years to calm my nerves. My analyst tells me I should stop taking this medication. How should I do this safely?

**A** If you abruptly stop taking your medication on your own you will experience two effects – a resurgence of anxiety and withdrawal symptoms. Talk to your doctor so that he or she can design a gradual withdrawal from the drug. It would also be advisable to make sure that your analyst can give you psychological support during this time, when you may possibly experience added stress because of the withdrawal from the medication.

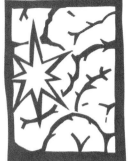

# DRUGS FOR DIGESTIVE DISORDERS

T HE DIGESTIVE TRACT consists of the mouth, esophagus, stomach, small intestine (including the duodenum), large intestine (including the colon and rectum), and anus. The purpose of the digestive tract is to digest food and absorb nutrients. The system is also referred to as the gastrointestinal or alimentary tract.

Digestion begins in the mouth, where enzymes in saliva begin to break down food. Food passes down the esophagus into the stomach, which stores and mixes food and secretes acids and enzymes that break down food to a semiliquid consistency. The food passes into the small intestine, where nutrients are absorbed into the bloodstream. The remaining undigested food enters the large intestine, where water is absorbed into the bloodstream; waste products are excreted through the anus.

## WHAT CAN GO WRONG?

Digestive disorders can be caused by inflammation or ulceration of the digestive tract or by disruption of the muscular contractions that move food through the digestive system. Drugs used to treat gastrointestinal disorders include antacids and other antiulcer drugs, antidiarrheals, anti-inflammatory drugs, drugs for gallstones, antispasmodics, and drugs for rectal and anal problems.

## DRUGS FOR GASTRIC DISORDERS

Gastric (stomach) disorders include gastroenteritis (inflammation of the lining of the stomach and intestines), dyspepsia (indigestion), and ulcers. Gastroenteritis may be caused by a bacterial or viral infection. Symptoms of gastroenteritis include severe nausea, vomiting, and diarrhea, which can lead to dehydration. Replacement of the body's fluids lost through severe vomiting and diarrhea can prevent dehydration (see WARNING on page 125). Stomach disorders may result from eating spicy food, drinking alcohol, ingesting caffeine, or taking nonsteroidal anti-inflammatory drugs (NSAIDs) such as aspirin and ibuprofen. Indigestion may be relieved by antacids (which neutralize stomach acids), which also effectively heal peptic ulcers of the esophagus, stomach, and duodenum if the antacids are taken regularly with your doctor's supervision.

**Prostaglandin analogues**
*Misoprostol is the first in a new drug group called prostaglandin analogues. This drug enhances the defense mechanisms of the stomach lining. The primary use of misoprostol is to prevent recurrent bleeding in the stomach caused by nonsteroidal anti-inflammatory drugs.*

Duodenal ulcer

Duodenum

**Mucosal protectors**
*Mucosal protectors, such as sucralfate and bismuth salts, coat the mucous membrane of the stomach with a protective layer to prevent acid from reaching an ulcer. Sucralfate can cause constipation and interfere with the absorption of some vitamins, so vitamin supplements may be recommended. Bismuth salts can cause the feces to turn black.*

Acid

Mucosal protector

Mucus

Stomach lining

Stomach wall

Gastric ulcer

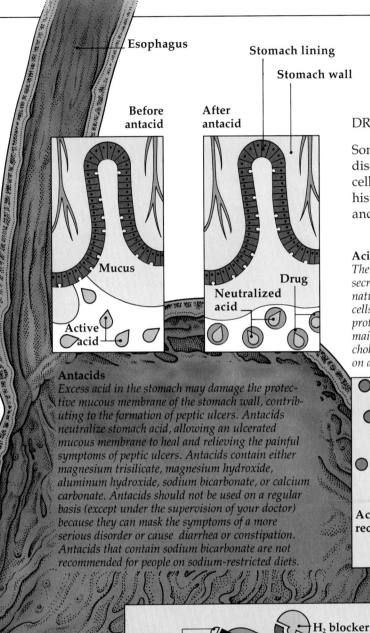

Esophagus

Stomach lining

Stomach wall

Before antacid

After antacid

Mucus

Drug

Neutralized acid

Active acid

Stomach

Stomach wall

## DRUGS THAT REDUCE ACID SECRETION

Some drugs that are used to treat digestive disorders work by reducing the acid secreted by cells in the stomach lining. These drugs include histamine ($H_2$) blockers, proton pump inhibitors, and anticholinergic agents.

### Acid secretion
*The diagram below shows three mechanisms involved in the secretion of acid by cells in the stomach lining. Histamine (a naturally occurring substance) acts on $H_2$ receptors on the cells to stimulate acid secretion. Tiny units in the cells called proton pumps release protons (which are hydrogen ions, the main constituent of acid) into the stomach channel. Acetylcholine (a neurotransmitter released by a cranial nerve) acts on acetylcholine receptors to promote acid secretion.*

### Antacids
*Excess acid in the stomach may damage the protective mucous membrane of the stomach wall, contributing to the formation of peptic ulcers. Antacids neutralize stomach acid, allowing an ulcerated mucous membrane to heal and relieving the painful symptoms of peptic ulcers. Antacids contain either magnesium trisilicate, magnesium hydroxide, aluminum hydroxide, sodium bicarbonate, or calcium carbonate. Antacids should not be used on a regular basis (except under the supervision of your doctor) because they can mask the symptoms of a more serious disorder or cause diarrhea or constipation. Antacids that contain sodium bicarbonate are not recommended for people on sodium-restricted diets.*

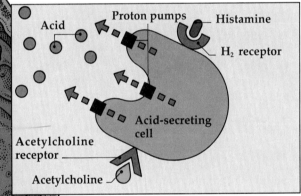

Acid

Proton pumps

Histamine

$H_2$ receptor

Acid-secreting cell

Acetylcholine receptor

Acetylcholine

### Proton pump inhibitors
*Omeprazole, the first drug in the new class of drugs called proton pump inhibitors, reduces gastric acid by blocking the release of protons by proton pumps. Omeprazole is approved by the Food and Drug Administration for treatment of esophagitis (inflammation of the esophagus) caused by regurgitation of acid from the stomach.*

### Histamine ($H_2$) blockers
*This group of drugs significantly reduces acid secretion by blocking histamine from reaching $H_2$ receptors. The drugs are mainly used to treat peptic ulcers. Peptic ulcers occur when the mucous layer and/or mucous membrane of the stomach or duodenum have been damaged, allowing hydrochloric acid and pepsin (a digestive enzyme) to erode underlying tissue. Reducing acidity allows peptic ulcers to heal in about 4 to 8 weeks. The $H_2$ blockers cause few side effects but some may cause confusion in older people or breast enlargement in men and may have interactions with some other drugs.*

$H_2$ blocker blocks $H_2$ receptor

Proton pump inhibitor blocks proton pumps

Acid

Anticholinergic drug blocks acetylcholine receptor

Acid-secreting cell

### Anticholinergic agents
*These drugs block acetylcholine receptors, thus reducing acid secretion. The use of these types of drugs has declined as more effective drugs to treat ulcers have become available.*

# DRUGS FOR INTESTINAL DISORDERS

Disorders of the small and large intestines include constipation, diarrhea, ulcerative colitis (inflammation and ulceration of the colon), Crohn's disease (inflammation of any part of the digestive tract), and rectal and anal problems. Medications prescribed for these disorders are often part of an overall treatment program, including changes in diet and control of stress.

## GALLSTONES

The gallbladder stores and concentrates bile. Bile is produced in the liver and contains ingredients that aid the breakdown and absorption of fat. Breakdown products that result from normal destruction and turnover of cells (such as pigments and cholesterol) are also present in bile. Most gallstones occur because the concentration of cholesterol has increased or bile acid levels have decreased, causing some of the undissolved cholesterol to accumulate and crystallize. These stones can be dissolved by drugs such as chenodiol and ursodiol. Stones can also be dissolved by injecting various ethers directly through the skin into the gall-bladder.

## ANTIDIARRHEALS

Diarrhea occurs when the large intestine is unable to absorb fluid brought to it from the upper digestive tract or when inflammation or tumor causes excess secretion of fluid. The most common cause of diarrhea is infection; diarrhea can also be caused by other illnesses, anxiety, or some drugs. The drugs most commonly used to treat diarrhea are codeine, loperamide, or diphenoxylate (which contain a narcotic drug) and adsorbent agents such as kaolin or methylcellulose (which absorb water and cause toxins to adsorb to them). Antispasmodic drugs such as belladonna are sometimes used to relieve cramps. It is vitally important to replace the body fluid that is lost through severe diarrhea (see WARNING on page 125).

### Narcotic antidiarrheals
*Narcotic drugs reduce the propulsive contractions of the intestine by reducing nerve signals sent to the intestinal muscles. This action slows the passage of the liquid stool, allowing more time for water to be absorbed and reducing the frequency and volume of bowel movements.*

### Adsorbent agents
*Adsorbent agents, which take up and hold other substances, are available in the form of pectin, kaolin, or methylcellulose products. Adsorbent agents are capable of absorbing many times their weight of water. Some of these agents may also absorb viral particles or bacterial toxins.*

**After narcotic**
Slowed propulsion allows more water to be absorbed.

**Before narcotic**
Rapid propulsion prevents water absorption.

**Water absorbed**

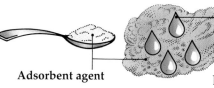

**Adsorbent agent**

**Gallstones (actual size)**

## DRUGS FOR RECTAL AND ANAL DISORDERS
Rectal and anal disorders include hemorrhoids, anal fissures (cracks), and pruritus ani (itching). These conditions are aggravated by constipation or factors such as tension. Treatment may include relieving constipation and reducing pain, inflammation, and itching with creams and ointments. Preparations may contain a soothing agent (such as zinc oxide) that has antiseptic or astringent properties and may also include a local anesthetic. Your doctor may also pre-scribe a topical corticosteroid to be applied as a cream or ointment or as a suppository to reduce inflammation.

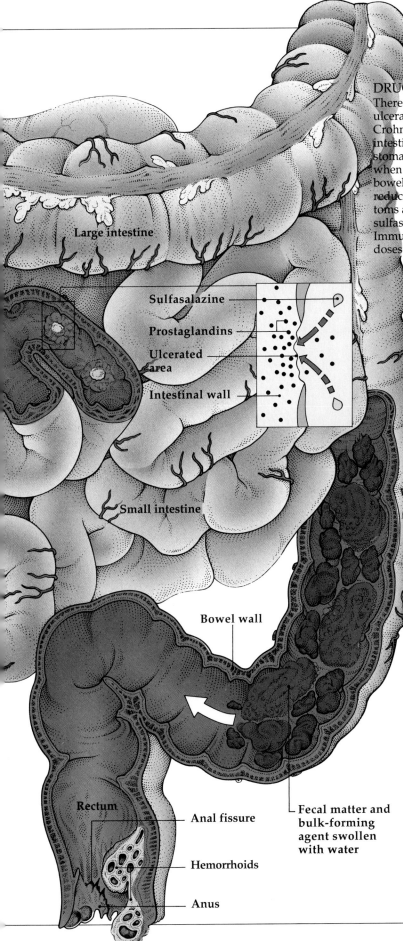

Large intestine

Sulfasalazine

Prostaglandins

Ulcerated area

Intestinal wall

Small intestine

Bowel wall

Rectum

Anal fissure — 

Hemorrhoids — 

Anus — 

└ Fecal matter and bulk-forming agent swollen with water

## DRUGS FOR INFLAMMATORY BOWEL DISEASE

There are two main types of inflammatory bowel disease – ulcerative colitis, which occurs in the large intestine, and Crohn's disease, which most often affects the small or large intestine, but also occurs in the mouth, esophagus, and stomach. Scientists believe that both diseases may occur when your body's immune system attacks the tissues of your bowel. These conditions can be treated with drugs that reduce the inflammation, which in turn controls the symptoms and prevents complications. Corticosteroid drugs and sulfasalazine (below left) are used to reduce inflammation. Immunosuppressant drugs may be prescribed so that lower doses of corticosteroids may be used.

### Sulfasalazine

*Inflammation is triggered by several naturally occurring chemicals, including the prostaglandins. Sulfasalazine prevents the formation of prostaglandins around the ulcerated area in the intestinal wall. This halts the inflammatory process and allows the ulcer to heal. Sulfasalazine can cause kidney problems or a rash. Derivatives of the salicylate portion of sulfasalazine have been introduced that cause fewer side effects.*

## LAXATIVES

Laxative drugs should almost never be used. Adequate intake of fruits, vegetables, unrefined grains, and fluids, along with proper toilet habits (including responding to the urge to have a bowel movement) and the use of glycerin suppositories (when needed) can prevent almost all constipation in most people. Types of laxatives include lubricants such as mineral oil and bulk-forming agents such as methylcellulose. Prolonged or regular use of laxatives can cause the bowel to be overemptied; the bowel can then become dependent on laxatives to achieve a bowel movement. Use of laxatives may be appropriate for very brief periods in preparation for some surgical and investigational procedures, during immobility from a fracture or during convalescence, or with the constipation that sometimes occurs after surgery.

### Bulk-forming agents

*Bulk-forming agents soften and increase the volume of feces by absorbing water in the bowel. The feces become more responsive to the pressure of the contracting bowel wall and are passed more easily. An increased intake of fluids is recommended when you are taking bulk-forming laxatives. You should not take bulk-forming laxatives for constipation associated with abdominal pain without first talking to your doctor.*

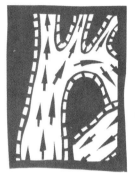

# DRUGS FOR THE HEART AND CIRCULATION

DISORDERS OF THE HEART and blood vessels are among the most common causes of death in developed countries, particularly for people over age 65. Some cardiovascular conditions can be improved by altering dietary and other habits. However, drug therapy is often required. Many different drugs are available for the treatment of heart and circulatory disorders.

Cardiovascular conditions that often require drug treatment include weakening of the heart's pumping action (heart failure), irregularity of the heartbeat (arrhythmia), fatty deposits in the blood vessels (atherosclerosis), angina (chest pain), and hypertension (high blood pressure). Drugs used for the treatment of heart conditions are always prescribed with caution, particularly for people with diabetes or a disorder of the liver or kidneys or for pregnant women.

## ANTI-ARRHYTHMICS

A broad range of drugs are used to regulate the heartbeat; all of them suppress the conduction of electrical signals in the heart. These drugs include cardiac glycosides, beta blockers, and calcium channel blockers. Specialized antiarrhythmic agents such as disopyramide, procainamide, and quinidine reduce the response of the heart muscle to electrical signals. All antiarrhythmic drugs can cause adverse effects; the most serious risk is that of causing potentially fatal abnormal heart rhythms. Therefore, treatment with these drugs is undertaken only when the benefits outweigh the risks.

## NITRATES

Nitrate drugs are often prescribed to treat angina (chest pain), which occurs when the blood supply to the heart is reduced by narrowing of the arteries.

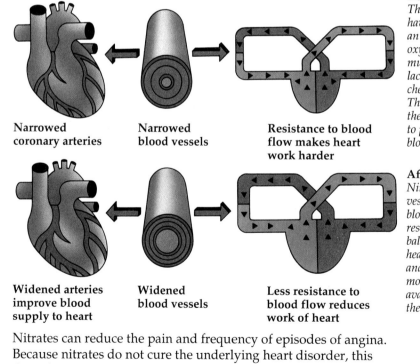

Narrowed coronary arteries

Narrowed blood vessels

Resistance to blood flow makes heart work harder

Widened arteries improve blood supply to heart

Widened blood vessels

Less resistance to blood flow reduces work of heart

**Before nitrate drugs**
*The coronary arteries have narrowed, causing an insufficient amount of oxygen to reach the heart muscle and allowing lactic acid and other chemicals to accumulate. This causes angina as the heart works harder to provide an adequate blood supply.*

**After nitrate drugs**
*Nitrates widen blood vessels to increase the blood flow to the heart, restoring the normal balance between the heart's need for oxygen and its availability. As more oxygen becomes available, the strain on the heart is reduced.*

Nitrates can reduce the pain and frequency of episodes of angina. Because nitrates do not cure the underlying heart disorder, this drug therapy must continue indefinitely in most cases. Nitrates rarely cause serious adverse effects, but minor side effects such as flushing, headache, dizziness, and fainting are common. Nitrates are sometimes used as part of the treatment of heart failure.

## CARDIAC GLYCOSIDES

Cardiac glycosides (also called digitalis drugs) are derived from the leaves of foxglove plants. These drugs are prescribed for a variety of heart disorders, including arrhythmias and heart failure. Cardiac glycosides slow the passage of electrical impulses through the heart muscle to reduce the heart rate. In most cases, treatment with cardiac glycosides must continue indefinitely. A diuretic is often prescribed with a cardiac glycoside to relieve the symptoms of fatigue, breathlessness, and swelling of the legs that result from heart failure. Cardiac glycosides can be poisonous if the level in your blood becomes too high or if your potassium level becomes too low. To prevent these complications, your doctor will periodically monitor the concentration of the drug in your blood. Potassium supplements may be recommended if you are taking both a cardiac glycoside and a diuretic.

## BETA BLOCKERS

Beta blockers are used in the treatment of hypertension, angina, arrhythmia, and hypertrophic cardiomyopathy (a disorder in which portions of the heart muscle become abnormally thick). These drugs are also sometimes prescribed to minimize the possibility of sudden death after a heart attack, but they should never be taken for treatment of heart failure. Beta blockers reduce the frequency and severity of episodes of angina. However, they also reduce circulation to the extremities, so you may experience cold hands and feet. Beta blockers are not usually prescribed for people with lung conditions such as asthma or bronchitis because these drugs can further narrow the airways. Withdrawal from treatment with beta blockers should be achieved with tapered dosages because sudden, complete withdrawal can cause a recurrence of angina or, rarely, a heart attack.

## ACE INHIBITORS

Angiotensin-converting enzyme (ACE) inhibitors are used to treat hypertension and heart failure. These medications block the enzyme that activates angiotensin (a naturally occurring substance involved in the narrowing of blood vessels) and lower blood pressure rapidly. ACE inhibitors are also effective in treating moderately severe and severe heart failure. These drugs may cause minor adverse reactions, including nausea, cough, dizziness, and a rash.

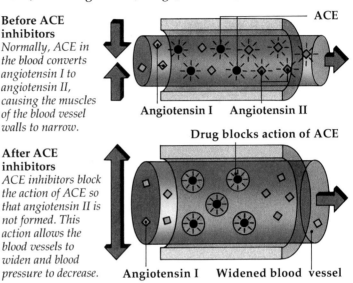

**Before ACE inhibitors**
*Normally, ACE in the blood converts angiotensin I to angiotensin II, causing the muscles of the blood vessel walls to narrow.*

**After ACE inhibitors**
*ACE inhibitors block the action of ACE so that angiotensin II is not formed. This action allows the blood vessels to widen and blood pressure to decrease.*

### ANTIRENINS

Renin is an enzyme produced by the kidney that converts inactive angiotensin in the blood to angiotensin I (still inactive). Angiotensin I may then be converted to angiotensin II (active form), which narrows blood vessels. Antirenins block the converting action of renin on angiotensin, thereby widening the blood vessels. The action of antirenins is similar to that of ACE inhibitors, but antirenins affect an earlier stage of the angiotensin conversion process.

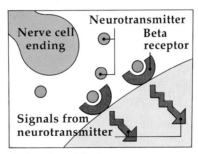

**Before beta blockers**
*The neurotransmitter norepinephrine attaches to a beta receptor (see DRUGS AND RECEPTORS on page 31), signaling widening of a blood vessel or an increase in the heart rate or in the strength of cardiac contraction.*

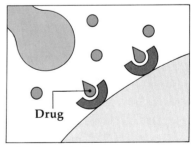

**After beta blockers**
*By occupying the beta receptors, beta blockers reduce the workload of the heart and decrease the amount of oxygen the heart requires. By this mechanism, blood pressure is reduced and heart rate is lowered.*

## DIURETICS

Diuretics help convert excess body fluid into urine. As this fluid is expelled, swelling of tissues caused by the retention of excess fluid is reduced. Diuretics increase sodium excretion, which leads to increased water excretion. The workload of the heart is decreased because the volume of circulating blood is reduced. Diuretics are most commonly used to treat excess fluid in the body as a result of heart, liver, or kidney disease and to treat high blood pressure.

Diuretics (thiazides and loop diuretics) act on different parts of the kidneys' collecting tubules. Both types of diuretics can cause a potassium deficiency and are used in conjunction with either potassium-sparing diuretics or potassium supplements. A decreased potassium level can cause arrhythmias, weakness, and confusion. With some diuretics, uric acid is retained and there is a risk of gout. Other side effects of diuretics include nausea, leg cramps, and a partial inability to metabolize sugar.

## LOVASTATIN – A LIPID-LOWERING DRUG

Lovastatin is a lipid-lowering drug that controls hyperlipidemia (a high level of fatty substances in the blood). The drug is used to treat people at high risk from atherosclerosis (thickening of the arterial wall, which reduces blood flow) and those who have other conditions caused by arteries that have become clogged with fatty deposits. Lovastatin only occasionally removes existing fatty deposits in the blood vessels but it does prevent buildup of excess cholesterol in the blood vessels. This drug acts on the liver, where it blocks coenzyme A reductase, an enzyme important in the formation of cholesterol. Other lipid-lowering drugs act in the intestine to bind with bile salts, which carry large amounts of cholesterol, thus preventing the cholesterol from being reabsorbed into the bloodstream. In most cases, treatment must continue indefinitely. Drug therapy is only part of the overall treatment, along with efforts to reduce fat in the diet and to lose excess weight.

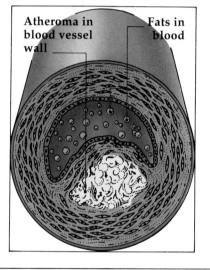

Atheroma in blood vessel wall

Fats in blood

## HOW DIURETICS WORK

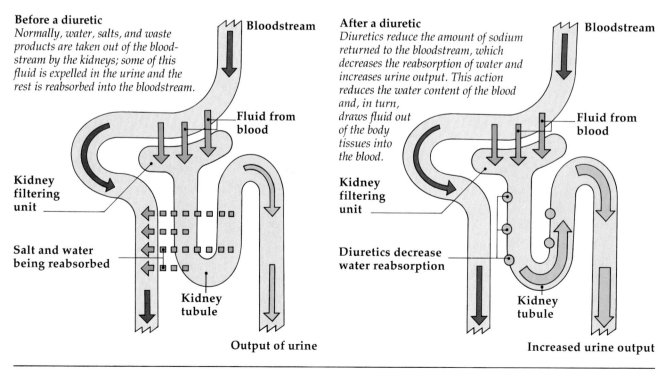

**Before a diuretic**
*Normally, water, salts, and waste products are taken out of the bloodstream by the kidneys; some of this fluid is expelled in the urine and the rest is reabsorbed into the bloodstream.*

Bloodstream

Fluid from blood

Kidney filtering unit

Salt and water being reabsorbed

Kidney tubule

Output of urine

**After a diuretic**
*Diuretics reduce the amount of sodium returned to the bloodstream, which decreases the reabsorption of water and increases urine output. This action reduces the water content of the blood and, in turn, draws fluid out of the body tissues into the blood.*

Bloodstream

Fluid from blood

Kidney filtering unit

Diuretics decrease water reabsorption

Kidney tubule

Increased urine output

**The action of sympatholytics**
*Messages from the sympathetic nervous system travel to muscle fibers in the walls of blood vessels and cause the muscles to contract, thereby narrowing the blood vessels. Sympatholytic drugs block the nerve signals that trigger narrowing of the blood vessels.*

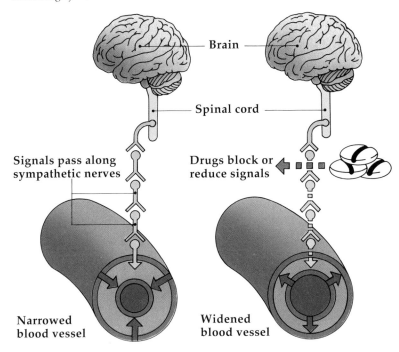

# SYMPATHOLYTICS

Sympatholytic drugs are sometimes used in the treatment of hypertension. These medications block or inhibit the function of the sympathetic nervous system (which controls many of the body's involuntary activities, such as narrowing of blood vessels). Because these drugs cause blood vessels to widen, they are known as vasodilators. Sympatholytics can act on control centers in the brain (clonidine), block the transmission of signals through the sympathetic nerve pathways (guanethidine), or stop the signals to the muscles of blood vessel walls (prazosin). Minor side effects include nausea, diarrhea, and fatigue or drowsiness, but sympatholytics can also cause a drop in blood pressure, making you feel dizzy when you stand up. If this occurs, contact your doctor immediately; he or she may wish to make an adjustment in the dosage of your medication or switch you to a different drug.

## CALCIUM CHANNEL BLOCKERS

Calcium channel blockers are used to treat hypertension and disorders that affect the blood supply to the heart. They also help prevent angina and are effective in the treatment of irregular heartbeats. Because these drugs do not cure the underlying disorder, therapy may be required indefinitely. There are few risks associated with prolonged use. Unlike the beta blockers, they can be used safely by people who have asthma.

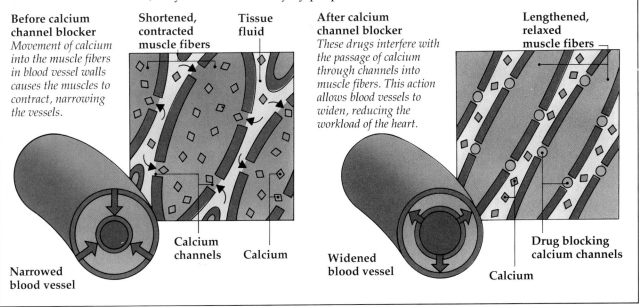

**Before calcium channel blocker**
*Movement of calcium into the muscle fibers in blood vessel walls causes the muscles to contract, narrowing the vessels.*

**After calcium channel blocker**
*These drugs interfere with the passage of calcium through channels into muscle fibers. This action allows blood vessels to widen, reducing the workload of the heart.*

# DRUGS THAT AFFECT BLOOD CLOTTING

When a blood clot forms in a blood vessel, it effectively shuts off the blood flow through that vessel to the tissue it supplies. This can lead to a stroke, heart attack, or other circulatory crises. You are at increased risk of clot formation if you have atherosclerosis; your doctor may prescribe a drug that prevents blood clots or causes them to disperse.

## ANTIPLATELETS

Antiplatelet drugs reduce the ability of platelets to stick together and form a clot. These drugs are used as a precautionary measure to prevent clot formation after heart surgery or a heart attack. The most commonly used antiplatelet drug is aspirin, which is taken in varying doses from 50 to 300 milligrams every day or every other day. Antiplatelet drug therapy must continue indefinitely in most cases. Minor side effects include rash, indigestion, and dizziness.

## ANTICOAGULANTS

Anticoagulant drugs such as warfarin help maintain normal blood flow in people who have an increased risk of clot formation, such as those who are bedridden or who have heart failure. Anticoagulants prevent extension of existing clots and formation of new clots. These drugs do not dissolve clots that have already formed, a task that is performed by substances in the body or by thrombolytic drugs. Anticoagulants are normally taken for at least 6 months and people who have artificial heart valves may have to take them indefinitely. Side effects include increased susceptibility to bruising; occasional bleeding from the nose, gums, or urinary tract; and nausea.

## THROMBOLYTICS

Thrombolytic medications are often used to treat heart attacks. These drugs dissolve blood clots, restoring the normal blood supply to the heart. The most commonly used thrombolytics are streptokinase and tissue plasminogen activator (TPA). The two medications are almost equally effective. TPA is produced by genetic engineering from a substance formed in the body and is less likely to produce an allergic reaction than streptokinase, which is produced by bacteria. Side effects of thrombolytics include greater susceptibility to bleeding, nausea, and vomiting.

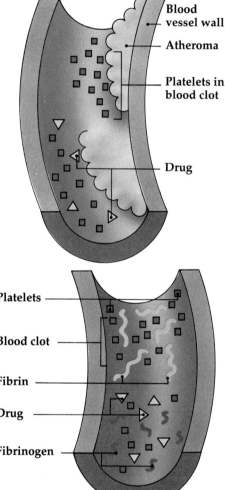

Blood vessel wall

Atheroma

Platelets in blood clot

Drug

**Effect of antiplatelets**
*If an atheroma (a fatty deposit on the inner lining of an artery) forms, small cells in the blood known as platelets may tend to clump together around this area, leading to a blood clot. Antiplatelet drugs reduce the ability of platelets to stick together, preventing the formation of a clot.*

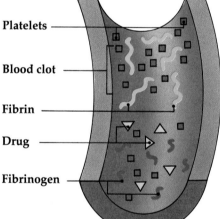

Platelets

Blood clot

Fibrin

Drug

Fibrinogen

**Effect of anticoagulants**
*A blood clot can form on a blood vessel wall as platelets bind together with the protein fibrin. Anticoagulants work by inhibiting the production of the blood-clotting substances that convert the inactive substance fibrinogen into fibrin, thereby preventing the formation of clots.*

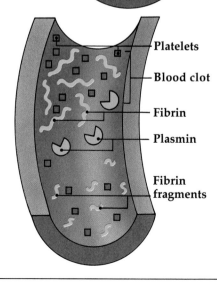

Platelets

Blood clot

Fibrin

Plasmin

Fibrin fragments

**Effect of thrombolytics**
*Thrombolytics act in the blood by stimulating the natural conversion of inactive plasminogen to plasmin. Plasmin is an enzyme that breaks down the fibrin that binds a clot together and allows the clot to dissolve.*

# CASE HISTORY
# RISING BLOOD PRESSURE

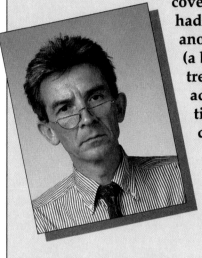

MICHAEL HAS HAD **moderately high blood pressure (hypertension) for 25 years. His condition had been treated effectively for many years with a combination of two antihypertensive drugs – a diuretic and a vasodilator. During a checkup Michael's doctor discovered that his blood pressure had risen. His doctor added yet another antihypertensive drug (a beta blocker) to his course of treatment. Shortly after the addition of this new medication, Michael returned to his doctor's office for follow-up.**

### PERSONAL DETAILS
**Name** Michael Sykova
**Age** 55
**Occupation** Personnel manager
**Family** Both parents have high blood pressure.

at which they are usually prescribed. Once this point is reached, further increases in dosage will not reduce the blood pressure and are likely to have an adverse effect.

## THE TREATMENT
Michael's doctor prescribes a newer type of antihypertensive drug called an angiotensin-converting enzyme (ACE) inhibitor to be added to his current drug treatment. The dosage of the ACE inhibitor will be increased gradually over a period of several weeks to reach the effective level, while the doses of his other antihypertensives will be gradually reduced until he can stop taking the other drugs entirely. The doctor's goal is to switch Michael's drug treatment program without causing wide fluctuations in his blood pressure.

## THE OUTCOME
Michael's hypertension is now controlled with just one drug instead of several. After 6 months his blood pressure has been reduced and has remained steady at 140 over 85.

## MEDICAL BACKGROUND
Michael has had only the usual childhood diseases; his hypertension developed at age 30. He does not smoke cigarettes or drink alcohol. Michael's doctor has monitored his blood pressure regularly and has found that Michael experienced no adverse effects from his previous drug treatment. Michael's blood pressure was at first regulated with hydralazine (a vasodilator). After a few months his doctor added the diuretic chlorthalidone to his therapy. When Michael's doctor discovered during a checkup that his blood pressure had risen, atenolol (a beta blocker) was prescribed in addition to his current medications.

## THE CONSULTATION
The doctor checks Michael's blood pressure after 15 minutes of rest and finds it is 180 (systolic) over 110 (diastolic), which is too high. She finds that Michael is otherwise well.

## THE DIAGNOSIS
Michael's doctor explains that a RE-ADJUSTMENT OF MEDICATION is necessary because the drugs he is taking have reached the maximum safe dose

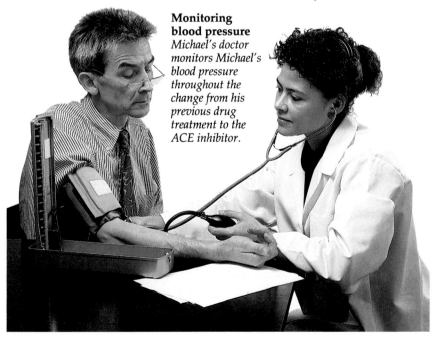

**Monitoring blood pressure**
*Michael's doctor monitors Michael's blood pressure throughout the change from his previous drug treatment to the ACE inhibitor.*

# DRUGS FOR RESPIRATORY DISORDERS

THE RESPIRATORY SYSTEM includes the nose, throat, trachea (windpipe), bronchial tubes, and lungs. Breathing enables the body to obtain the oxygen it needs for energy production and to expel carbon dioxide. Breathing difficulties can be caused by blockage or narrowing of the airways and damage to or destruction of the alveoli (tiny air sacs in the lungs).

Problems that affect the lungs include contraction or chronic inflammation of the muscles in the bronchial walls, causing narrowing of the small airways (bronchioles) in the lungs. Breathing difficulties can also be aggravated by the release of mucus into the airways. Examples of these conditions are asthmatic bronchitis and emphysema. Emphysema results from the breakdown of the walls of the alveoli, which reduces the surface available for the exchange of oxygen and carbon dioxide between air and blood. Medications that influence the lung's air passages have a variety of actions; they may be used to clear the air passages, to reduce inflammation, or to reduce the production of mucus.

**Alveoli**

**Oxygen** flowing from alveoli to red blood cells

**Carbon dioxide** flowing from red blood cells to alveoli

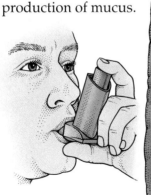

**Corticosteroids**
*Corticosteroids are powerful drugs that can be used to prevent minor asthma attacks or to treat severe attacks. The drugs relieve inflammation in the air passages and indirectly cause relaxation of the muscles in the walls of the air passages. Corticosteroids are taken by inhaler. Because inhalation is thought to deliver the drug directly to the bronchioles, only very small doses of a corticosteroid are required. In severe attacks, an appropriate dose of a corticosteroid may be given by injection or in tablet form.*

## WARNING

Occasionally, bronchodilators do not relieve asthma even when (or especially when) the dosage is increased. Taking more medication can be dangerous and even fatal because it may mask underlying inflammatory changes. If you feel that your bronchodilator medication is not working – even if you take more of it – call your doctor.

**Trachea (windpipe)**

**Bronchi**

**Lung**

**Bronchioles in spasm**

**Normal bronchioles**

**Mast cell**

**Airway**

**Drug**

**Chemicals that narrow the airway**

**Airway**

**Bronchiole**

### Sympathomimetics

*Sympathomimetics are bronchodilators that are used to prevent or to treat bronchospasm (narrowing of the lung's air passages). These drugs relax smooth muscles and widen the bronchioles, allowing air to move through the passages more freely. Sympathomimetics, such as albuterol, can be taken as tablets or by injection, but are most commonly inhaled in pressurized aerosols or taken by nebulizer. Nebulizers pump compressed air through a drug solution, which is inhaled through a face mask.*

### Xanthines

*Xanthine bronchodilators (such as theophylline and aminophylline) are used for the prevention and treatment of bronchospasm. They are usually taken as tablets or by injection. Xanthines act directly on the muscles in the walls of the air passages, causing the muscles to relax.*

### Anticholinergics

*Anticholinergic bronchodilators produce relaxation and widening of the bronchioles by blocking the action of acetylcholine, the neurotransmitter that causes bronchial muscle to contract. Anticholinergics are usually used in combination with sympathomimetics or xanthines and are prescribed in the form of inhalers.*

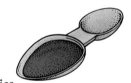

### Cough remedies

*Mucolytics and expectorants are cough remedies that are believed to act directly on the lungs and airways. Mucolytics alter the consistency of phlegm, making it easier to cough up; expectorants are designed to help cough up the phlegm. The best way to get rid of phlegm is to drink plenty of water. Cough suppressants are taken orally and act on the cough center in the brain. They are useful if you are trying to suppress a dry cough (a cough that does not produce phlegm).*

### Mast cell stabilizers (antiallergics)

*As their name suggests, mast cell stabilizers act on the mast cells in the bronchiole walls – the cells that release chemicals that narrow the airway. Drugs such as cromolyn sodium are useful for the prevention (but not the treatment) of bronchospasm. Cromolyn sodium prevents the release of these chemicals from the mast cells and also has a direct anti-inflammatory effect. Although effective as a preventive treatment in children, it is often less effective in adults. This drug is effective only if inhaled because it cannot be absorbed in the gastrointestinal tract. It can be taken by aerosol and by inhalation of powder from a cartridge.*

## ASK YOUR DOCTOR
# DRUGS FOR RESPIRATORY DISORDERS

**Q I use an albuterol inhaler for asthma. Recently, I have needed to use it more often. What should I do?**

**A** See your doctor at once. Increasing your doses of medication is ineffective and may be dangerous because it can mask underlying inflammatory changes in your lungs. Your doctor may prescribe a corticosteroid to be inhaled regularly to control your asthma.

**Q I have heard that corticosteroids cause side effects. Is my corticosteroid inhaler dangerous?**

**A** No. Corticosteroid tablets can produce side effects because the corticosteroid is absorbed into the bloodstream. An inhaled corticosteroid is given in doses far smaller than the doses given in tablets because the inhaled drug is delivered directly to the airways in the lungs and only a very small amount is absorbed into the bloodstream.

**Q My friend says that you can have injections for hay fever. What are they and do they work?**

**A** If drugs such as antihistamines prove ineffective against hay fever, desensitization injections may be recommended before the start of the hay-fever season. Your doctor will give you a series of injections with gradually increased doses of an allergen extract (the substance that causes your allergic reaction). The injections desensitize your body to the allergen, reducing the reaction when you are exposed to it naturally. In some cases, desensitization may not work completely.

## DRUGS FOR CONGESTION

Nasal congestion is caused by inflammation of the mucous membrane that lines the nasal passages (rhinitis), due to engorgement of the underlying blood vessels. The condition is further aggravated by excessive production of mucus. These symptoms may be caused by an infection such as the common cold or an allergy such as hay fever. Congestion caused by inflammation may also occur in the air spaces in the skull (the sinuses), a condition known as sinusitis. Decongestant drugs may be used to relieve nasal congestion and sinusitis by promoting drainage of mucus.

### Decongestants
Decongestants such as oxymetazoline, phenylephrine, and phenylpropanolamine are available in the form of tablets, aerosols, or nose drops. Decongestant drops start to relieve congestion within a few minutes. Oral decongestants take a little longer to act, but the effects of the drug may last longer. These drugs may be used to treat common colds, sinusitis, and hay fever. However, do not use decongestant sprays or drops for more than 6 to 8 days. If you use a decongestant excessively for a long time you may notice stuffiness when you suddenly stop using it; the congestion may recur and symptoms may become more severe.

**Corticosteroids and cromolyn sodium**
*Both corticosteroid drugs and cromolyn sodium can be used to reduce and prevent the symptoms of an allergy. They are available as nasal sprays and eye drops.*

### ANTIALLERGICS
Hay fever, the best known allergy affecting the respiratory system, occurs when pollen is inhaled and irritates the lining of the nose. This irritation is caused by the pollen triggering the release of histamine from the mast cells. Histamine causes swelling and widening of the blood vessels that leak fluid into the lining of the nose. The result is increased production of mucus. Widespread irritation also causes sneezing and often redness and watering of the eyes. Drug treatment for allergic reactions includes antihistamines, decongestants, corticosteroids, and cromolyn sodium.

# DRUGS TO TREAT ALLERGIES AND CONGESTION

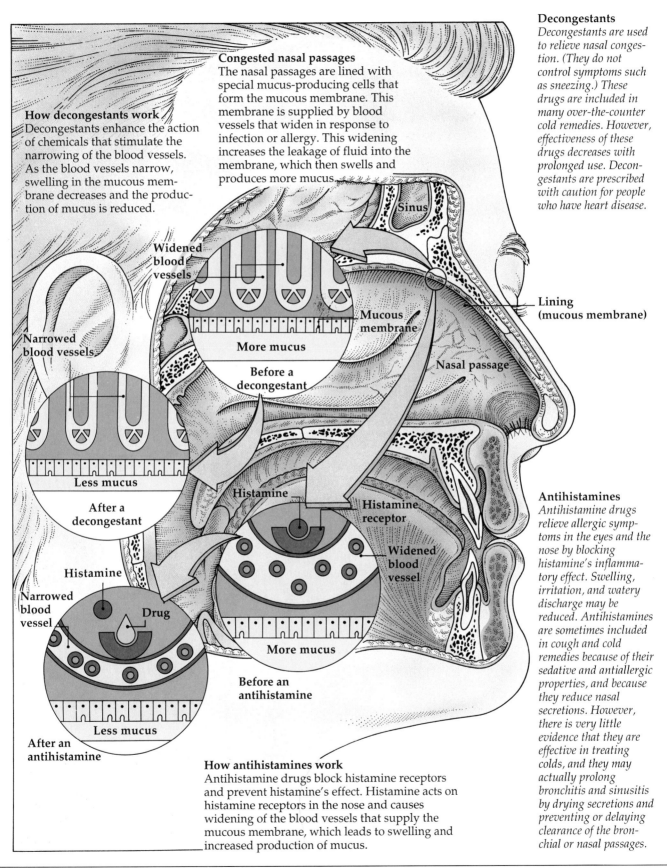

**How decongestants work**
Decongestants enhance the action of chemicals that stimulate the narrowing of the blood vessels. As the blood vessels narrow, swelling in the mucous membrane decreases and the production of mucus is reduced.

**Congested nasal passages**
The nasal passages are lined with special mucus-producing cells that form the mucous membrane. This membrane is supplied by blood vessels that widen in response to infection or allergy. This widening increases the leakage of fluid into the membrane, which then swells and produces more mucus.

Widened blood vessels

Sinus

Mucous membrane

More mucus

Before a decongestant

Lining (mucous membrane)

Narrowed blood vessels

Nasal passage

Less mucus

After a decongestant

Histamine

Histamine receptor

Widened blood vessel

More mucus

Before an antihistamine

Histamine

Drug

Narrowed blood vessel

Less mucus

After an antihistamine

**How antihistamines work**
Antihistamine drugs block histamine receptors and prevent histamine's effect. Histamine acts on histamine receptors in the nose and causes widening of the blood vessels that supply the mucous membrane, which leads to swelling and increased production of mucus.

**Decongestants**
*Decongestants are used to relieve nasal congestion. (They do not control symptoms such as sneezing.) These drugs are included in many over-the-counter cold remedies. However, effectiveness of these drugs decreases with prolonged use. Decongestants are prescribed with caution for people who have heart disease.*

**Antihistamines**
*Antihistamine drugs relieve allergic symptoms in the eyes and the nose by blocking histamine's inflammatory effect. Swelling, irritation, and watery discharge may be reduced. Antihistamines are sometimes included in cough and cold remedies because of their sedative and antiallergic properties, and because they reduce nasal secretions. However, there is very little evidence that they are effective in treating colds, and they may actually prolong bronchitis and sinusitis by drying secretions and preventing or delaying clearance of the bronchial or nasal passages.*

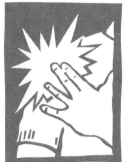

# DRUGS FOR PAIN AND INFLAMMATION

P AIN IS A LOCALIZED sensation, ranging from mild discomfort to an unbearable, excruciating experience, that is caused by the chemical or physical stimulation of sensory nerve endings in the course of a disease or injury. Inflammation is the redness, swelling, heat, and pain in an organ or tissue that is caused by a chemical reaction in the body or by a physical injury.

## NSAIDs AND OSTEOARTHRITIS

NSAIDs reduce the inflammation, pain, and stiffness in joints affected by osteoarthritis (degeneration of the cartilage and bones of the joints).

**Before treatment**
*The protective layers of cartilage on the surface of a joint are ragged and worn away and the joint tissue has become inflamed and painful.*

**Worn cartilage**
**Inflamed joint tissue**

**Inflamed tissue**
*Inflammation occurs when white blood cells are attracted to the site of injury by natural substances produced there. Swelling and stiffness occur in the affected area if large numbers of white blood cells accumulate.*

**Inflammation**
**White blood cells**
**Blood vessel**

**After an NSAID**
*NSAIDs reduce pain and inflammation in the affected joint, but any resulting damage remains. Symptoms are likely to recur some time after treatment has stopped.*

**Drug**
**Reduced inflammation**

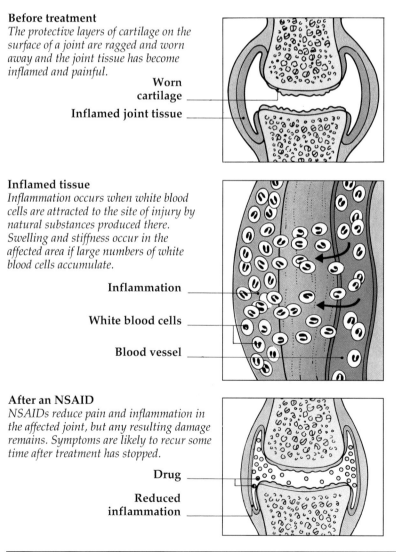

The sensation of pain is caused by the stimulation of pain-sensitive nerve endings in the skin, tissues, and internal organs. Pain signals then travel along nerve pathways to the brain. Pain-sensitive nerves can be either directly stimulated, as when your hand touches something very hot, or indirectly stimulated by the release of prostaglandins, which occurs in rheumatoid arthritis. Prostaglandins are naturally occurring chemicals released as a result of tissue damage that act on nerves to trigger pain and cause inflammation. Medications used to suppress pain and reduce inflammation can act directly on the brain or interfere with the production of prostaglandins in the skin, tissues, and organs.

## NONSTEROIDAL ANTI-INFLAMMATORY DRUGS

Nonsteroidal anti-inflammatory drugs (NSAIDs) inhibit the production of enzymes that are necessary for the synthesis of prostaglandins, thus reducing pain and inflammation. NSAIDs reduce stiffness and improve the function of an injured joint. NSAIDs have no effect on the underlying disease or condition but do reduce the effects of the inflammation. They relieve symptoms rapidly (in hours or days) but have their peak effect over a longer period (days to weeks). These drugs are absorbed rapidly from the digestive system and vary in their duration of action. Some have a short duration of action and need to be taken every 4 to 6 hours; others need to be taken only once a day. Because there is considerable variability among patients in both effectiveness and tolerance of NSAIDs, you may have to try several types to find the one that is most effective for you.

## ANTIRHEUMATICS

Antirheumatic drugs are used to treat rheumatic diseases (generalized disorders causing stiff, painful muscles and joints). Unlike anti-inflammatory drugs, some antirheumatics seem to stop progression of the underlying disease. Gold derivatives, penicillamine, and methotrexate suppress the body's immune response (believed to be partly responsible for rheumatoid arthritis), thereby preventing more tissue damage and stopping progressive disability. Antirheumatics are generally slow-acting, so NSAIDs may also be used during the initial phase of treatment. Antirheumatics can also have severe adverse effects, ranging from allergic reactions to potentially fatal organ damage. Because of their side effects, antirheumatics are never prescribed initially or without close medical supervision; NSAIDs are the first choice for treatment.

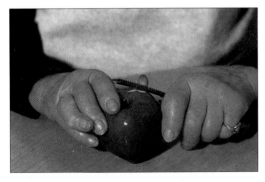

**Rheumatoid arthritis**
*Rheumatoid arthritis is usually thought to occur when the body's immune system causes antibodies to be produced against the body's own tissues. The disease makes the joints become swollen, stiff, and painful, sometimes leading to disability and deformity. The joints of the hands and fingers are among those affected earliest and most often.*

## PIROXICAM

Piroxicam is an NSAID (see page 98) used in the treatment of rheumatoid arthritis and osteoarthritis. A high level of piroxicam remains in the blood many hours after the drug has been taken, so it needs to be taken only once daily. Piroxicam (like every other NSAID) gives relief from the symptoms of arthritis but does not cure the underlying disease. You and your doctor will have to select the NSAID with the most benefits and the fewest side effects. Possible side effects of piroxicam include nausea, indigestion, abdominal pain, peptic ulcer, and swollen ankles.

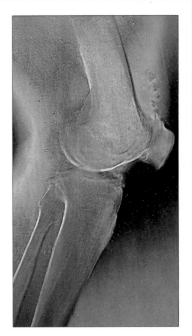

**Arthritis in the knee**
*This color-enhanced X-ray shows a knee joint that has been damaged by arthritis.*

## MUSCLE RELAXANTS

Several drugs are available to treat involuntary, painful contraction of muscles. Muscle relaxants such as diazepam and orphenadrine act on the brain and central nervous system to slow the passage of the nerve signals that cause muscles to contract. Other muscle relaxants, such as baclofen and methocarbamol, act on the spinal nerves, blocking the signals that cause muscles to go into spasm. Dantrolene acts directly on the skeletal muscle itself. Use of muscle relaxants has not been extensive because of limited effectiveness and adverse reactions that outweigh the benefits.

Muscle relaxants that act on the spinal nerves have been utilized to improve the use of limbs that have been impaired by severe muscle spasm. The muscle relaxants that act on the brain and central nervous system, such as diazepam, can cause drowsiness, and a dosage that is too high can cause weakness.

### IMMUNO-SUPPRESSANTS

Immunosuppressants are useful in the treatment of rheumatoid arthritis when treatment with other drugs has not provided a satisfactory degree of relief and when the pain is severe and disabling. Immunosuppressants reduce the immune system's production of antibodies that attack the body's own tissues, which reduces or stops tissue destruction. Close medical supervision of treatment with immunosuppressants is required because of serious adverse effects.

# PAIN AND ANALGESICS

Pain can be temporarily relieved by an analgesic drug (a painkiller). There are two main classes of analgesic drugs – nonnarcotics and narcotics. Nonnarcotic drugs include acetaminophen and the NSAIDs (nonsteroidal anti-inflammatory drugs, which include aspirin). Narcotic drugs include morphine, meperidine, and codeine. Some painkilling drugs are injected or applied to the skin or mucous membranes to prevent nerves or nerve endings from being stimulated.

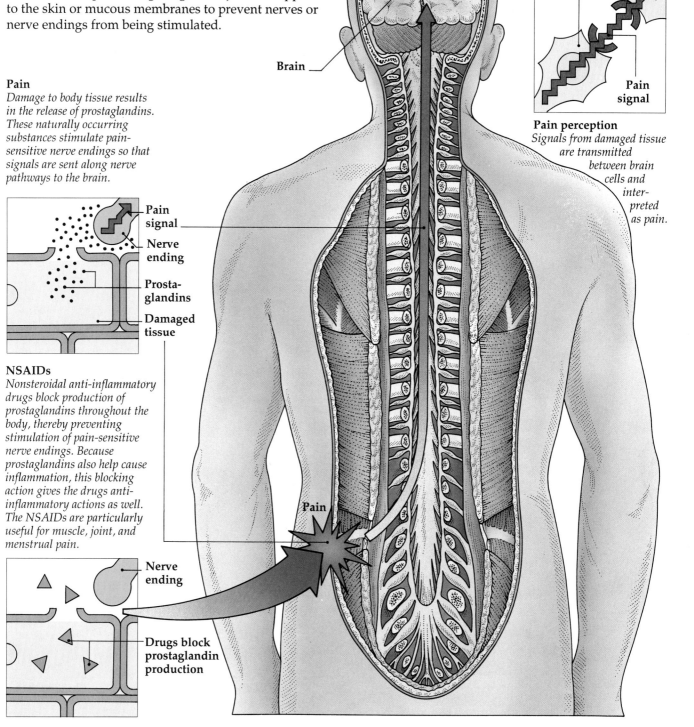

**Brain**

**Brain cells**

**Pain signal**

**Pain perception**
*Signals from damaged tissue are transmitted between brain cells and interpreted as pain.*

**Pain**
*Damage to body tissue results in the release of prostaglandins. These naturally occurring substances stimulate pain-sensitive nerve endings so that signals are sent along nerve pathways to the brain.*

**Pain signal**

**Nerve ending**

**Prosta-glandins**

**Damaged tissue**

**NSAIDs**
*Nonsteroidal anti-inflammatory drugs block production of prostaglandins throughout the body, thereby preventing stimulation of pain-sensitive nerve endings. Because prostaglandins also help cause inflammation, this blocking action gives the drugs anti-inflammatory actions as well. The NSAIDs are particularly useful for muscle, joint, and menstrual pain.*

**Pain**

**Nerve ending**

**Drugs block prostaglandin production**

### Acetaminophen

*Acetaminophen blocks the production of prostaglandins in the brain. However, unlike aspirin, acetaminophen does not block the production of prostaglandins in the rest of the body, so it does not reduce inflammation. It can be used for everyday aches and pains such as headaches and toothaches.*

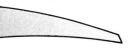

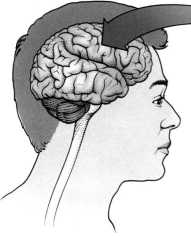

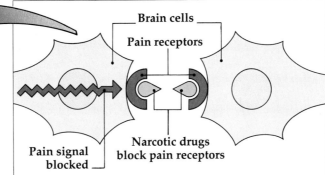

Brain cells

Pain receptors

Pain signal blocked

Narcotic drugs block pain receptors

### Narcotic analgesics

*Narcotic analgesics diminish our perception of pain by combining with special pain receptors on brain cells and blocking the transmission of pain signals within the brain and spinal cord. Opioids are the most effective narcotic analgesics and are used to treat severe pain such as occurs with the movement of a kidney stone and bone cancer. Some narcotics, such as morphine, are extremely powerful and are given only under medical supervision to avoid the risk of dependence and abuse. Others, such as codeine, are less potent and more widely used for moderately severe pain.*

## CORTICOSTEROIDS

Corticosteroids are drugs that mimic the effects of natural hormones made in the outer portions of the adrenal glands. These drugs are useful for treating inflammatory conditions. Corticosteroids, considered miracle agents when they were introduced about 40 years ago, are now known to be limited in effect. In most instances they do not stop progression of the underlying disorder. The serious adverse effects encountered with prolonged use have substantially reduced use of corticosteroids by the medical profession.

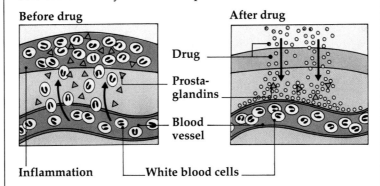

Before drug

After drug

Drug

Prosta-glandins

Blood vessel

Inflammation

White blood cells

### Action of corticosteroids

*Corticosteroids suppress inflammation by blocking the synthesis of prostaglandins (the naturally occurring chemicals that trigger pain), which results in decreased production of white blood cells.*

---

### DRUGS FOR GOUT

Gout is a metabolic disorder that is accompanied by abnormally high blood levels of uric acid (a substance excreted in the urine). Uric acid may crystallize in a joint and surrounding tissues, causing pain and inflammation. Allopurinol, which suppresses the production of uric acid, is administered to prevent attacks of gout. NSAIDs and corticosteroids are used to treat the pain and inflammation of an acute attack of gout. Medications such as probenecid help reduce uric acid by increasing its output in the urine.

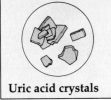

**Uric acid crystals**

---

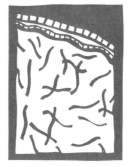

# DRUGS FOR INFECTIONS AND INFESTATIONS

OUR ENVIRONMENT CONTAINS many microorganisms capable of causing disease, but we are usually protected by our body's natural defenses such as the skin, mucous membranes, and immune system. Infections occur when these defenses break down or we have not developed resistance to a microorganism as a result of earlier exposure (by immunization or previous infection). Infestations occur when parasites are present on or inside the body.

Drugs used to treat infections and infestations are usually effective against one type of organism, such as bacteria, viruses, fungi, or protozoa. For example, both antibiotic and antibacterial drugs are effective against bacteria; they either kill the bacteria (bactericidal drugs) or prevent reproduction of the bacteria by stopping their growth process (bacteriostatic drugs). With growth halted, the body's natural defenses can fight off the infection. However, antibiotics and antibacterials are different in origin. The original antibiotics were derived from molds and fungi. Antibacterials have always been produced synthetically.

## WARNING

Common side effects of antibiotic drugs include nausea, diarrhea, or rash. Fungal infections in the mouth, gastrointestinal tract, and vagina may also occur because antibiotics can destroy the normal protective bacteria that usually suppress the growth of the fungi. Some people are allergic to antibiotics, particularly to penicillins. Always tell your doctor if you have ever had an adverse reaction to any drug.

**Antibiotic action**
*Some antibiotics kill bacteria by interfering with the formation of cell walls. In the photograph (right), the wall of the upper bacterium has been weakened by an antibiotic, causing the organism to disintegrate; the lower bacterium has not yet been affected. Other antibiotics kill by disrupting growth inside bacteria.*

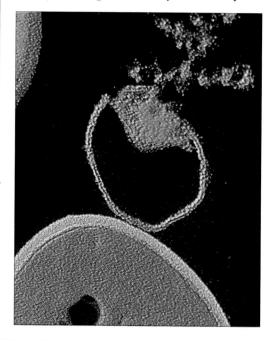

## ANTIBIOTICS

Many types of antibiotics are available. Some of these drugs are effective against a wide range of bacteria; they are called broad-spectrum agents. Other antibiotics have a more specific range of use; these drugs are effective against only one or two types of bacteria and are called narrow-spectrum agents.

Antibiotics are usually taken orally but can also be given by injection or applied to the affected part of the body (such as the skin, eyes, or ears). The drugs begin to stop most infections within a

### SOME COMMON ANTIBIOTICS

**Penicillins** – the first antibiotics to be developed; still widely used to treat many commonly occurring infections; may cause allergic reactions (examples: ampicillin, cloxacillin, penicillin G)

**Cephalosporins** – useful in the treatment of a wide variety of infections; some kill many different types of bacteria; may interfere with normal blood clotting (examples: cefaclor, cefazolin, cefoxitin)

**Tetracyclines** – effective against a broad range of bacteria, although some strains of bacteria have become increasingly resistant; can discolor developing teeth; should be avoided by pregnant women and young children; some people have an increased sensitivity to sunlight when taking a tetracycline (examples: doxycycline, oxytetracycline, tetracycline)

few hours. However, it is vital to take all of your medication to prevent a recurrence of the infection. Sometimes organisms become resistant to the antibiotic you have been taking (see AN INCOMPLETE COURSE OF ANTIBIOTICS on page 53).

# ANTIBACTERIALS

Sulfonamides are the oldest group of antibacterial drugs. These drugs are effective in treating urinary tract infections because they reach high concentrations in the urine. Sulfonamides are also often used to treat eye, ear, and skin disorders. Sulfonamides prevent bacteria from producing folic acid, a chemical they need for growth.

## SOME COMMON ANTIBACTERIALS

**Sulfonamides** – useful for acute urinary tract infections (examples: sulfacetamide, sulfamethoxazole, sulfisoxazole)
**Urinary antiseptics** – used primarily for chronic bladder infections (examples: methenamine, nitrofurantoin)
**Quinolones** – used to treat urinary tract infections (examples: cinoxacin, ciprofloxacin, nalidixic acid)
**Others** – metronidazole, used to treat genital and intestinal infections

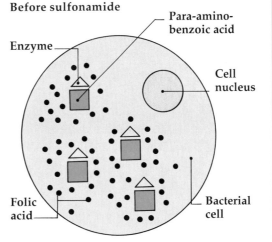

**Before sulfonamide**

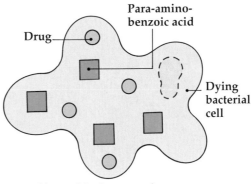

**After sulfonamide**

**How sulfonamide drugs work**
*Sulfonamides block the release of an enzyme that acts on the chemical para-aminobenzoic acid to produce folic acid inside bacterial cells. The bacteria are unable to function properly without folic acid and cannot reproduce. In this way, growth of bacteria is stopped and infection is halted.*

## WARNING

Antibacterials, like antibiotics, can cause an allergic reaction (a rash or fever, for example). Tell your doctor about any previous adverse reactions to these drugs. Sulfonamide antibacterials have been shown in rare cases to cause severe side effects, including formation of crystals in the kidneys (which can cause blood in the urine, irritation, or obstruction) and liver damage. Bacteria can develop resistance to sulfonamides, which has limited the usefulness of these drugs.

# RESISTANCE TO ANTIBIOTICS

The use of antibiotics over time has led to the proliferation of resistant bacteria. Doctors now select the fastest-acting and most effective antibiotic whenever possible. If bacterial resistance to an antibiotic develops, your doctor will prescribe a different type of antibiotic.

**Neutralizing enzymes**
*Production of a bacterial enzyme that causes a change in the chemical structure of an antibiotic drug is one method by which bacteria develop resistance to previously effective antibiotics. This change in chemical structure makes the drug inactive and ineffective against the bacteria.*

**Evaluating resistance**
*Bacteria can be grown on a culture dish containing antibiotic-impregnated paper discs. Bacteria will grow near discs containing antibiotics to which the bacteria are resistant, but will not grow near discs that contain antibiotics to which the bacteria are sensitive.*

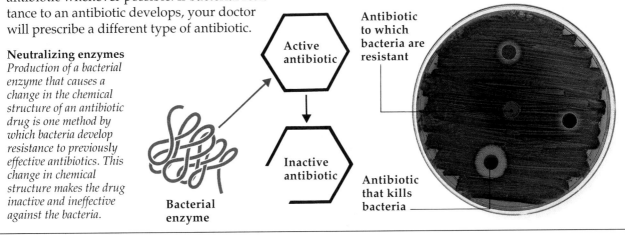

# CASE HISTORY
## SENSITIVITY TO ANTIBIOTICS

EMILIO WAS RECENTLY **admitted to the hospital for treatment of bacterial endocarditis (inflammation of the heart valves). This infection of his heart appeared to be linked to a tooth extraction that Emilio had the week before. Emilio's doctor started him on a course of penicillin to kill the bacteria that were causing the inflammation. After the second dose, the attending nurse noticed that a rash had developed on Emilio's face and neck. The nurse called Emilio's doctor immediately.**

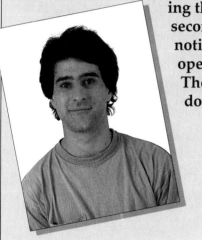

### PERSONAL DETAILS
**Name** Emilio Sanchez-Garcia
**Age** 30
**Occupation** Taxi driver
**Family** Emilio's parents are both healthy. He has one older sister who is in good health.

### MEDICAL BACKGROUND
Emilio's only illness of any note was an episode of swelling and pain in his joints and a fever when he was 11. His joint pain and swelling and the fever subsided without medical treatment (except for bed rest and taking aspirin) after a few months.

### THE CONSULTATION
Emilio's doctor comes to see him immediately. The rash on his face and neck is light red and raised, with clearly defined edges. Emilio is not feeling any major discomfort, only mild itching of the rash.

### THE DIAGNOSIS
The doctor believes that Emilio's rash is an ALLERGIC REACTION TO PENICILLIN. He considers replacing the penicillin with cefazolin, which belongs to the cephalosporin class of antibiotics. However, he decides against prescribing cefazolin because the penicillins and the cephalosporins have similar chemical properties. Substituting cefazolin would probably cause Emilio's rash to recur.

Emilio's doctor believes that the fever Emilio had at age 11 was probably a case of rheumatic fever. Rheumatic fever may have caused permanent damage to Emilio's heart valves. This damage facilitated the recent development of the endocarditis. Emilio's doctor arranges for an echocardiogram (ultrasound examination of the heart), which shows a small crust on a narrowed heart valve. Along with a positive test result from a blood culture, this confirms the diagnosis of endocarditis.

### THE TREATMENT
The doctor decides to substitute vancomycin because this antibiotic does not cause allergic reactions in people who are sensitive to penicillin and it is effective against a broader range of bacteria than penicillin.

### THE OUTCOME
The rash caused by Emilio's allergic reaction to penicillin disappears within a few days and he is released from the hospital. He experiences no adverse reactions to vancomycin during 6 weeks of treatment. Emilio recovers completely.

**Allergy to penicillin**
*Emilio is told by his doctor that his rash was an allergic reaction to penicillin. He is advised to always carry a warning card with him that states he is allergic to penicillin.*

# ANTIVIRAL DRUGS

Conditions caused by viruses range from the common cold to serious infections such as pneumonia (inflammation of the lungs) and meningitis (inflammation of the membranes that cover the brain and spinal cord). Unlike bacteria, viruses can reproduce only by using the genetic material (DNA) inside the cells of their host. It has been difficult to develop antiviral drugs because any drug that can damage a virus is also likely to damage both diseased and normal cells.

## Uses of antiviral drugs

With the advent of AIDS, much more time and money have been invested in a search for drugs to treat severe viral infections. Some of the earlier antivirals (such as amantadine for type A influenza) had limited success in preventing viral infections. Although these antivirals did reduce the severity of viral infections, they did not cure the conditions in the way antibiotics cure bacterial infections. The newer antivirals have been more effective, with fewer adverse effects. For example, acyclovir is used for herpesvirus infections and zidovudine (the first antiviral drug licensed for the treatment of human immunodeficiency virus infection) has been used with some success in treating people with AIDS.

## How antivirals work

The processes of viral and host cell reproduction are similar in some respects. However, some processes in the viral system of reproduction are different and can be used as targets for virus-specific drugs. Most antiviral drugs block the activity of the viral enzymes that are essential for reproduction, halting the rapid growth of the viruses.

> **WARNING**
>
> The use of antiviral drugs has some drawbacks. Although an outbreak of herpesvirus infection can be cleared up within a few days with a drug such as acyclovir, a recurrence is likely. Most antivirals must be given early in the course of an infection or used preventively to achieve the desired effect. Some antivirals adversely affect the kidneys; others disrupt the activity of healthy cells, especially those in the bone marrow.

---

## ACYCLOVIR

Acyclovir is the first antiviral drug that has a specific action against herpesviruses. A drug that causes few adverse effects, acyclovir is used in the treatment of herpesvirus infections such as genital herpes and severe or complicated cases of shingles (a painful rash of small, crusting blisters). Acyclovir resembles a nucleotide base, one of the basic structural units for making genetic material (DNA) that the virus and human cell would normally use to reproduce. Acyclovir is activated by an enzyme present only in cells infected by the virus. It has no effect on uninfected cells; thus it is not harmful to healthy human cells.

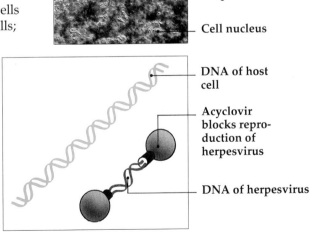

**The herpesvirus**
*This slide shows herpesvirus moving from the nucleus of a cell (where the DNA is stored) toward the cell surface.*

- Cell cytoplasm
- Herpesvirus
- Cell nucleus

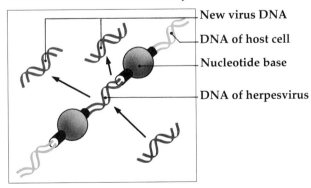

- New virus DNA
- DNA of host cell
- Nucleotide base
- DNA of herpesvirus

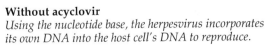

- DNA of host cell
- Acyclovir blocks reproduction of herpesvirus
- DNA of herpesvirus

**Without acyclovir**
*Using the nucleotide base, the herpesvirus incorporates its own DNA into the host cell's DNA to reproduce.*

**With acyclovir**
*The herpesvirus uses acyclovir instead of the host cell's nucleotide base; thus reproduction of the herpesvirus is prevented.*

## ANTIPROTOZOAL DRUGS

Protozoa are single-celled organisms that are transmitted to humans by animals, contaminated food or water, or insect bites. Protozoa cause diseases such as giardiasis (an intestinal infection), trichomoniasis (a vaginal infection), amebic dysentery (an infection of the colon), and malaria (a mosquito-borne disease). Some antiprotozoal drugs are effective against more than one type of protozoa; for example, metronidazole may be used for amebiasis or trichomoniasis, and chloroquine for amebiasis or malaria. Because protozoa are often difficult to eradicate from the body, prolonged treatment may be needed to prevent recurrence of the disease. Antiprotozoals can cause a range of side effects. Some of these side effects, such as nausea or diarrhea, are minor; some, such as blood disorders, rash, or damage to the eye, are potentially more serious and must be monitored by your doctor.

### ANTIMALARIAL DRUGS

Malaria causes more sickness and death worldwide than any other infectious disease. Visitors to areas of the world where malaria is known to occur are at high risk of infection and require treatment with preventive antimalarial drugs before and during travel. Selecting an appropriate drug or drugs depends on whether the parasites are resistant or sensitive to the standard drug chloroquine. Most areas of the world report the presence of chloroquine-resistant falciparum malaria (the most severe form of malaria). In chloroquine-resistant areas, mefloquine (a newly approved antimalarial drug) is recommended. However, some resistance to mefloquine has already been reported. The treatment of malaria depends on the type of malaria and on its sensitivity to the drugs currently in use. Falciparum malaria may cause a fatal illness. In such cases, treatment may include new antimalarials and quinine, the original antimalarial drug.

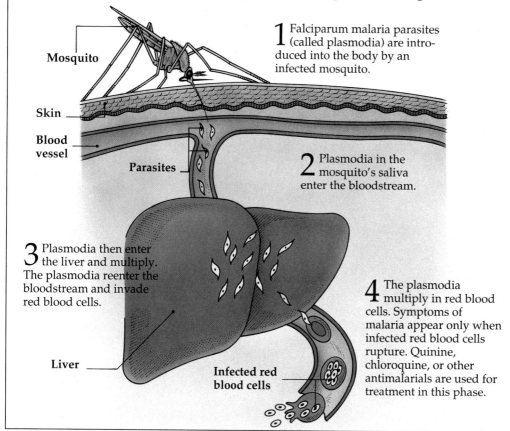

**Mosquito**

**Skin**

**Blood vessel**

**Parasites**

**Liver**

**Infected red blood cells**

1 Falciparum malaria parasites (called plasmodia) are introduced into the body by an infected mosquito.

2 Plasmodia in the mosquito's saliva enter the bloodstream.

3 Plasmodia then enter the liver and multiply. The plasmodia reenter the bloodstream and invade red blood cells.

4 The plasmodia multiply in red blood cells. Symptoms of malaria appear only when infected red blood cells rupture. Quinine, chloroquine, or other antimalarials are used for treatment in this phase.

#### WARNING

Possible side effects of antimalarial treatment include nausea, diarrhea, dizziness, disturbances in vision or hearing, and blood disorders. Although antimalarial drugs can cause these side effects, it is essential to begin preventive treatment before traveling to areas where malaria is known to occur; the risks of severe illness and death outweigh the inconvenience of these side effects. Antimalarial drugs must be taken for the entire period recommended by your doctor.

**Scabies mites and lice**
*Infestations of scabies mites and lice spread rapidly, causing severe skin irritation. These infestations should be treated with an appropriate topical antiparasitic drug to kill adult insects and their eggs as soon as possible. There are three types of lice – the head louse, the body or clothes louse, and the crab (pubic) louse. Lice lay their eggs near the base of hair shafts and mites burrow into the skin to lay their eggs. Scabies mites or lice are transmitted by direct contact with an infested person or by contact with infested clothing or bedding.*

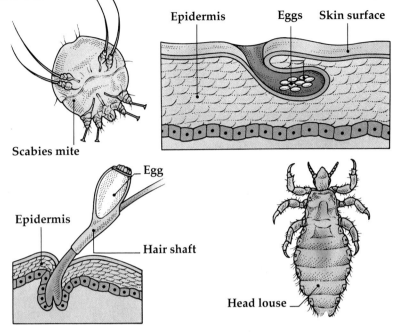

Epidermis    Eggs    Skin surface

Scabies mite

Egg

Epidermis

Hair shaft

Head louse

## TREATMENTS FOR SKIN PARASITES

The most common skin parasites are scabies mites and lice. Lindane or permethrin lotions are used for scabies mite infestations. These lotions are applied to all areas of the body except the head and neck. They must be left on the skin for the time recommended by your doctor (usually for several hours) and then thoroughly washed off. One to two treatments are usually sufficient to kill the scabies mite. Your doctor may recommend using a soothing cream to relieve the itching that usually persists for up to 2 weeks after treatment.

Head and pubic lice are usually eradicated with a shampoo containing pyrethrins or permethrin. The shampoo is rinsed out after 10 to 15 minutes; dead lice can then be combed out. The comb must be washed immediately in hot water. If the skin has become infected from scratching, an antibiotic may be applied to the affected area. Lindane was once widely used in shampoos. However, in some areas of the world, lice have become resistant to lindane.

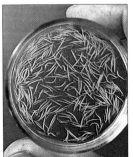

**Pinworm**
*The pinworm* Enterobius vermicularis *is highly contagious; all members of an infested household should be treated with anthelmintic drugs simultaneously. Towels and sheets should be laundered daily.*

## ANTHELMINTICS

Drugs used to treat parasitic worms are called anthelmintics. Most types of parasitic worms live in the intestines or bile ducts. Often they cause few or no symptoms. In some cases, the worms attach themselves to the bowel wall and cause anemia and nutritional deficiencies. Anthelmintics either kill or paralyze the worms, which then pass out of the body in the feces; laxatives are given to hasten expulsion of the worms. The most commonly prescribed anthelmintic drugs are mebendazole and pyrantel. Mebendazole is effective against a broad range of parasites, so it is called a broad-spectrum anthelmintic. However, it is not effective against worm larvae that have spread into tissues. Pyrantel is effective against the common roundworm and the pinworm; both of these infestations are usually cleared up by a single dose of this drug. Praziquantel is a new, effective broad-spectrum anthelmintic drug that is used to treat a parasitic disease called schistosomiasis. Your doctor may recommend an over-the-counter anthelmintic drug to treat common parasitic infestations such as pinworms.

### ANTIFUNGAL DRUGS

Most fungal infections occur on the skin. However, thrush (a commonly occurring infection caused by the fungus *Candida albicans*) can affect the mouth, esophagus, intestines, or vagina. Oral thrush can be treated with a mouthwash containing an antifungal drug such as nystatin or amphotericin. Vaginal thrush is usually treated with suppositories or creams. A new antifungal drug taken by mouth, fluconazole, has been introduced to treat thrush that occurs in the intestines. Fluconazole acts rapidly and causes fewer side effects than the previously available antifungal drugs.

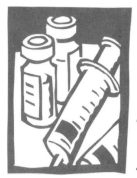

# DRUGS FOR HORMONAL DISORDERS

**H**ORMONES ARE RELEASED into the bloodstream by glands and have specific effects in various parts of the body. When hormone production is insufficient or excessive, disease can result. Some hormonal disorders are present from birth; others result from inflammation, autoimmune disease (an inappropriate reaction of the body's immune system), injury, or cancer.

## OSTEOPOROSIS

Osteoporosis is a condition in which the density of bone decreases. This condition occurs naturally as part of the aging process but is far more common in women than men. Women are especially vulnerable just after menopause because the ovaries stop producing estrogen, a hormone that helps to maintain bone mass. Although osteoporosis can become severe after menopause, bone fractures rarely occur until a woman is over 60. Estrogen, with or without a progestin (a synthetic form of progesterone), is used to treat this disorder in women. Medications called diphosphonates (including etidronate) seem to restore some bone mass by inhibiting the activity of osteoclasts – large cells on bone surfaces that are associated with bone thinning.

If the body does not produce enough of a particular hormone, doctors can prescribe a natural hormone or a synthetic version to make up for the deficiency. In other cases, drugs are given to stimulate production of hormones or to reduce the activity of the gland that is producing too much of a hormone.

## DIABETES MELLITUS

Diabetes mellitus is a condition in which the pancreas produces insufficient amounts of insulin or none at all. Insulin is the hormone responsible for the absorption of glucose into cells and its conversion to glycogen for storage.

There are two forms of diabetes. Insulin-dependent (type I) diabetes is the more severe form and can be treated only by lifelong injections of insulin. Non-insulin-dependent (type II) diabetes develops gradually, usually in people older than 40, and can generally be treated without insulin. If diet alone fails to improve the non-insulin-dependent condition, sulfonylurea drugs such as tolbutamide and chlorpropamide may be prescribed. The main action of these drugs is to stimulate the production of insulin by the pancreas.

**Insulin today**
*Insulin must be given by injection. Today's insulin is manufactured to rigorous standards of purity that allow highly accurate regulation of dosage. The diabetic is able to control his or her diabetes and lead a normal, active life. Some insulin is derived from the pancreas glands of cattle and pigs. Another source is bacteria that have been altered by genetic engineering to produce pure human insulin.*

## THYROID DISORDERS

Hormones produced by the thyroid gland regulate the body's metabolism; these hormones are an essential part of the body's release and use of energy. Thyrotoxicosis (with symptoms such as weight loss, intolerance to heat, and increased appetite) is caused by excessive secretion of the thyroid hormones by an overactive thyroid gland (hyperthyroidism). Antithyroid drugs act directly on the cells of the thyroid gland and stop the chemical processes that lead to the production of thyroid hormones. These drugs do not always cure the underlying disorder and are often used in conjunction with surgery or treatment with radioactive iodine to restore the normal functioning of the thyroid gland. Underproduction of hormones by the thyroid gland causes hypothyroidism (with symptoms such as weight gain and lethargy). The condition usually requires lifelong treatment with synthetic thyroid hormone preparations.

## ADRENAL DISORDERS

The adrenal glands produce two sets of hormones – the catecholamines (epinephrine and norepinephrine) and the corticosteroids. The catecholamines are vital for an appropriate response to physical and emotional stress. The corticosteroids include hydrocortisone, aldosterone, and the androgens. Overproduction of hydrocortisone causes Cushing's syndrome (characterized by obesity and muscle weakness). Corticosteroid drugs are used to treat insufficient production of hormones by the adrenal glands or pituitary gland.

### WARNING

Because thyroid hormone drugs supply a substance that is normally produced by the body, they do not usually produce adverse effects if taken in the appropriate dosage. Drug treatment of hypothyroidism is begun with a low dosage; the dosage is adjusted if necessary, based on results of regular testing for levels of the drug in the blood. Thyroid drugs are prescribed with caution for people who have a history of heart disease.

## DRUGS FOR PITUITARY DISORDERS

The pituitary gland, located at the base of the brain, is responsible for the production of many hormones, including those that regulate growth, sexual development, and metabolism. Any change in the levels of the hormones produced in the pituitary gland causes changes elsewhere in the body. Drugs are the treatment of choice for many pituitary gland disorders.

**Excess lactation**
*In women, the hormone prolactin controls the secretion of breast milk (lactation) after childbirth. Overproduction of prolactin causes several conditions, including lactation unassociated with pregnancy, lack of menstruation, and infertility. The drug bromocriptine is used to inhibit the production of prolactin.*

**Diabetes insipidus**
*Antidiuretic hormone (vasopressin) is produced by the pituitary gland and acts on the tubules of the kidneys, where it controls the amount of water reabsorbed into the blood. Insufficient production of vasopressin is usually caused by damage to the pituitary gland and leads to diabetes insipidus, in which the kidneys are unable to retain water. Large volumes of urine are passed, leading to constant thirst. Treatment may include vasopressin or a synthetic version of the hormone, such as lypressin.*

Excess lactation

Diabetes insipidus

**Growth hormone disorders**
*Lack of growth hormone inhibits growth, a condition known as pituitary dwarfism. Genetically engineered human growth hormone is administered to replace a lack of this naturally produced hormone. Treatment should be started in childhood while bone growth is still possible. In contrast, excess production of growth hormone in early life (before bone growth ceases) causes gigantism or, in adult life, acromegaly (enlargement of the skull, hands, and feet). Drug treatment may include bromocriptine or somatostatin, both of which lower the levels of growth hormone. Somatostatin is also used to shrink tumors of the pituitary gland.*

# ORAL CONTRACEPTIVES

There are two main types of oral contraceptives – the combined pill and the minipill. The combined pill contains synthetic forms of both female hormones – estrogen and progesterone (synthetic progesterone is called progestin) – and is the most efficient form of contraception available. The minipill contains only a progestin. The pill reduces the risk of ovarian and uterine cancer and the risk of pelvic inflammatory disease (infection of the reproductive organs). Most studies have not shown any connection between pill use and subsequent breast or cervical cancer, although there is some concern that long-term use may slightly increase the risk. Problems with blood clotting may occur in smokers over 35 who have been taking the pill for many years. If you are concerned about any aspect of oral contraceptive use, ask your doctor for his or her opinion.

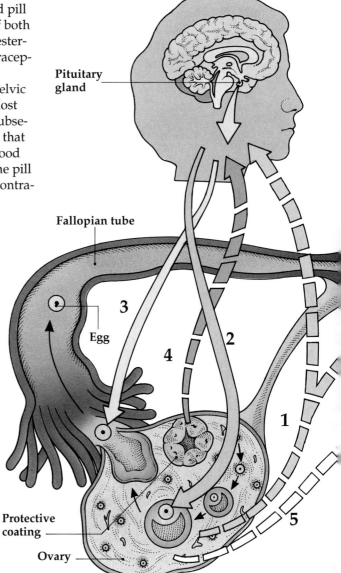

Pituitary gland

Fallopian tube

Egg

Protective coating

Ovary

3

2

4

1

5

## THE NORMAL FEMALE REPRODUCTIVE CYCLE

**1** The ovaries produce estrogen, which causes the lining of the uterus (endometrium) to thicken and stimulates the pituitary gland in the brain.

**2** In response, the pituitary gland secretes a hormone called follicle-stimulating hormone (FSH). FSH causes the maturation of an unripened egg in the ovary. As the egg develops, the ovary releases more estrogen.

**3** Increased levels of estrogen in the blood stimulate the pituitary gland to produce large amounts of luteinizing hormone (LH). The increased levels of LH cause the release of the ripened egg from the ovary (ovulation).

**4** After ovulation, the egg passes down the fallopian tube toward the uterus. The egg's protective coating (left behind in the ovary) starts to produce both estrogen and progesterone. The combination of these two hormones stops the pituitary gland from producing any more FSH and LH. This process is known as negative feedback.

**5** Unless the egg is fertilized, levels of estrogen and progesterone decrease, and the reproductive cycle begins again. Because estrogen and progesterone are necessary to maintain the endometrium, a decrease in the levels of these hormones causes the endometrium and the unfertilized egg to be shed through the cervix into the vagina and expelled. This process is known as menstruation.

---

**IMPLANTS : AN ALTERNATIVE**

A new implantable contraceptive that is effective for 5 years is now available in the US. The implant, which has had a 96 percent success rate, is composed of six small capsules that release a progestin (a synthetic form of progesterone) to suppress ovulation. Common side effects include change in menstrual patterns, weight gain, acne, mood changes, and headaches.

---

# THE EFFECT OF THE COMBINED PILL

**1** The oral contraceptive pill has a negative-feedback effect on the pituitary gland by providing constant levels of synthetic estrogen and a synthetic form of progesterone called a progestin in the blood. This suppresses the release of both LH and FSH from the pituitary gland.

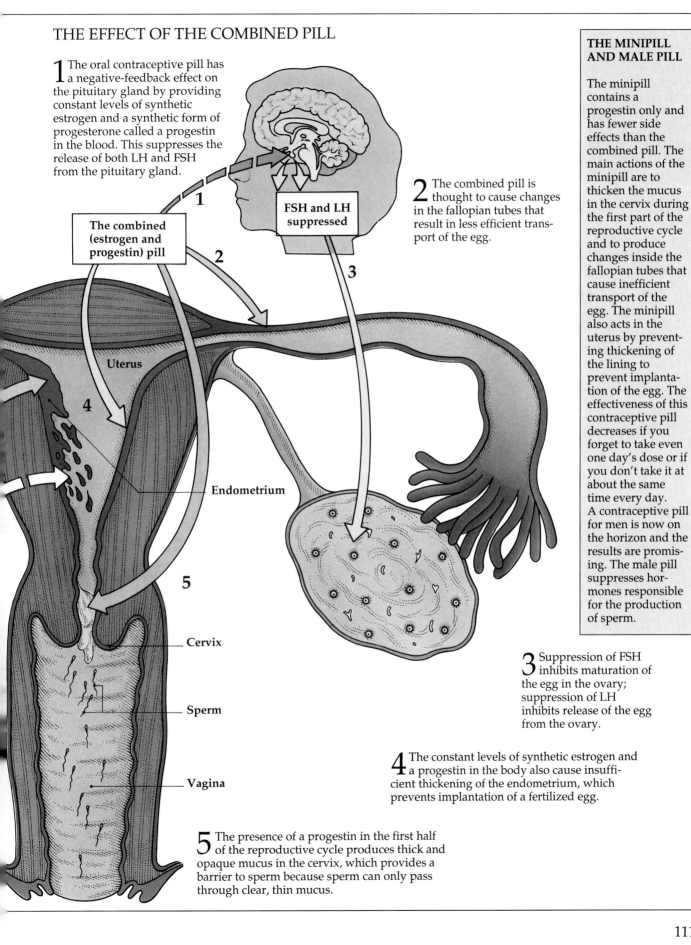

FSH and LH suppressed

The combined (estrogen and progestin) pill

**2** The combined pill is thought to cause changes in the fallopian tubes that result in less efficient transport of the egg.

Uterus

Endometrium

Cervix

Sperm

Vagina

**3** Suppression of FSH inhibits maturation of the egg in the ovary; suppression of LH inhibits release of the egg from the ovary.

**4** The constant levels of synthetic estrogen and a progestin in the body also cause insufficient thickening of the endometrium, which prevents implantation of a fertilized egg.

**5** The presence of a progestin in the first half of the reproductive cycle produces thick and opaque mucus in the cervix, which provides a barrier to sperm because sperm can only pass through clear, thin mucus.

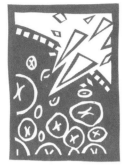

# ANTICANCER DRUGS

THE TERM CANCER covers many different types of related disorders. Anticancer treatment using drugs (chemotherapy) relies mostly on drugs that are cytotoxic – that is, the drugs kill or damage cells. Chemotherapy is often used in combination with surgery or radiation therapy and is useful in treating many types of cancers, especially lymphomas (cancer of the lymph glands), leukemias (overproduction of white blood cells by the bone marrow), and cancers of the breasts, ovaries, and testicles.

The cells of the healthy body grow and divide in an organized, controlled way, with old or damaged cells constantly being replaced by new, healthy cells. Sometimes, for reasons that are not completely understood, this regulated mechanism of growth breaks down and the cells begin to reproduce rapidly in an abnormal way. This process leads to the formation of a tumor, which can be benign (unlikely to spread) or malignant (likely to spread and life-threatening).

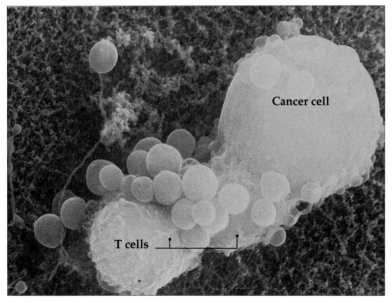

**Natural defenses**
*This photograph shows the body's natural response to cancer cells. The body recognizes certain proteins on the surface of a cancer cell and sends in cells from the immune system, called T cells. These T cells then destroy the abnormal cell by binding to it and altering its chemical growth process. However, the body's defenses against cancer do not consistently and effectively eliminate developing tumor cells. In the future, successful treatment may be possible with drugs that boost the activity of the body's immune system.*

## CANCER TREATMENT

Malignant tumors are usually called cancers; they tend to spread to and grow in other parts of the body. Cancerous cells block and distort blood vessels and other vital body structures and cause progressive impairment of normal functions. Anticancer drugs (chemotherapy) slow down or halt the reproduction of cancerous cells. The choice of drug depends on the form of cancer, the cancer's stage of development, and the patient's condition. Several anticancer drugs may be given in combination to maximize the effect. Some cancers respond to drug treatment alone, while others are treated with drugs in combination with surgery or radiation therapy.

### Problems of selectivity

Chemotherapy is useful in temporarily controlling some incurable tumors. However, the anticancer drugs available today are relatively nonselective in their action. This means that, in addition to attacking cancer cells, the anticancer drugs damage healthy cells, especially fast-growing types such as those in the bone marrow (causing increased susceptibility to infection), hair follicles (causing hair loss), and ovaries and testicles (causing infertility). Because of the risks associated with chemotherapy, anticancer drugs are usually given only in

# HOW ANTICANCER DRUGS WORK

There are several different types of anticancer drugs, and all of these drugs affect more than one type of cancer. All the anticancer drugs work by preventing cancer cells from growing and dividing. Some anticancer drugs damage the cancer cells' DNA (genetic material) while others block the essential chemical growth processes in the cells. Since the activity in healthy cells is also adversely affected by anticancer drugs, these drugs are not prescribed unless the tumor is known to be susceptible. Sex hormones, and drugs that block the production of sex hormones, are also used to treat some types of cancer.

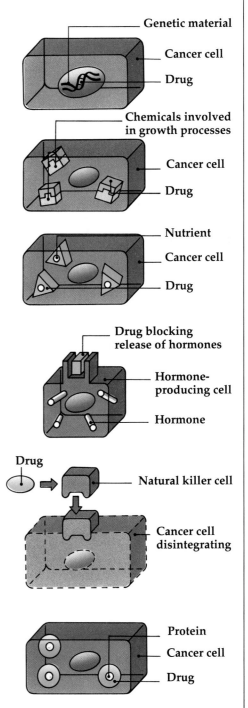

| NAME OF GROUP | HOW THEY WORK |
|---|---|
| **Cytotoxic antibiotics**<br>bleomycin, doxorubicin | Originally intended for use against microorganisms, cytotoxic antibiotics were found to effectively inhibit the growth of tumors by interfering with the genetic material of cancer cells. These drugs are useful in treating leukemias, lymphomas, and a variety of other tumors. |
| **Alkylating agents**<br>chlorambucil, cisplatin, cyclophosphamide, melphalan | These drugs are mainly used for cancers of the white blood cells such as leukemias and lymphomas. They work in a similar way to radiation therapy by interfering with the chemical growth processes of cancer cells. |
| **Antimetabolites**<br>azathioprine, cytarabine, fluorouracil, mercaptopurine, methotrexate | These drugs prevent cancer cells from metabolizing nutrients and other essential substances, thus blocking processes within the cell that lead to cell division. They are used for childhood leukemias, lymphomas, and some other tumors. |
| **Hormone treatment**<br>aminoglutethimide, diethylstilbestrol, ethinyl estradiol, luteinizing hormone–releasing hormone, medroxyprogesterone, megestrol, nandrolone, tamoxifen | Some types of cancers, such as prostate cancer and some forms of breast cancer, are dependent on hormones because their growth is stimulated by testosterone, estrogen, or progesterone. Some anticancer drugs inhibit tumor growth by chemically blocking the release of the hormone in the body or by binding to hormone receptors on the tumor cells. |
| **Interferons**<br>interferon alfa, interferon beta, interferon gamma | Interferons are antiviral substances produced naturally by the body. Currently under investigation for the treatment of a variety of cancers, the anticancer activity of interferons stems from their ability to stimulate natural killer cells in the body to attack cancer cells. Interferons have achieved some success against hairy-cell leukemia, AIDS-related Kaposi's sarcoma (malignant skin tumors), and Wilms' tumor (a malignant tumor of the kidney). |
| **Vinca alkaloids**<br>vinblastine, vincristine | Vinca alkaloids are highly poisonous substances derived from the periwinkle plant and are used to a very limited extent in cancer treatment. These drugs interfere with the reproduction of cancer cells by binding with proteins inside cancer cells. |

short courses (cyclic chemotherapy), allowing time between each treatment course to enable noncancerous cells to recover from the effects of the drugs.

Much larger doses of some of these drugs may be used in the treatment of some cancers. However, in these cases, the patient's bone marrow is destroyed by the drug. The bone marrow is then restored by bone marrow replacement (transplantation). Although deaths have occurred during the recovery period, the success rate for bone marrow transplantation in the treatment of a limited number of cancers is encouraging.

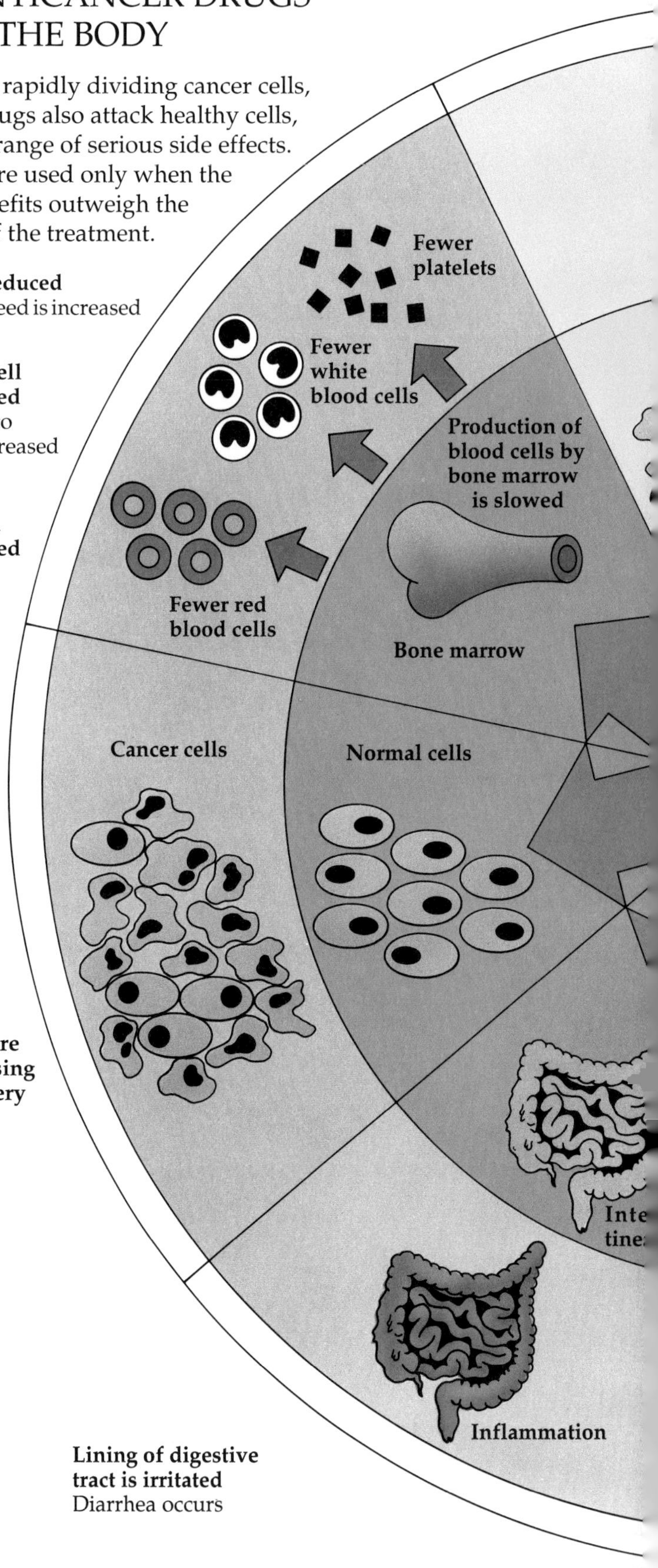

## WHICH CANCERS RESPOND TO TREATMENT WITH ANTICANCER DRUGS?

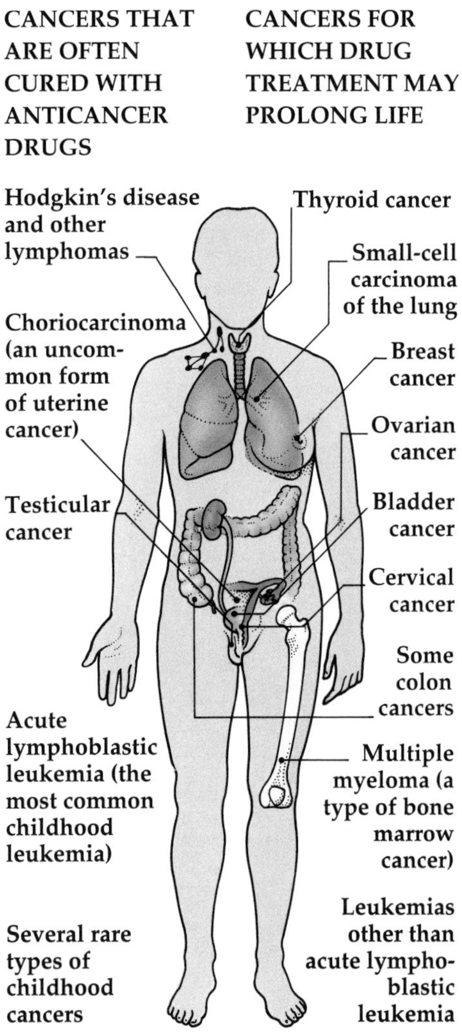

**CANCERS THAT ARE OFTEN CURED WITH ANTICANCER DRUGS**

**CANCERS FOR WHICH DRUG TREATMENT MAY PROLONG LIFE**

Hodgkin's disease and other lymphomas

Choriocarcinoma (an uncommon form of uterine cancer)

Testicular cancer

Acute lymphoblastic leukemia (the most common childhood leukemia)

Several rare types of childhood cancers

Thyroid cancer

Small-cell carcinoma of the lung

Breast cancer

Ovarian cancer

Bladder cancer

Cervical cancer

Some colon cancers

Multiple myeloma (a type of bone marrow cancer)

Leukemias other than acute lymphoblastic leukemia

# HOW ANTICANCER DRUGS AFFECT THE BODY

While killing rapidly dividing cancer cells, anticancer drugs also attack healthy cells, producing a range of serious side effects. Such drugs are used only when the potential benefits outweigh the drawbacks of the treatment.

**Platelets are reduced**
Tendency to bleed is increased

**White blood cell count is reduced**
Susceptibility to infection is increased

**Red blood cell count is reduced**
Anemia

Fewer platelets

Fewer white blood cells

Production of blood cells by bone marrow is slowed

Fewer red blood cells

Bone marrow

Cancer cells

Normal cells

Normal cells are damaged, causing leukemia in very rare cases

Intestine

**Lining of digestive tract is irritated**
Diarrhea occurs

Inflammation

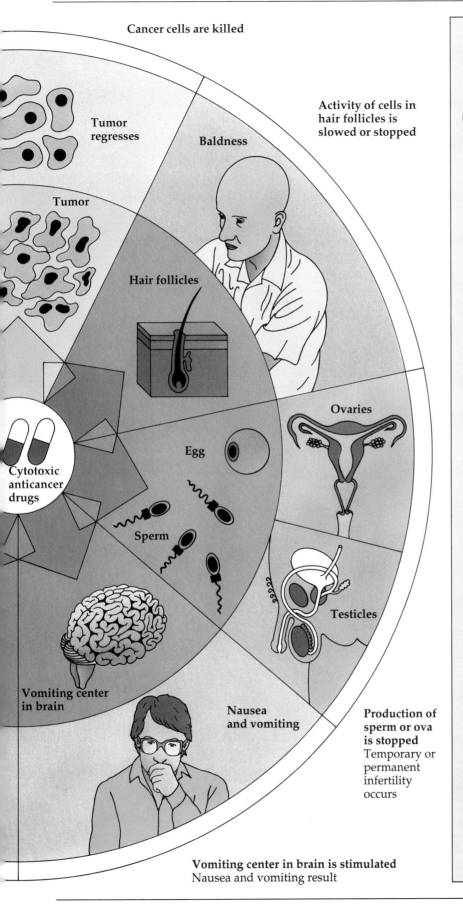

Cancer cells are killed

Tumor regresses

Tumor

Cytotoxic anticancer drugs

Baldness

Activity of cells in hair follicles is slowed or stopped

Hair follicles

Ovaries

Egg

Sperm

Testicles

Vomiting center in brain

Nausea and vomiting

Production of sperm or ova is stopped
Temporary or permanent infertility occurs

**Vomiting center in brain is stimulated**
Nausea and vomiting result

## ASK YOUR DOCTOR
## ANTICANCER DRUGS

**Q** I have been diagnosed as having Hodgkin's disease. My doctor has told me I must have chemotherapy in addition to radiation therapy and surgery. Can't I have just the radiation therapy and surgery to avoid the unpleasant side effects of chemotherapy?

**A** Chemotherapy substantially improves your chances of being cured of the disease. Many people with Hodgkin's disease are now completely cured after being treated with surgery, radiation therapy, and chemotherapy. After radiation therapy and surgery, anticancer drugs are given to prevent the spread of any remaining cancer cells.

**Q** A few years ago, I read about the development of new drugs called interferons. The report suggested that they were going to be standard treatment for many cancers. Are they widely available now?

**A** Interferons are still being researched but have not yet fulfilled the early claims made. Results of clinical trials have shown that interferons are effective against some forms of cancer. It remains to be seen whether interferons will be effective anticancer drugs in the future.

**Q** Will scientists ever discover a miracle drug that is capable of curing all types of cancers?

**A** Most current research is directed to finding drugs to treat individual types of cancer more effectively or devising more effective ways of combining drugs, surgery, and radiation therapy. However, the possibility of a single "wonder" drug cannot be ruled out.

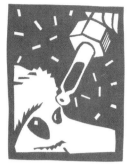

# DRUGS FOR EYE, EAR, AND SKIN DISORDERS

A GREAT NUMBER of visits to the doctor occur as a result of symptoms that involve the eyes, ears, and skin. The most common disorders are infection, inflammation, and irritation. In each case the most widely used treatment is a topical preparation.

For minor disorders of the eyes, ears, and skin, antibiotics can be prescribed for bacterial infections, antifungals for fungal infections, corticosteroids for inflammation, and antihistamines for inflammation caused by allergy. A variety of over-the-counter medications are available to treat these types of disorders.

## DRUGS FOR GLAUCOMA

Glaucoma in general is an eye disorder caused by a build-up of pressure due to reduced drainage of fluid from the eye. It can result in loss of vision. Eye drops containing a beta blocker (such as timolol) can be used to reduce the secretion of fluid in the eye. Miotic drugs, such as pilocarpine, cause the pupil in the center of the colored part of the eye (the iris) to constrict. These drugs are used to improve fluid drainage and reduce pressure within the eye. Acetazolamide blocks the enzyme carbonate dehydratase, resulting in reduced production of fluid. However, acetazolamide frequently causes side effects. When necessary, an osmotic agent, which induces the rapid drainage of fluid from the eye tissues, may be given to reduce the pressure in the eye.

## EYE DISORDERS

The drug chosen to treat an eye disorder depends on the cause and severity of the problem and the area of the eye that is affected. Drugs for eye disorders are formulated for use on the eye only.

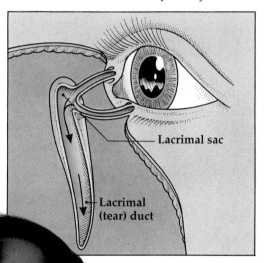

Lacrimal sac

Lacrimal (tear) duct

**How vision is lost**
*In glaucoma, rising pressure inside the eye results in compression of blood vessels that supply the optic nerve. This reduces blood supply and can cause damage to the nerve fibers and permanent loss of vision.*

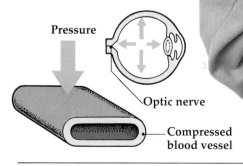

Pressure

Optic nerve

Compressed blood vessel

**Applying eye drops**
*When applying eye drops, press firmly on the lacrimal (tear) sac in the inner corner between your eye and nose to reduce the amount of the medication that might pass out through the lacrimal (tear) duct. Maintain the pressure for a few minutes after the eye drops have been applied.*

Mydriatics, which cause the pupil to dilate, are most commonly used for diagnostic purposes because they allow doctors to view the inside of the eye. Topical preparations (drops or ointments) of antibiotics are used to treat conjunctivitis (inflammation of the membrane covering the inside of the eyelids and part of the outside of the eyeballs) caused by bacterial infections. The development of inflammation caused by an allergy may be prevented by cromolyn sodium eye drops. Keratitis (inflammation of the cornea) caused by herpesvirus can be treated with antiviral drops or ointments.

## EAR DISORDERS

Infection and inflammation of the middle and outer ear are often treated with antibiotic or antibacterial drugs. The choice of drug and method of treatment depend on the cause of the problem, the severity of the problem, and the site within the ear that is affected.

### The outer ear

Otitis externa (inflammation of the outer ear) may be treated with ear drops containing a weak solution of a corticosteroid drug. Itching and swelling are usually reduced within a day or two. The risk of infection is increased by swimming in dirty water, the accumulation of earwax, poking objects (including cotton swabs) into the ear canal, or scratching the ear. When otitis externa is caused by or complicated by bacteria, an antibiotic is the appropriate treatment. Sometimes a combination of a corticosteroid and an antibiotic is prescribed. Fungal infections in the outer ear are rare and respond better to cleaning and application of antiseptics than to antifungal drugs.

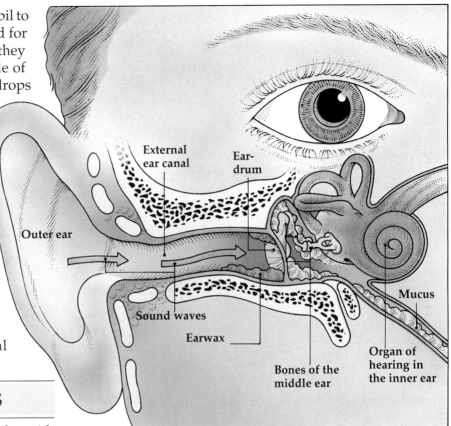

Labels: External ear canal · Ear-drum · Outer ear · Sound waves · Earwax · Bones of the middle ear · Mucus · Organ of hearing in the inner ear

**Inflammation of the outer or middle ear**
*Middle-ear infections are common among children. Obstruction of the transmission of sound waves through the air in the external ear canal or via the tiny bones of the middle ear (which transmit sound vibrations to the inner ear) decreases the ability to hear.*

### The middle ear

Otitis media is a bacterial infection of the middle ear that primarily affects infants and children, particularly those younger than 3. It usually occurs following a viral infection of the upper respiratory tract. Otitis media should be treated with antibiotics such as amoxicillin or trimethoprim with sulfamethoxazole. Acetaminophen may be given to reduce pain. Before the use of antibiotics and antibacterials, infection of the middle ear was commonly complicated by mastoiditis (infection of the air cells of the mastoid process – a part of the skull behind the ear), which required surgical drainage. If fluid or pus is present in the middle ear, hearing is impaired. It is sometimes necessary to temporarily place drainage tubes in the middle ear.

### WARNING

Although the corticosteroid drugs used for ear infections are unlikely to affect other parts of the body, long-term treatment is not advised for infants or during pregnancy. Prolonged use of topical antibiotics should also be avoided because of the risks of damage to hearing and the development of resistance by bacteria. If sensitivity develops, contact your doctor.

# HOW SKIN DISORDERS ARE TREATED

Many people visit their doctors seeking treatment for skin disorders. The cause and severity of their disorders are usually immediately apparent, and most skin conditions respond to treatment. Some doctors discourage self-treatment with over-the-counter drugs, especially hydrocortisone, because these preparations can aggravate certain skin conditions such as fungal infections (ringworm).

## Other skin treatments

*Oral antihistamines act within a few hours to reduce allergy-related skin inflammation. Taken orally, an antihistamine acts on the brain, reducing its response to signals sent from irritated skin. Dermatologists do not often recommend antihistamine lotions because they frequently cause an allergic rash. Coal tar preparations restore abnormally thickened skin to normal and have an antiseptic and soothing effect. Emollients reduce itching and prevent dryness by lubricating the skin.*

## Antifungal drugs

*Infections caused by fungi, such as athletes' foot and ringworm, rarely improve without treatment. Antifungal drugs can be applied topically for skin infections or taken orally for nail infections. Most antifungal drugs cause alterations in the fungal cell wall that enable essential chemicals to leak out of the fungal cell. Without these chemicals, the cell dies.*

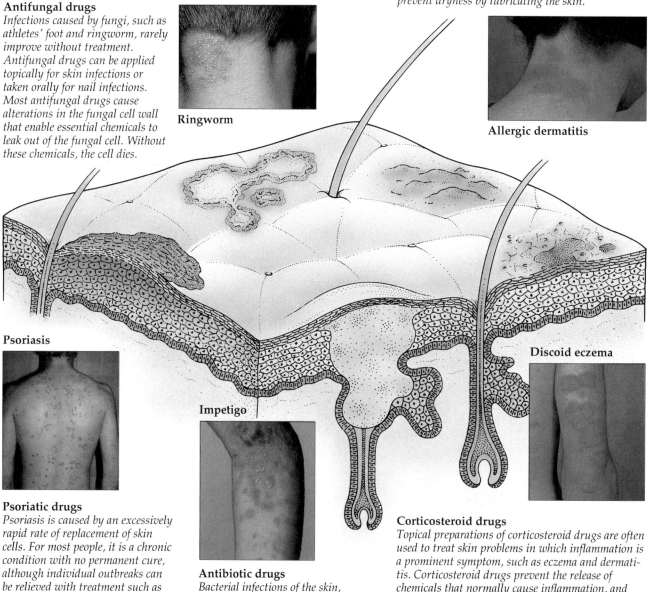

**Ringworm**

**Allergic dermatitis**

**Psoriasis**

**Discoid eczema**

**Impetigo**

## Psoriatic drugs

*Psoriasis is caused by an excessively rapid rate of replacement of skin cells. For most people, it is a chronic condition with no permanent cure, although individual outbreaks can be relieved with treatment such as corticosteroid lotions or creams, coal tar, anthralin, salicyclic acid (which loosens and removes scales), etretinate, methotrexate, and psoralen drugs and ultraviolet light. Most of these drugs slow down the reproduction of skin cells. Your doctor should supervise treatment.*

## Antibiotic drugs

*Bacterial infections of the skin, including boils and impetigo, can usually be treated by thorough cleansing and the application of antiseptic creams. Mupirocin cream is very effective in the treatment of impetigo and causes few side effects. For serious skin infections, an oral antibiotic may also be prescribed.*

## Corticosteroid drugs

*Topical preparations of corticosteroid drugs are often used to treat skin problems in which inflammation is a prominent symptom, such as eczema and dermatitis. Corticosteroid drugs prevent the release of chemicals that normally cause inflammation, and most skin conditions improve within a few days of treatment. Topical corticosteroids are generally not used on broken or infected skin (though they may be used on eczema that has been scratched). Prolonged use of corticosteroids can lead to permanent changes in the skin such as thinning, the appearance of fine blood vessels under the skin surface, easy bruising, and increased susceptibility to infection.*

# CASE HISTORY
## RESISTANCE TO DRUG TREATMENT

JANE HAS BEEN DIAGNOSED as having acne. Her dermatologist had prescribed various treatments, including benzoyl peroxide and chlorhexidine lotions, and then the antibiotics tetracycline and erythromycin to be taken orally. Jane followed her dermatologist's instructions but none of the drugs produced much improvement in her acne. Jane made another appointment with her dermatologist.

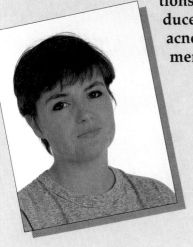

### PERSONAL DETAILS
**Name** Jane Green
**Age** 17
**Occupation** Student
**Family** Jane's parents are both healthy; neither of them has any skin disorders.

### THE TREATMENT
The doctor tells Jane to continue taking the tetracycline orally and using the benzoyl peroxide lotion. In addition, he prescribes tretinoin cream, a vitamin A derivative. He explains that tretinoin cream works by speeding up the turnover and reducing the stickiness of skin cells, thereby unblocking the pores. The doctor tells Jane that she may experience some minor skin irritation, dryness, and peeling during the first few days of treatment. Jane's doctor could have prescribed oral isotretinoin, which is also a vitamin A derivative. However, although the drug is very effective, it is used only in very severe cases of acne because of a relatively high risk of harmful side effects. Jane's doctor explains that there is no "cure" for acne. Treatment is aimed at controlling the acne until the body stops producing it.

### THE OUTCOME
After 2 months of her new drug therapy, Jane's acne improves dramatically. Her doctor advises her to continue taking the tetracycline and using both the lotion and the cream until maximum improvement is seen. Jane sees her dermatologist regularly so he can check on the condition of her acne.

### MEDICAL BACKGROUND
Jane had not experienced any skin problems until a year ago, when her acne developed. She does not have any allergies. Jane's dermatologist originally prescribed benzoyl peroxide, an antibacterial lotion, to unblock her pores and remove sebum (oil secreted by sebaceous glands). He also prescribed chlorhexidine, an antiseptic lotion. When no noticeable improvement occurred, Jane's dermatologist added oral antibiotics (first tetracycline, then erythromycin) to her treatment. Tetracycline and erythromycin are antibiotics that, like chlorhexidine, kill the bacteria that infect the sebaceous ducts and glands; the drugs also may have an anti-inflammatory effect.

### THE CONSULTATION
Jane's dermatologist examines her face and neck, as well as shoulders and back. He reviews the medications she is taking and confirms that she is using each as he had prescribed.

### THE DIAGNOSIS
Jane's dermatologist diagnoses a case of PERSISTENT ACNE. Her acne has not improved because it is resistant to the various medications that have been prescribed so far.

**Persistent acne**
*Jane's doctor explains that severe forms of acne may be resistant to treatment with oral antibiotics, antibacterial lotions, and antiseptic lotions.*

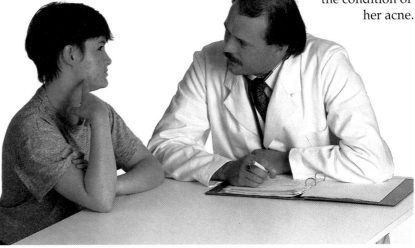

# CHAPTER FIVE

# OVER-THE-COUNTER MEDICATIONS

INTRODUCTION

NONPRESCRIPTION DRUGS

VITAMINS AND MINERALS

MANY PRODUCTS of the US pharmaceutical industry are available over-the-counter. Millions of Americans go to the pharmacy every year to purchase remedies for a wide range of common symptoms. A drug may be sold over-the-counter only after the Food and Drug Administration (FDA) has determined that it is effective and safe for use without medical supervision. Easy availability should not be equated with absolute safety, however; many drugs can cause allergic reactions or can be dangerous if taken in excessive dosages. It is important to be absolutely sure of the cause of your symptoms when you select a nonprescription medication. For example, sneezing and a runny nose in midsummer, or nausea during a car ride, are often symptoms of hay fever and motion sickness, respectively. If you experience sudden and inexplicable symptoms, or if after a few days your symptoms have not disappeared or have worsened, you should stop self-treatment and seek medical advice from your doctor.

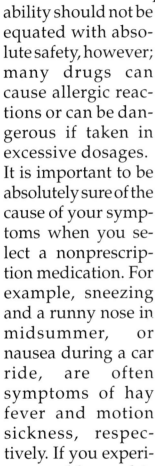

Most people suffer no ill effects when using over-the-counter drugs, but before taking any such medications pregnant women and people who are taking any prescription drug should consult their doctor. Although the FDA requires that all active ingredients be listed on product labels, medications may also contain inactive chemicals or dyes that are capable of causing allergic reactions. If you are sensitive to a chemical and are unsure whether that chemical is contained in an over-the-counter medication, check with your pharmacist or the manufacturer of the medication before taking it.

Many over-the-counter medications have identical active ingredients. Generic drugs usually contain identical active ingredients and are just as effective and less expensive than their brand-name equivalents. However, manufacturing methods may affect the rate at which a drug is absorbed into your bloodstream and the amount of the drug that becomes available for use by your body. This chapter discusses the advertised claims and the usual therapeutic benefits of over-the-counter medications. The first section gives advice on the most appropriate medications for treating pain, coughs, colds, sore throats, headaches, indigestion, and skin irritations, and how to use these medications safely and effectively. The second section describes risk factors for, and symptoms of, vitamin and mineral deficiencies and warns against taking excessive doses of vitamin and mineral supplements.

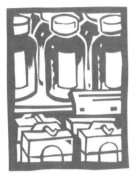

# NONPRESCRIPTION DRUGS

MANY MINOR AILMENTS can be treated with medications that are available without a prescription. These medications can be purchased primarily at drugstores, although some can also be found in supermarkets and other stores. Nonprescription drugs are also called over-the-counter medications.

Over-the-counter medications are used to relieve symptoms of common conditions, which, as a rule, go away by themselves. Some of these conditions are pain, coughs, colds, sore throats, headaches, indigestion, and skin irritations. There are several different types of remedies for these symptoms and ailments, and this chapter is designed to help you decide which one is most appropriate for you. An explanation of the actions and side effects of most of the drugs mentioned can be found in Chapter Four.

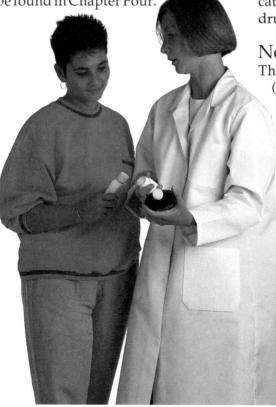

### SORE THROATS

A number of mouthwashes, sprays, and lozenges are available to soothe the pain of a sore throat. These preparations contain a variety of ingredients, some of which have a partial, temporary painkilling effect. There is absolutely no scientific evidence that any of these preparations effectively cures the cause of the sore throat. Gargling with a solution of salt and warm water may produce just as much (or more) pain relief. Preparations that contain phenol may cause swelling of the throat. If sore throat pain lasts for more than 48 hours, call your doctor.

## THE SAFETY FACTOR

Even though over-the-counter medications can be obtained without a prescription, these preparations can be harmful if they are misused. Over-the-counter medications are unlikely to cause side effects when taken according to the directions on the label, but it is very important that you read and follow all instructions. You should take the same precautions with over-the-counter medications that you do with prescription drugs (see USING DRUGS WISELY on page 46).

### New nonprescription drugs

The Food and Drug Administration (FDA) determines whether a drug can be sold directly to the public or whether a prescription is needed. The FDA may change the status of a prescription drug to that of an over-the-counter medication if the drug has been used safely by large numbers of people and use of the drug does not require a doctor's supervision. For example, some topical (used on the surface of the skin) antibiotics have been designated as nonprescription drugs.

**Seeking advice**
*Your pharmacist can help you select the most suitable over-the-counter medication for your ailment. He or she may also advise you to seek medical advice from your doctor.*

# PAINKILLERS

Although there are more than 100 over-the-counter oral medications with analgesic (painkilling) properties, the active ingredient in most of these products is one of three analgesic drugs – acetaminophen, aspirin, or ibuprofen. Some preparations contain a mixture of analgesics and may contain other drugs, such as antacids, antihistamines, or decongestants. Such combination products are not any more effective in relieving a particular symptom than single-ingredient medications. In addition, these combination products increase the risk of having an adverse reaction. Single-ingredient preparations are also usually less expensive.

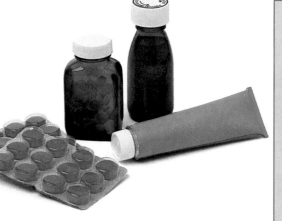

**Analgesic drugs**
*Acetaminophen, aspirin, and ibuprofen relieve mild to moderate pain and reduce fever. Aspirin and ibuprofen also have an anti-inflammatory effect and can be used for the treatment of arthritis. Ibuprofen is particularly effective against menstrual pain and pain caused by soft-tissue injuries such as tendon sprains and muscle strains.*

**WARNING**

You should use over-the-counter painkillers for only 48 hours before seeking medical advice.
◆ Do not take aspirin for a few weeks before surgery.
◆ Do not give aspirin to children or teenagers.
◆ Do not take ibuprofen if you are allergic to aspirin; you may be allergic to both.
◆ Do not take ibuprofen if you have kidney disease.

## COUGH AND COLD PREPARATIONS

There is no cure for the common cold. Yet an overwhelming number of cough and cold remedies can be found on drugstore shelves. Some remedies help relieve symptoms; others probably neither help nor hinder your body's natural process of recovery. This chart describes the main drug groups used in cough and cold preparations. Many preparations contain a mixture of drugs. It can be dangerous for you to take more than one cough or cold medication because they may include the same or very similar ingredients.

| CLASSIFICATION | | SYMPTOMS | FORM | ADVICE |
|---|---|---|---|---|
| Decongestants | | Stuffy nose | Tablets, capsules, nasal sprays and drops | Decongestant sprays and drops are most effective. However, long-term use of a decongestant can cause an increase in congestion. Decongestants taken orally can cause blood pressure to increase. |
| Antihistamines | | Stuffy or runny nose, sneezing, watery and itchy eyes caused by an allergy | Tablets, capsules, nasal sprays and drops | Effective in relieving symptoms caused by allergy; often included in cough and cold medications to dry up nasal secretions; may cause drowsiness or dizziness. |
| Analgesics | | Pains, muscle aches, fever | Tablets, capsules, liquids, creams, gums, lozenges | Effective. Do not give aspirin to children or teenagers. |
| Cough suppressants | | Dry cough | Liquids, lozenges, tablets | Effective. Do not take for a productive (phlegm-producing) cough because this will prevent you from getting rid of phlegm and possibly delay your recovery. |
| Expectorants, mucolytics | | Productive (phlegm-producing) cough | Liquids, lozenges, tablets | Effectiveness unproven. Increasing your fluid intake is more helpful. |
| Bronchodilators | | Shortness of breath, cough, wheezing, feeling of tightness in chest | Inhalers, tablets, capsules, liquids | Do not use unless recommended by your doctor. |

## KITS FOR QUITTING SMOKING

Over-the-counter kits are available to help smokers kick the habit. Some of these kits contain tablets of lobeline, a drug that resembles nicotine in structure and action. The tablets reduce withdrawal symptoms of nicotine dependence. Other kits contain silver acetate lozenges. Silver acetate gives cigarette smoke its bitter taste. The lozenges produce an unpleasant taste if a cigarette is smoked, reinforcing the smoker's desire to quit. Kits that contain filters of increasing strength are also available. These filters attach to cigarettes and are intended to reduce the smoker's intake of nicotine slowly, usually over 2 weeks. None of these kits has been conclusively shown to help substantial numbers of people quit smoking.

**Side effects**
*Prolonged use of silver acetate can cause a permanent bluish discoloration of body tissues, so silver acetate lozenges should not be taken for more than 3 weeks. Lobeline is not addictive, but should not be taken for longer than 6 weeks. Neither drug should be taken by women who are pregnant or breast-feeding.*

## DIGESTIVE DISORDERS

Hundreds of over-the-counter preparations are available to treat disorders of the digestive tract. These preparations include antacids for indigestion, antigas medications, antinausea drugs, laxatives, and antidiarrheal drugs.

## Antacids

Antacids relieve the symptoms of indigestion and heartburn; they neutralize stomach acid and effectively heal peptic ulcers. Use of antacids can mask the symptoms of more serious disorders. Call your doctor if you have stomach pain for longer than 2 weeks. Excessive, prolonged use of antacids may result in serious disorders of the kidneys or the bones or may cause retention of fluids.

## Antigas medications

Simethicone (alone or combined with antacid preparations) is used to treat flatulence (expulsion of intestinal gas). There is no conclusive evidence that simethicone is effective, however. Simple measures such as chewing your food well, eating slowly, and avoiding carbonated drinks and foods known to cause gas (such as cabbage) can help prevent formation of gas in the stomach.

## Antinausea drugs

Nausea remedies (antiemetics) that are available without a prescription are also appropriate for treating motion sickness. Medications for motion sickness frequently contain an antihistamine, which can cause drowsiness. Antiemetics should not be taken while driving or with alcohol. Talk to your doctor before taking any drug that contains an antihistamine if you have glaucoma, are taking sedatives, or have asthma, emphysema, or prostate problems.

If you vomit, do not eat or drink for an hour or two. If your nausea subsides, try taking frequent 1- to 3-ounce sips of flu-

**Indigestion remedies**
*Indigestion remedies are sold in forms ranging from tablets or powders that dissolve in water to chewable tablets or liquids. Most antacids contain one or more of only four active ingredients – sodium bicarbonate, calcium carbonate, magnesium hydroxide (or trisilicate), and aluminum hydroxide. Talk to your doctor before taking any antacid if you have kidney, heart, or liver disease.*

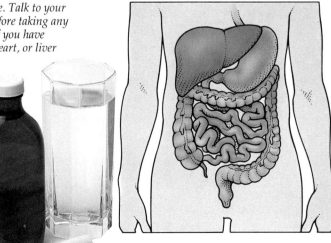

ids before eating any solid foods. If you cannot control vomiting after 3 or 4 hours or if you have other symptoms such as drowsiness, fever, or sensitivity to bright lights, call your doctor immediately.

## Laxatives

In most cases, constipation can be relieved by eating high-fiber foods and drinking plenty of fluids. Glycerin suppositories can help reestablish the urge to have a bowel movement. Mild bulk-forming or lubricant laxatives may be used for constipation that does not respond to an increased intake of fiber and fluids. Talk to your doctor about any change in your bowel habits. Long-term use of laxatives can lead to dependence and, occasionally, loss of potassium (resulting in muscle weakness).

**Constipation, enemas, and suppositories**
*The occasional use of an 8-ounce tap-water enema can relieve constipation. Enemas that introduce a large amount of fluid far into the colon can be harmful and do not "promote health" as claimed. Glycerin suppositories may be used for occasional relief of constipation or in a program of treatment for constipation that also includes changing your toilet habits (that is, responding to the urge to have a bowel movement).*

## Antidiarrheal drugs

Most bouts of diarrhea last only a day or two; the best treatment is to abstain from food and to drink small quantities of clear fluids, including water, juice, and broth, every 20 to 60 minutes. However, among the antidiarrheal drugs, the weak narcotic preparations of loperamide or diphenoxylate are more likely to stop bowel activity than bulk-forming and adsorbent agents such as methylcellulose, kaolin, and charcoal. Loperamide is available over-the-counter in liquid form. Consult your doctor if you or your child has diarrhea that lasts for more than 48 hours, if there is severe abdominal pain, if the diarrhea contains blood or pus, if there are signs of dehydration (such as drowsiness, sunken eyes, or dry skin), or if your child is under age 2.

### WARNING

Persistent diarrhea or vomiting can lead to dehydration, which can be life-threatening. Babies, young children, and elderly people are at particular risk. For persistent diarrhea, drink an oral rehydration solution to replace lost body fluids. Premixed packets of ingredients can be added to water to promote rehydration; instructions are on the label. You can make a solution by mixing $3/4$ teaspoon of salt, 1 tablespoon of sugar, $1/2$ teaspoon of baking soda, and $1/4$ teaspoon of potassium chloride in a quart of water. Ask your doctor or pharmacist for dosage instructions.

---

## WEIGHT-LOSS PRODUCTS

The best and most healthy way to lose weight and keep it off is to eat a balanced diet containing fewer calories than you have been consuming, and to exercise regularly. Taking appetite suppressants or other types of diet pills, eating or drinking diet foods or drinks, or eating large amounts of fiber may help you lose weight but can have serious side effects. Many doctors believe that losing weight quickly may slow down your metabolism so that when you start eating normally again you quickly regain the weight you had lost.

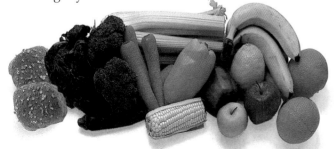

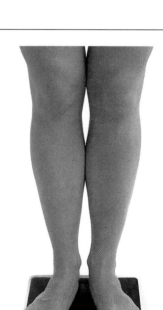

**Diet pills**
*Most over-the-counter appetite suppressants contain the stimulant phenylpropanolamine, a drug also found in some cold remedies. There is no convincing evidence that phenylpropanolamine can help you lose weight and keep it off. It can be dangerous to take diet pills if you have high blood pressure, heart disease, glaucoma, diabetes, thyroid disease, or kidney problems. Diuretic drugs increase your output of urine and can cause loss of essential minerals from the body.*

# REMEDIES FOR EXTERNAL CONDITIONS

Many over-the-counter remedies are available for treating conditions that affect external parts of the body. These preparations usually affect only the part of the body to which they are applied.

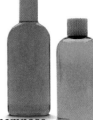

**Dandruff shampoos**
*Medicated shampoo may help control dandruff (shedding of dead skin from the scalp). Ingredients for these shampoos considered to be safe and effective by the Food and Drug Administration include coal tar, sulfur, salicylic acid, selenium sulfide, and zinc pyrithione. Dandruff shampoos are also used to treat seborrheic dermatitis (rash) and psoriasis (thickened patches of red, inflamed skin) of the scalp.*

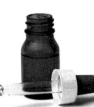

**Ear preparations**
*A variety of over-the-counter ear drops are available to soothe minor irritation or to soften earwax. Some of these drops can cause allergic reactions. If you have perforated eardrums, do not use nonprescription ear drops. Call your doctor if you have any persistent ear problems.*

**Eye preparations**
*Eye drops containing a decongestant drug can relieve mild redness, itching, stinging, and minor eye irritations. Prolonged use can increase redness and mask symptoms of more serious problems. Consult your doctor if any eye irritation does not clear up within 2 days, or if there is any blurring of vision. You can purchase eye solutions for flushing out chemicals or particles from the eye. However, if such solutions are not available, flush the chemicals out with tap water and call your doctor immediately.*

**Antihistamines**
*Topically applied antihistamines reduce skin inflammation and itching caused by an allergic reaction.*

**Acne preparations**
*Mild cases of acne can usually be controlled with twice-daily washing with soap and water to remove any excess natural skin oil (sebum). Preparations containing benzoyl peroxide, which kills bacteria, provide effective treatment for more severe cases of acne. Cleansers containing salicylic acid, sulfur, or resorcinol are less effective. Abrasive cleansers containing fine particles can irritate inflamed areas of the skin.*

**Toothpastes and oral rinses**
*It is important to brush and floss your teeth at least once a day, limit your intake of sugar, and visit your dentist every 6 months. Drinking fluoridated water and using toothpastes containing fluoride help prevent tooth decay. However, fluoride has a minimal effect on gums. Some over-the-counter mouthwashes for bad breath are effective in controlling plaque and maintaining healthy gums. Over-the-counter rinses designed to reduce plaque are not much more effective than rinsing with water before brushing and flossing.*

## Moisturizers

*Moisturizers (sometimes known as emollients) can be used to soothe dry skin conditions such as dermatitis and eczema (inflammatory skin conditions) and psoriasis (thickened patches of red, inflamed skin) by lubricating the skin surface and preventing water evaporation. Simple preparations of moisturizing cream or petroleum jelly can be just as effective as expensive, perfumed products.*

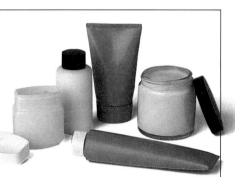

## Sunscreens

*Use a sunscreen to protect your skin from the sun's harmful ultraviolet rays. Sunscreens are graded according to the amount of protection they provide. It is best to use a sunscreen with a protection factor of 15 or higher; apply it frequently to maintain protection. Sunscreens containing para-aminobenzoic acid or a benzophenone derivative may cause a rash.*

## Antiseptics and antibiotics

*Preparations containing an antiseptic such as chlorhexidine can be used to clean minor cuts, scrapes, and burns and to prevent minor bacterial infection. Topical antibiotics such as neomycin can be used to treat minor infection. However, self-medication with antibiotics carries a risk of using the wrong antibiotic or using inadequate amounts of the correct antibiotic. Boils and serious infections, deep wounds, animal or human bites, or serious burns should always be treated by your doctor. Avoid getting any antiseptic in your eyes; some antiseptics can cause serious eye injury.*

## Preparations for hemorrhoids

*Over-the-counter preparations for the relief of hemorrhoids and other irritations of the skin surrounding the anus include creams, pastes, ointments, foams, suppositories, and cleansers to use after bowel movements. These preparations often include a soothing agent with antiseptic or astringent properties, such as zinc oxide, bismuth, or witch hazel. Many of these treatments contain an anesthetic drug to relieve pain and itching. However, these preparations can cause an allergic reaction and may increase the irritation.*

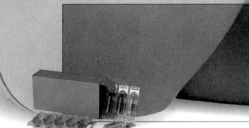

## Hydrocortisone

*Creams, ointments, sprays, and lotions containing 0.5 percent hydrocortisone are available over-the-counter for the temporary relief of minor skin irritations. However, such preparations should be used sparingly and should never be applied to broken or infected skin. If your skin condition worsens or persists for longer than a week, consult your doctor.*

## Fungicides

*Preparations containing fungicidal drugs such as clotrimazole and miconazole can be effective for fungal infections of the skin, including athletes' foot. However, if you do not see improvement within 2 to 4 weeks, call your doctor. Candidiasis, a fungal infection of the mouth or vagina, is resistant to most over-the-counter antifungal preparations and must be treated with an antifungal cream or suppository prescribed by your doctor.*

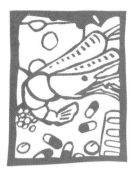

# VITAMINS AND MINERALS

A BALANCED DIET should supply all the vitamins and minerals your body needs if you are physically fit and healthy. In developed countries, deficiencies generally occur only in individuals whose diets might be compromised by choice (such as some low-calorie or vegetarian diets) or by an illness that decreases appetite or intestinal absorption of nutrients. In recent years, an enthusiastic pursuit of good health has led some people to consume an excessive amount of vitamin supplements.

## SELENIUM

Low intake of the mineral selenium has been implicated in the development of breast cancer. However, a recent study of more than 60,000 women showed no such relationship. Also, claims regarding the antiaging properties of selenium are unproven. Fish and shellfish; kidney, liver, and other meat; and whole grains are good dietary sources of selenium. Intake of excessive amounts of selenium supplements can be fatal.

**Intake of vitamins and minerals**
*If you suspect that your diet is lacking in nutrients, talk to your doctor about how to select foods for a well-balanced diet. Ask his or her advice on whether you need to take vitamin or mineral supplements.*

Many people mistakenly take vitamin and mineral supplements to "safeguard" their health or as a substitute for a balanced diet. Supplements are usually required only for women who are pregnant or breast-feeding, infants, young children, people who are on diets deficient in some ingredients, and the elderly. Nutritional deficiencies can also be caused by prolonged cooking of food, which destroys some water-soluble vitamins. People who have an addiction to alcohol, impaired absorption of nutrients from the digestive tract, or a severe illness or injury may have a deficiency of one or more vitamins or minerals. Consult your doctor if you think you need a vitamin or mineral supplement.

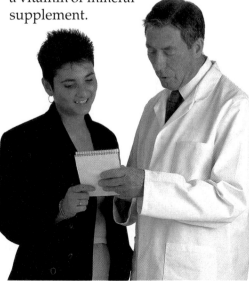

## VITAMINS

Vitamins are chemicals that are essential for our bodies to function normally. With the exceptions of vitamin D (formed by the action of sunlight on the skin), vitamin K and biotin (synthesized in small amounts by intestinal bacteria), and niacin (produced from the amino acid tryptophan), vitamins cannot be produced by the body; instead, they are absorbed from the foods we eat. The commonly known vitamins are the fat-soluble vitamins A, D, E, and K (stored in the liver and fatty tissues) and the water-soluble vitamins C and B complex (excesses are excreted in the urine). The B-complex vitamins include thiamine (vitamin $B_1$), riboflavin (vitamin $B_2$), niacin, vitamin $B_6$, folic acid, pantothenic acid, and biotin. Vitamin $B_{12}$ is not usually considered part of the B complex.

## MINERALS

Some minerals (basic chemical elements) are also vital. The major minerals needed are calcium, phosphorus, sodium, potassium, magnesium, chlorine, and sulfur. Others that are essential in smaller amounts are iron, copper, fluorine, iodine, selenium, zinc, chromium, cobalt, manganese, and molybdenum.

# VITAMIN DEFICIENCY

| VITAMINS AND GOOD DIETARY SOURCES | RISK FACTORS FOR AND SYMPTOMS OF DEFICIENCY |
|---|---|

**VITAMIN A**
Dark green leafy vegetables; orange and yellow fruits and vegetables; liver; fortified milk; eggs

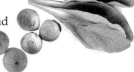

**Risk factors** Low-fat diet; intestinal malabsorption disorders; obstruction of bile duct; growth spurts in adolescents; hyperthyroidism (overactive thyroid gland); long-term use of some lipid-lowering drugs
**Symptoms** Poor vision in dim light; dry, rough, itchy skin; lowered resistance to infection; poor appetite; diarrhea

**THIAMINE (VITAMIN B₁)**
Whole grains; cereals; pork; organ meats; spinach; peas; lima beans; nuts

**Risk factors** Pregnancy and breast-feeding; hemodialysis (removal of waste products from the blood by an artificial kidney); long-term intravenous feeding; chronic liver disease; chronic alcoholism; intestinal malabsorption disorders
**Symptoms** Fatigue; weakness; confusion; depression; nausea; constipation; paralysis of eye muscles; dementia; memory loss

**RIBOFLAVIN (VITAMIN B₂)**
Milk; cheese; yogurt; eggs; liver and other meats; green leafy vegetables; whole grains; nuts; peas; beans

**Risk factors** Intestinal malabsorption disorders; severe illness or injury; surgery; chronic alcoholism; aging; pregnancy and breast-feeding; long-term use of phenothiazine antipsychotic drugs, tricyclic antidepressants, or oral contraceptives; excessive exercise
**Symptoms** Cracks in corners of mouth; ulcers in the mouth; red, sore tongue; seborrheic dermatitis (rash)

**NIACIN**
Whole grains; nuts; peanut butter; peas; beans; liver, poultry, and other meats; fish; milk; eggs

**Risk factors** Low-protein diet; intestinal malabsorption disorders; liver disease; chronic alcoholism; pregnancy and breast-feeding
**Symptoms** Inflammation of mouth and tongue; upset stomach; nausea; diarrhea; anxiety; depression; dementia (decline of mental abilities); dermatitis (inflammation of the skin)

**PANTOTHENIC ACID**
Broccoli; lima beans; whole-grain cereals; meat; eggs; milk

**Risk factors** Severe illness or injury; surgery; prolonged periods of stress; intestinal malabsorption disorders; chronic alcoholism
**Symptoms** Fatigue; respiratory infections; headaches; abdominal pain; numbness or tingling in arms and legs; muscle cramps; dizziness; confusion; lack of coordination; low blood sugar level

**VITAMIN B₆**
Whole grains; poultry, liver, and other meats; bananas; eggs; fish; potatoes; green leafy vegetables

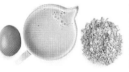

**Risk factors** Long-term use of oral contraceptives; long-term treatment with isoniazid, penicillamine, and hydralazine; drugs used to treat parkinsonism (muscle tremor, stiffness, and weakness) or epilepsy; chronic alcoholism; aging; intestinal malabsorption disorders
**Symptoms** Anemia; weakness; nervousness; irritability; skin disorders

**VITAMIN B₁₂**
Poultry, liver, and other meats; fish; shellfish; cheese; milk; eggs

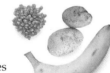

**Risk factors** Intestinal malabsorption disorders; surgical removal of large parts of stomach; lack of intrinsic factor (substance produced in the stomach that is necessary for absorption of vitamin B₁₂); strict vegetarian diet; chronic alcoholism
**Symptoms** Anemia; sore tongue and mouth; numbness and tingling of arms and legs; memory loss; depression

**BIOTIN**
Liver; eggs; nuts; beans; cauliflower

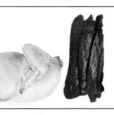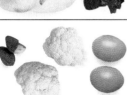

**Risk factors** Long-term treatment with antibiotics or sulfonamide antibacterials; long-term use of oral contraceptives; consumption of large amounts of alcohol; excessive intake of raw eggs
**Symptoms** Weakness; tiredness; nausea; depression; hair loss; eczema (inflammation of the skin); inflammation of the tongue

## VITAMIN DEFICIENCY (continued)

| VITAMINS AND GOOD DIETARY SOURCES | RISK FACTORS FOR AND SYMPTOMS OF DEFICIENCY |
|---|---|
| **FOLIC ACID** 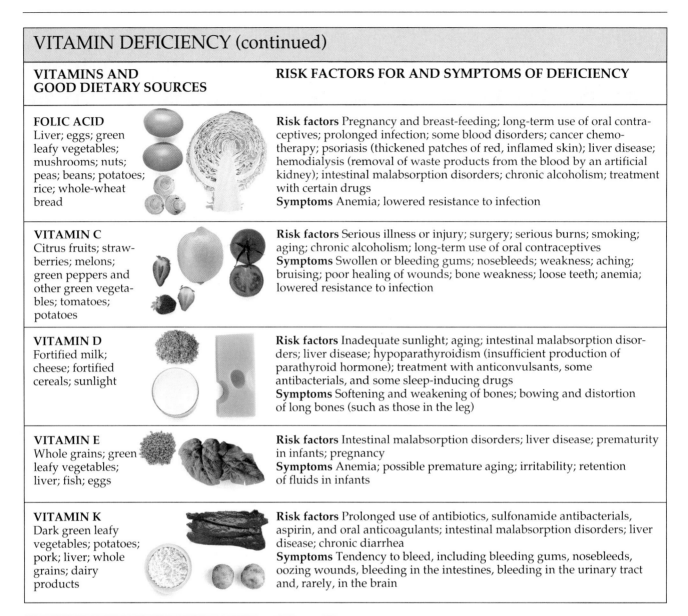 Liver; eggs; green leafy vegetables; mushrooms; nuts; peas; beans; potatoes; rice; whole-wheat bread | **Risk factors** Pregnancy and breast-feeding; long-term use of oral contraceptives; prolonged infection; some blood disorders; cancer chemotherapy; psoriasis (thickened patches of red, inflamed skin); liver disease; hemodialysis (removal of waste products from the blood by an artificial kidney); intestinal malabsorption disorders; chronic alcoholism; treatment with certain drugs <br> **Symptoms** Anemia; lowered resistance to infection |
| **VITAMIN C** Citrus fruits; strawberries; melons; green peppers and other green vegetables; tomatoes; potatoes | **Risk factors** Serious illness or injury; surgery; serious burns; smoking; aging; chronic alcoholism; long-term use of oral contraceptives <br> **Symptoms** Swollen or bleeding gums; nosebleeds; weakness; aching; bruising; poor healing of wounds; bone weakness; loose teeth; anemia; lowered resistance to infection |
| **VITAMIN D** Fortified milk; cheese; fortified cereals; sunlight | **Risk factors** Inadequate sunlight; aging; intestinal malabsorption disorders; liver disease; hypoparathyroidism (insufficient production of parathyroid hormone); treatment with anticonvulsants, some antibacterials, and some sleep-inducing drugs <br> **Symptoms** Softening and weakening of bones; bowing and distortion of long bones (such as those in the leg) |
| **VITAMIN E** Whole grains; green leafy vegetables; liver; fish; eggs | **Risk factors** Intestinal malabsorption disorders; liver disease; prematurity in infants; pregnancy <br> **Symptoms** Anemia; possible premature aging; irritability; retention of fluids in infants |
| **VITAMIN K** Dark green leafy vegetables; potatoes; pork; liver; whole grains; dairy products | **Risk factors** Prolonged use of antibiotics, sulfonamide antibacterials, aspirin, and oral anticoagulants; intestinal malabsorption disorders; liver disease; chronic diarrhea <br> **Symptoms** Tendency to bleed, including bleeding gums, nosebleeds, oozing wounds, bleeding in the intestines, bleeding in the urinary tract and, rarely, in the brain |

## VITAMIN SUPPLEMENTS AND OVERDOSE

The idea that taking a vitamin supplement can do no harm, even if it is not doing any good, is dangerously misguided. Fat-soluble vitamins are not promptly excreted from the body and can build up to toxic levels if taken in high doses for prolonged periods of time. An excess of vitamin A, for example, can cause headache, bone pain, enlargement of the spleen, and severe liver damage; high doses of vitamin D can eventually lead to kidney damage. Excess amounts of some of the water-soluble vitamins can also cause problems. Sustained doses of vitamin $B_6$ may lead to permanent damage of the nervous system, excessive vitamin C can cause diarrhea, and an excess of niacin has been associated with high blood sugar levels.

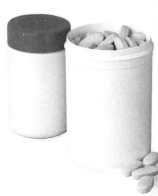

**False vitamins**
*The substances amygdalin, bioflavonoid, carnitine, choline, inositol, orotic acid, pangamic acid, and para-aminobenzoic acid are often sold in supplement form. However, these substances are not true vitamins, either because the body can produce them or because there is no evidence that they are needed by the body to promote growth or sustain life.*

## MINERAL DEFICIENCY

| MINERALS AND GOOD DIETARY SOURCES | RISK FACTORS FOR AND SYMPTOMS OF DEFICIENCY |
|---|---|
| **CALCIUM** Dairy products; dried peas; dried beans; green leafy vegetables; soybeans | **Risk factors** Intestinal malabsorption disorders; use of fiber supplements; pregnancy and breast-feeding <br> **Symptoms** Osteoporosis (loss of bone density, with increased tendency to fracture); abnormal stimulation of nervous system leading to cramps in muscles throughout the body, especially the hands, feet, and face |
| **CHROMIUM** Meat; dairy products; whole grains; green leafy vegetables | **Risk factors** Food grown in chromium-deficient soil; a diet containing too many processed foods <br> **Symptoms** High blood glucose levels |
| **FLUORIDE** Fish; shellfish; tea; fluoridated drinking water | **Risk factors** Lack of fluoride in local drinking water <br> **Symptoms** Tooth decay, especially in children who do not use a fluoride toothpaste |
| **IODINE** Fish; shellfish; bread; dairy products; iodized table salt | **Risk factors** Food grown in iodine-deficient soil <br> **Symptoms** Goiter (enlargement of thyroid gland); hypothyroidism (underactive thyroid gland) in adults; cretinism (mental retardation, stunted growth, coarse facial features) in infants |
| **IRON** Red meat; liver; egg yolk; shellfish; green leafy vegetables; nuts; fortified grains; dried fruit | **Risk factors** Pregnancy; heavy menstrual periods or between-period bleeding; chronic blood loss due to disorders or diseases such as hemorrhoids or inflammatory bowel disease <br> **Symptoms** Anemia; sore mouth; nail changes; apathy; irritability; lowered resistance to infection |
| **MAGNESIUM** Dark green vegetables; nuts; dry peas; dry beans; whole grains; bananas | **Risk factors** Intestinal malabsorption disorders; severe diarrhea; advanced kidney disease; chronic alcoholism; long-term treatment with some diuretic drugs <br> **Symptoms** Nausea; tremors; muscle weakness; muscle spasm; anxiety; palpitations (awareness of heartbeat) |
| **POTASSIUM** Green leafy vegetables; oranges; bananas; potatoes; whole grains; beans; nuts; meat; milk; fish | **Risk factors** Severe diarrhea; vomiting; kidney disease; consumption of large amounts of coffee, alcohol, or salt; treatment with insulin, diuretics, or corticosteroid drugs; excessive use of laxatives <br> **Symptoms** Muscle weakness; fatigue; dizziness; confusion; disturbances of heart rhythm; constipation |
| **SODIUM** Almost all foods, especially processed foods; smoked, pickled, or cured meats; fish; vegetables; table salt | **Risk factors** Prolonged vomiting; diarrhea; very excessive perspiration; kidney disorders; insufficient production of hormones by the adrenal glands; severe bleeding; use of diuretic drugs <br> **Symptoms** Lethargy; muscle cramps; dizziness; fall in blood pressure causing confusion and palpitations (awareness of heartbeat) |
| **ZINC** Lean meat; fish; shellfish; whole grains; dry peas; dry beans; nuts; eggs | **Risk factors** Growth spurts in adolescents; aging; pregnancy and breast-feeding; liver damage due to chronic alcoholism <br> **Symptoms** Loss of appetite; poor growth and delayed sexual development in children; delayed wound healing; lowered resistance to infection |

# DEALING WITH DRUG POISONING EMERGENCIES

This section gives important practical advice on how to react to a drug poisoning emergency. Emergency action may be required if you suspect that a person has taken an overdose of any drug. Symptoms of drug overdose include any signs of drowsiness, unconsciousness, breathing that is shallow or irregular or has stopped, vomiting, or seizures. Administer any necessary first aid and call an ambulance. If possible, ask the overdose victim what drug he or she took; if the victim is unconscious, look for any leftover drug. Report the information about the drug taken to the paramedics or the doctor in the emergency room.

## MOUTH-TO-MOUTH RESUSCITATION

When there is no rise and fall of the chest and you can feel no movement of exhaled air, immediately start mouth-to-mouth resuscitation. In cases of a neck injury, do not move the victim; call for help immediately.

1 Quickly clear the mouth and airway of any foreign material with your fingers.

2 (Not shown.) To open the victim's airway, tilt his or her head backward by placing your palm on the victim's forehead and then placing the fingers of your other hand under the bony part of his or her chin.

3 Using the hand that is placed on the victim's forehead, pinch the nostrils closed. Take a deep breath, seal your mouth over the victim's mouth, and exhale. Blow two quick breaths into the victim's mouth.

4 Turn to watch the victim's chest rise. Stop blowing when the chest expands. If the victim's chest does not fall as the air is exhaled, sweep your fingers around his or her mouth again to check for blockage of the airway.

## EMERGENCY CHECK LIST

1 Is the victim breathing? If he or she is not breathing, begin MOUTH-TO-MOUTH RESUSCITATION (see below). If the victim does not respond after two breaths, check his or her heartbeat. If you cannot detect a heartbeat or pulse at the wrist or neck, begin CARDIOPULMONARY RESUSCITATION (see page 133). Call for medical help immediately.

2 Is the victim conscious? If he or she is unconscious but breathing, make the person as comfortable as possible and keep him or her warm. Call for medical help immediately.

3 Is the victim drowsy? If so, keep the person awake and talking if possible. Call for medical help immediately.

## DEALING WITH A SEIZURE

Some types of drug poisoning can provoke seizures. Seizures are uncontrolled muscle movements of the body. The person may be partially or totally unconscious. If you witness a seizure, do not try to hold the person down, and do not put anything into his or her mouth. Move hazards, such as furniture, out of the way to ensure that the person is not injured. Once the seizure is over, make the person as comfortable as possible.

5 (Not shown.) Begin mouth-to-mouth resuscitation again. Be sure to take a deep breath between each of your breaths. Continue at the rate of 12 breaths per minute until you can see the victim beginning to breathe on his or her own.

## CARDIOPULMONARY RESUSCITATION

If a person's heart has stopped beating, he or she will be unresponsive, skin color will be gray, you will feel no pulse at the wrist or neck, and no heartbeat will be audible in the chest. If a person is breathing, then the heart is beating, even if you cannot feel a pulse. Cardiopulmonary resuscitation is a technique carried out in conjunction with MOUTH-TO-MOUTH RESUSCITATION (see page 132) to restart a stopped heart.

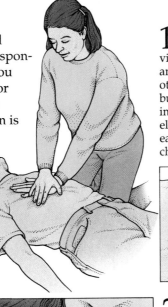

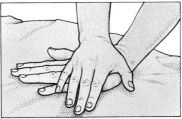

**1** Place the heel of one hand two finger-widths above where the victim's ribs meet the breastbone and cover with the heel of the other hand. Push down forcefully but smoothly about 1 1/2 to 2 inches without bending your elbows. Release pressure following each compression to allow the chest to expand.

**2** Repeat step 1 at the rate of 80 compressions per minute, giving two breaths by mouth-to-mouth resuscitation after every 15 compressions.

**3** As soon as you detect a pulse or heartbeat, resume mouth-to-mouth resuscitation and continue until the victim is breathing on his or her own.

## DEALING WITH ANAPHYLACTIC SHOCK

Anaphylactic shock sometimes occurs as the result of a severe allergic reaction. Blood pressure drops dramatically and the airways may become narrowed. The reaction usually occurs within minutes of taking the drug. Danger symptoms are pallor, tightness in the chest, difficulty breathing, nausea and vomiting, rash, swelling of the face, and collapse.

**1** If the victim has stopped breathing, perform MOUTH-TO-MOUTH RESUSCITATION (see page 132). If the victim is breathing, lie him or her down and raise the legs above the level of the heart to ensure adequate circulation of blood.

**2** Loosen any tight clothing and cover the victim with a blanket or coat. Call for medical help and do not give the victim anything to eat or drink.

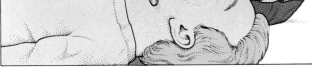

### WARNING

Do not attempt to perform cardiopulmonary resuscitation unless you have clear written instructions or, ideally, have been thoroughly trained in the technique. The information at left explains the basic techniques of cardiopulmonary resuscitation.

### INDUCING VOMITING

When dealing with a drug poisoning emergency, call your doctor, a hospital emergency room, or a poison control center for medical advice. Follow all instructions carefully, especially those with regard to inducing vomiting. It is sometimes necessary to induce vomiting to expel the drug from the stomach, thus preventing the drug from being absorbed into the bloodstream. If the person is conscious, you may give him or her syrup of ipecac. To avoid choking and inhalation of vomit, make sure the person leans well forward before he or she begins vomiting.

# DRUG GLOSSARY

## How to use the glossary

This glossary catalogs more than 700 prescription and over-the-counter drugs that are available in the US. The listings give (1) the generic name of the drug (brand names of drugs are not included) and, in most cases, (2) the drug group to which the drug belongs (set in italics) and/or (3) a brief explanation of the drug or its primary uses (for drugs with several actions, only the most important use or uses are given). For more information on a drug or a drug group, refer to the comprehensive Index (pages 142 to 144). If your doctor has prescribed or you have purchased a brand-name product, you can determine the generic name of the drug by asking your doctor or pharmacist or by reading the package insert. The drug that you have been prescribed or have purchased may not be discussed elsewhere in this book. If the drug is not listed in the Index, you can look it up in this glossary to determine the drug group to which it belongs, and then use the Index to learn more about that group. Drugs that are still being tested for efficacy and safety and are not yet approved by the Food and Drug Administration are listed here as "investigational."

## A

**acebutolol** a *beta blocker* primarily used to treat high blood pressure and angina

**acecainide** an *antiarrhythmic* used to treat irregular heartbeat

**acetaminophen** a nonnarcotic *analgesic* (painkiller)

**acetazolamide** a weak *diuretic* used to treat glaucoma

**acetohexamide** a *sulfonylurea drug* used to treat diabetes mellitus

**acetophenazine** an *antipsychotic* used to treat acute psychosis

**acetylcysteine** a *mucolytic* (mucus thinner); also used as an antidote for acetaminophen poisoning

**acyclovir** an *antiviral* primarily used to treat herpesvirus and cytomegalovirus infections

**adenosine** an *antiarrhythmic* used to treat irregular heartbeat

**albuterol** a *bronchodilator* primarily used to treat asthma

**allopurinol** a drug used to prevent attacks of gout

**alprazolam** a *benzodiazepine* primarily used to treat panic disorders and anxiety

**alprostadil** a *prostaglandin* used to treat congenital heart disease and Raynaud's disease (disorder of the blood vessels)

**alteplase** a *thrombolytic* used to dissolve blood clots

**aluminum carbonate** a drug used to reduce phosphate levels in the blood; occasionally used as an *antacid*

**aluminum chloride** an antiperspirant

**aluminum hydroxide** an *antacid*

**amantadine** an *antiviral*; also used to treat parkinsonism

**ambenonium** a drug used to treat myasthenia gravis (muscle disorder)

**amcinonide** a topical *corticosteroid* used to treat skin disorders

**amikacin** an aminoglycoside *antibiotic*

**amiloride** a weak *diuretic* primarily used to treat high blood pressure

**aminocaproic acid** a drug used to prevent abnormal bleeding

**aminoglutethimide** an *anticancer drug*

**aminophylline** a *bronchodilator* used to treat narrowing of the airways in the lung

**amiodarone** an *antiarrhythmic* used to treat life-threatening irregular heartbeat

**amitriptyline** a tricyclic *antidepressant*

**amobarbital** a *barbiturate* primarily used as a *sedative*

**amoxapine** a tricyclic *antidepressant*

**amoxicillin** a penicillin *antibiotic*

**amphetamine** a central nervous system *stimulant* used to treat narcolepsy (sleep disorder) and attention deficit disorder

**amphotericin B** an *antifungal*

**ampicillin** a penicillin *antibiotic*

**amrinone** a drug used to treat heart failure

**anisindione** an *anticoagulant* used to prevent blood clots

**anistreplase** a *thrombolytic* primarily used to dissolve blood clots

**anthralin** a drug used to treat psoriasis (skin disease)

**antihemophilic factor** a substance used to promote clotting of blood in hemophiliacs

**apraclonidine hydrochloride** a drug used to treat glaucoma

**aprobarbital** a *barbiturate* used as a *sedative*

**aspirin** an NSAID *analgesic* used to treat pain, stiffness, and inflammation (especially arthritis)

**astemizole** a nonsedating *antihistamine* used to prevent symptoms of allergies

**atenolol** a *beta blocker* primarily used to treat angina, irregular heartbeat, heart attack, and high blood pressure

**atropine** an *anticholinergic antispasmodic* used to treat irregular heartbeat; also used as an antidote for some pesticide poisonings

**auranofin** an *antirheumatic* gold compound used to treat arthritis

**aurothioglucose** an *antirheumatic* gold compound used to treat arthritis

**azathioprine** an *immunosuppressant* used to treat immune disorders and prevent rejection of transplanted organs

**azlocillin** a penicillin *antibiotic*

**aztreonam** an *antibiotic*

## B

**bacampicillin** a penicillin *antibiotic*

**bacitracin** a topical *antibiotic*

**baclofen** a *muscle relaxant* primarily used in the treatment of spastic conditions that occur with multiple sclerosis (disorder of central nervous system) and dystonias (abnormal muscle rigidity)

**beclomethasone** a topical *corticosteroid* used to treat inflammation and allergic skin disorders

**belladonna** an *anticholinergic antispasmodic* primarily used to reduce cramping of the intestines

**bendroflumethiazide** a *diuretic* primarily used to treat high blood pressure

**benzalkonium chloride** a topical *antiseptic* (prevents infection)

**benzocaine** a topical *anesthetic* (causes loss of sensation)

**benzonatate** a *cough suppressant*

**benzoyl peroxide** a topical *antibacterial* used to treat acne

**benzquinamide** an *antiemetic* used to treat nausea and vomiting

**benztropine** an *anticholinergic* used to treat parkinsonism

**benzyl alcohol** a topical *anesthetic* (causes loss of sensation)

**benzyl benzoate** a topical drug used to treat scabies (skin infestation)

**betamethasone** a topical *corticosteroid* used to treat inflammation and allergic skin disorders

**betaxolol** a *beta blocker* used to treat glaucoma

**bethanechol** a drug used to treat retention of urine after an operation

**bichloracetic acid** a corrosive substance used topically for removal of warts, corns, and calluses

**biperiden** an *anticholinergic* used to treat parkinsonism

**bismuth** a *mucosal protector* primarily used in the treatment of peptic ulcers

**bitolterol** a *bronchodilator* used to treat asthma

**bleomycin** an *anticancer drug*

**botulinum A toxin** a substance used to treat spasmodic muscle disorders

**bretylium** an *antiarrhythmic* used to treat irregular heartbeat

**bromocriptine** a *dopamine-boosting drug* used to treat parkinsonism and to regulate ovarian function and breast milk secretion

**bromodiphenhydramine** an *antihistamine* primarily used in cold preparations

**brompheniramine** an *antihistamine* primarily used in cold preparations

**buclizine** an *antiemetic* used to treat nausea and vomiting

**bumetanide** a *diuretic* used to treat high blood pressure

**buprenorphine** a narcotic *analgesic* (painkiller)

**buspirone hydrochloride** a drug used to treat anxiety

**busulfan** an *anticancer drug*

**butabarbital** a *barbiturate* primarily used as a *sedative*

**butamben** a topical *anesthetic* (causes loss of sensation)

**butoconazole nitrate** an *antifungal* used to treat fungal infections of the vagina

**butorphanol** a narcotic *analgesic* (painkiller)

# C

**calamine** a lotion used to soothe irritated skin

**calcitonin** a *hormone drug* used to treat bone disorders

**cantharidin** a blistering agent used to remove warts

**capreomycin** an *antibacterial* used to treat tuberculosis

**captopril** an *ACE inhibitor* used to treat high blood pressure and congestive heart failure

**carbachol** a *miotic* used to treat glaucoma

**carbamazepine** an *anticonvulsant* used to treat epilepsy; also used to reduce pain in neuralgias

**carbamide peroxide** a topical drug used to soften earwax and as a mouthwash

**carbenicillin** a penicillin *antibiotic*

**carbidopa** a drug used to treat parkinsonism

**carbinoxamine** an *antihistamine* primarily used to treat allergies

**carboplatin** an *anticancer drug*

**carboprost** a *prostaglandin* used to stimulate contractions of the uterus

**carisoprodol** a *sedative* used to promote muscle relaxation

**carmustine** an *anticancer drug*

**carprofen** an NSAID *analgesic* used to treat pain, stiffness, and inflammation (especially arthritis)

**carteolol** a *beta blocker* used to treat high blood pressure

**cefaclor** a cephalosporin *antibiotic*

**cefadroxil** a cephalosporin *antibiotic*

**cefazolin** a cephalosporin *antibiotic*

**cefoxitin** a cephalosporin *antibiotic*

**cefuroxime** a cephalosporin *antibiotic*

**cephalexin** a cephalosporin *antibiotic*

**charcoal, activated** primarily used to absorb and inactivate poisons or as an antidote for drug overdoses

**chenodiol** a drug used to dissolve gallstones

**chloral hydrate** a *sedative* and *hypnotic* used to induce sleep

**chlorambucil** an *anticancer drug*

**chloramphenicol** an *antibiotic*

**chlordiazepoxide** a *benzodiazepine* primarily used to treat anxiety and symptoms of alcohol withdrawal

**chlorhexidine** a topical *antiseptic* (prevents infection)

**chlormezanone** a drug used to treat anxiety

**chloroquine** an *antimalarial*; also used to treat liver abscess that has developed from infection caused by a parasite

**chlorotrianisene** a *hormone drug* primarily used to treat cancer of the prostate gland

**chlorphenesin** a *sedative* primarily used to promote muscle relaxation

**chlorpheniramine** an *antihistamine* primarily used to treat allergies and cold symptoms

**chlorpromazine** an *antiemetic* used to treat nausea and vomiting; and an *antipsychotic* used to treat psychoses

**chlorpropamide** a *sulfonylurea drug* used to treat diabetes mellitus

**chlorprothixene** an *antipsychotic* used to treat acute psychosis

**chlortetracycline** a tetracycline *antibiotic*

**chlorthalidone** a *diuretic* primarily used to treat high blood pressure

**chlorzoxazone** a *sedative* primarily used to promote muscle relaxation

**cholestyramine** a *lipid-lowering drug* used to reduce levels of cholesterol in the blood

**choline salicylate** a nonnarcotic *analgesic* (painkiller)

**ciclopirox** an *antifungal*

**cilastatin/imipenem** a combination *antibiotic*

**cimetidine** an $H_2$ *blocker* primarily used to treat peptic ulcers

**cinnamates** a group of sunscreens

**cinoxacin** an *antibacterial* primarily used to treat urinary tract infections

**ciprofloxacin** an *antibacterial*

**cisplatin** an *anticancer drug*

**clavulanic acid** a drug used to inactivate bacterial enzymes that destroy some penicillin antibiotics

**clemastine** an *antihistamine* primarily used to treat allergies

**clidinium bromide** an *anticholinergic antispasmodic* primarily used to treat irritable bowel syndrome

**clindamycin** a lincosamide *antibiotic*

**clioquinol** a topical *antibacterial* and *antifungal*

**clobetasol** a topical *corticosteroid* used to treat inflammation and allergic skin disorders

**clocortolone** a topical *corticosteroid* used to treat inflammation and allergic skin disorders

**clofazimine** an *antibacterial* used in the treatment of leprosy

**clofibrate** a *lipid-lowering drug* used to reduce levels of fatty substances in the blood

**clomiphene** a drug used to treat infertility

**clomipramine** a tricyclic *antidepressant* used to treat obsessive-compulsive disorders

**clonazepam** an *anticonvulsant* primarily used to treat epilepsy

**clonidine** a *sympatholytic* primarily used to treat high blood pressure

**clorazepate** a *benzodiazepine* primarily used to treat anxiety and symptoms of alcohol withdrawal

**clotrimazole** an *antifungal*

**cloxacillin** a penicillin *antibiotic*

**clozapine** an *antipsychotic* primarily used to treat schizophrenia

**coal tar** a substance used topically to treat psoriasis (skin disease) and dandruff

**cocaine** a central nervous system *stimulant* and local anesthetic (causes loss of sensation)

**codeine** a narcotic *analgesic* (painkiller)

**colchicine** a drug used to treat and prevent attacks of gout

**colestipol** a *lipid-lowering drug* used to reduce levels of fatty substances in the blood

**colistin** an *antibiotic*

**corticotropin** a *hormone drug* used to stimulate the adrenal glands to produce more hydrocortisone

**cortisone** a *corticosteroid* used to treat inflammation

**cromolyn sodium** a drug used in the preventive treatment of asthma and hay fever

**crotamiton** a topical drug used to treat scabies (skin infestation) and itching

**cyclacillin** a penicillin *antibiotic*

**cyclizine** an *antiemetic* used to treat nausea and vomiting

**cyclobenzaprine** a *muscle relaxant* used to treat muscle spasms

**cyclophosphamide** an *anticancer drug*

**cycloserine** an *antibiotic* used to treat tuberculosis

**cyclosporine** an *immunosuppressant* primarily used to prevent rejection of transplanted organs

**cyclothiazide** a *diuretic* used to treat high blood pressure and edema

**cyproheptadine** an *antihistamine* primarily used to treat itching and hives

**cytarabine** an *anticancer drug*

# D

**dacarbazine** an *anticancer drug*

**dactinomycin** an *anticancer drug*

**danazol** a drug with hormone-like action used to treat endometriosis (fragments of the lining of the uterus present in the abdominal cavity) and cystic breast disease

**dantrolene** a *muscle relaxant* primarily used to treat muscle spasticity caused by stroke and malignant hyperthermia (life-threatening drug reactions with high fever and muscle spasms)

**dapsone** an *antibacterial* used to treat leprosy

**deferoxamine** a drug used to treat iron poisoning

**demecarium** a *miotic* used to treat glaucoma

**demeclocycline** a tetracycline *antibiotic*

**desipramine** a tricyclic *antidepressant*

**desmopressin** a drug used to prevent excess water loss from the kidney

**desonide** a topical *corticosteroid* used to treat inflammation and allergic skin disorders

**desoximetasone** a topical *corticosteroid* used to treat inflammation and allergic skin disorders

**dexamethasone** a *corticosteroid* used to treat inflammation

**dexbrompheniramine** an *antihistamine* used to treat symptoms of allergies

**dexchlorpheniramine** an *antihistamine* used to treat symptoms of allergies

**dextroamphetamine** a central nervous system *stimulant* primarily used to treat narcolepsy (sleep disorder) and attention deficit disorder

**dextromethorphan** a *cough suppressant*

**dextrothyroxine** a *lipid-lowering drug* used to reduce levels of fatty substances in the blood

**diazepam** a *benzodiazepine* primarily used to treat anxiety; also used as an *anticonvulsant*

**diazoxide** an *antihypertensive* used to treat high blood pressure; also used to treat hypoglycemia (low blood sugar level) and hyper-insulinemia (excessive secretion of insulin)

**dichlorphenamide** a weak *diuretic* primarily used to treat glaucoma

**diclofenac** an NSAID *analgesic* used to treat pain, stiffness, and inflammation (especially arthritis)

**dicloxacillin** a penicillin *antibiotic*

**dicumarol** an *anticoagulant* used to prevent blood clots

**dicyclomine** an *anticholinergic antispasmodic* used to treat irritable bowel syndrome

**dienestrol** a *hormone drug* primarily used to treat atrophic vaginitis (dry, irritated mucosal lining of the vagina)

**diethylpropion** a *stimulant* used to suppress appetite

**diethylstilbestrol** a *hormone drug* used to treat advanced prostate cancer and as a form of contraceptive

**diflorasone** a topical *corticosteroid* primarily used to treat inflammation and allergic skin disorders

**diflunisal** an NSAID *analgesic* used to treat pain, stiffness, and inflammation (especially arthritis)

**digitoxin** a *digitalis drug* primarily used to treat congestive heart failure and irregular heartbeat

**digoxin** a *digitalis drug* primarily used to treat congestive heart failure and irregular heartbeat

**dihydrocodeine** a narcotic *analgesic* primarily used as a cough suppressant

**dihydroergotamine** a drug used to treat migraine headache

**dihydroxyaluminum** an *antacid*

**diltiazem** a *calcium channel blocker* primarily used to treat angina and high blood pressure

**dimenhydrinate** an *antiemetic* used to treat nausea and vomiting

**dimercaprol** a drug used as an antidote for metal poisoning

**dimethicone** a water repellent used in barrier creams

**dinoprostone** a *prostaglandin* used to stimulate contractions of the uterus

**diphenhydramine** an *antihistamine* used to treat allergies and in cold preparations; an *antiemetic* used to treat nausea and vomiting; also used to treat insomnia

**dipivefrin** a *sympathomimetic* used to treat glaucoma

**dipyridamole** an *antiplatelet* used to prevent blood clots

**disopyramide** an *antiarrhythmic* used to treat irregular heartbeat

**disulfiram** an alcohol abuse deterrent

**dobutamine** a *sympathomimetic* used to treat severe heart failure

**dopamine** a naturally occurring neurotransmitter (chemical messenger) used to treat shock syndrome

**doxapram** a *stimulant* used to stimulate respiration after anesthesia or drug overdose

**doxepin** a tricyclic *antidepressant*

**doxorubicin** an *anticancer drug*

**doxycycline** a tetracycline *antibiotic*

**doxylamine** an *antihistamine* primarily used to induce sleep

**dronabinol** an *antiemetic* used to treat nausea and vomiting induced by anticancer drugs

**dyclonine** a topical *anesthetic* (causes loss of sensation)

**dyphylline** a *bronchodilator* used to treat narrowing of airways in the lungs

# E

**echothiophate** a drug used in the treatment of glaucoma

**econazole** an *antifungal*

**edetate calcium disodium** a drug used to treat lead poisoning

**edetate disodium** a drug used to reduce calcium levels in the blood

**emetine** an *antiprotozoal*

**enalapril** an *ACE inhibitor* used to treat high blood pressure and heart failure

**encainide** an *antiarrhythmic* used to treat life-threatening irregular heartbeat

**ephedrine** a drug primarily used to treat asthma; also used as a *decongestant*

**epinephrine** a drug primarily used in emergency treatment of cardiac arrest, anaphylactic shock (life-threatening allergic reaction), and acute asthma attacks; also used to treat persons with glaucoma and cataracts

**epoetin alfa** a drug used to stimulate production of red blood cells in the treatment of anemia associated with chronic renal failure (inability of kidneys to filter waste products from blood)

**ergonovine** a drug used to stop bleeding after childbirth

**ergotamine** a drug used to treat migraine headache

**erythrityl** a *nitrate* used to treat angina

**erythromycin** an *antibiotic*

**esmolol** a *beta blocker* used to treat irregular heartbeat

**estradiol** a *hormone drug* used to treat estrogen deficiency in menopausal women and to treat some types of prostate and breast cancer

**estramustine** an *anticancer drug*

**estrogens, conjugated** used as hormone replacement therapy in postmenopausal women

**estrogens, esterified** *hormone drugs* used in hormone replacement therapy

**estrone** a *hormone drug* used to treat symptoms of menopause, underactivity of ovaries or testes, and prostate cancer

**estropipate** a *hormone drug* used to treat symptoms of underactivity of ovaries

**ethacrynate sodium** a *diuretic* used to treat edema

**ethacrynic acid** a *diuretic* used to treat edema

**ethambutol** an *antibacterial* used to treat tuberculosis

**ethchlorvynol** a *sedative* used to induce sleep

**ethinamate** a *sedative* used to induce sleep

**ethinyl estradiol** a *hormone drug* (estrogen) used in oral contraceptives

**ethionamide** an *antibacterial* used to treat tuberculosis and leprosy

**ethopropazine** a drug used to treat parkinsonism

**ethosuximide** an *anticonvulsant* primarily used to treat epilepsy

**ethotoin** an *anticonvulsant* used to treat epilepsy

**etidronate** a drug used to treat Paget's disease (bone formation disorder) and osteoporosis (decreased bone density)

**etoposide** an *anticancer drug*

**etretinate** a vitamin A derivative used to treat psoriasis (skin disorder)

# F

**famotidine** an $H_2$ *blocker* used to treat peptic ulcers

**fenfluramine** a *stimulant* used to suppress appetite

**fenoprofen** an NSAID *analgesic* used to treat pain, stiffness, and inflammation (especially arthritis)

**ferrous sulfate** a mineral used to treat iron deficiency anemia

**flecainide** an *antiarrhythmic* used to treat life-threatening irregular heartbeat

**floxuridine** an *anticancer drug*

**fluconazole** an *antifungal*

**flucytosine** an *antifungal*

**fludarabine** an *anticancer drug*

**fludrocortisone** a *corticosteroid* used in the treatment of Addison's disease (underactive adrenal glands)

**flunisolide** a *corticosteroid* primarily used to treat asthma and hay fever

**fluocinolone** a topical *corticosteroid* used to treat inflammation and allergic skin disorders

**fluocinonide** a topical *corticosteroid* used to treat inflammation and allergic skin disorders

**fluorometholone** a topical *corticosteroid* used to treat eye disorders

**fluorouracil** an *anticancer drug*

**fluoxetine** an *antidepressant*

**fluoxymesterone** a *hormone drug* used for underactive testes and delayed puberty in men

**fluphenazine** an *antipsychotic* used to treat mental disorders

**flurandrenolide** a topical *corticosteroid* used to treat inflammation and allergic skin disorders

**flurazepam** a *benzodiazepine* primarily used to induce sleep

**flurbiprofen** an NSAID *analgesic* used to treat pain, stiffness, and inflammation (especially arthritis)

**flutamide** a *hormone drug* used to treat prostate cancer

**furosemide** a *diuretic* used to treat high blood pressure and edema

# G

**gemfibrozil** a *lipid-lowering drug* used to reduce levels of fatty substances in the blood

**gentamicin** an aminoglycoside *antibiotic*

**gentian violet** an *antiseptic* skin preparation

**glipizide** a *sulfonylurea drug* used to treat diabetes mellitus

**glucagon** a *hormone drug* used in emergency treatment of very low blood sugar levels in people with diabetes mellitus

**glutethimide** a *sedative* used to induce sleep

**glycerin** ingredient in cough mixtures, skin preparations, laxative suppositories, and earwax softening drops

**gold sodium thiomalate** an *antirheumatic* gold compound used in the treatment of arthritis

**gonadotropin, human chorionic** a *hormone drug* used to treat infertility

**goserelin acetate** a *hormone drug* used to treat prostate cancer

**gramicidin** an *antibiotic* used topically to treat eye infections

**griseofulvin** an *antifungal*

**growth hormone** a *hormone drug* used to treat short stature in children due to a disorder of the pituitary gland

**guanabenz** a *sympatholytic* used to treat high blood pressure

**guanadrel** a *sympatholytic* used to treat high blood pressure

**guanethidine** a *sympatholytic* used to treat high blood pressure

**guanfacine** a *sympatholytic* used to treat high blood pressure

# H

**halazepam** a *benzodiazepine* used to treat anxiety

**halcinonide** a topical *corticosteroid* used to treat inflammation and allergic skin disorders

**haloperidol** an *antipsychotic* used to treat agitated dementia; also used to treat Tourette's syndrome (disorder of body movement)

**haloprogin** a topical *antifungal*

**heparin** an *anticoagulant* used to prevent blood clots

**hydralazine** a *vasodilator* used to treat high blood pressure

**hydrochlorothiazide** a *diuretic* used to treat high blood pressure and edema

**hydrocodone** a narcotic *cough suppressant*

**hydrocortisone** a *hormone drug* used to treat Addison's disease (underactive adrenal glands) and to treat inflammation

**hydroflumethiazide** a *diuretic* used to treat high blood pressure and edema

**hydromorphone** a narcotic *analgesic* (painkiller)

**hydroquinone** a topical drug used to bleach the skin in people with pigmentation disorders

**hydroxychloroquine** an *antimalarial*; an *antirheumatic* used to treat arthritis

**hydroxyprogesterone** a *hormone drug* used to treat a variety of menstrual disorders

**hydroxyurea** an *anticancer drug*

**hydroxyzine** an *antihistamine* used to treat allergic skin conditions; also used as a *sedative* to induce sleep and occasionally to treat anxiety

**hyoscyamine** an *anticholinergic antispasmodic* used to treat irritable bowel syndrome

# I

**ibuprofen** an NSAID *analgesic* used to treat pain, stiffness, and inflammation (especially arthritis)

**idoxuridine** an *antiviral* used topically to treat herpes simplex infections of the eye

**ifosfamide** an *anticancer drug*

**imipenem/cilastatin** a combination *antibiotic*

**imipramine** a tricyclic *antidepressant*; also used in treatment of bed-wetting in children

**indapamide** a *diuretic* used to treat high blood pressure and edema

**indomethacin** an NSAID *analgesic* used to treat pain, stiffness, and inflammation (especially arthritis)

**insulin** a *hormone drug* used to treat diabetes

**interferon** an *antiviral* and *anticancer drug*

**interleukin-2** a protein (alters the immune response) and an *anticancer drug*

**iodoquinol** an *antiprotozoal*

**ipecac** a drug used to induce vomiting in cases of drug poisoning

**ipratropium** a *bronchodilator* primarily used to treat narrowing of airways of the lungs

**isocarboxazid** an MAO inhibitor *antidepressant*

**isoetharine** a *bronchodilator* primarily used as an inhalant to treat narrowing of airways of the lungs

**isoflurophate** a *miotic* used to treat glaucoma

**isoniazid** an *antibacterial* used to treat tuberculosis

**isopropyl alcohol** a topical *antiseptic* (prevents infection)

**isoproterenol** a *bronchodilator* primarily used to treat irregular heartbeat and narrowing of airways of the lungs

**isosorbide dinitrate** a *nitrate* used to treat angina

**isotretinoin** a derivative of vitamin A used topically to treat severe acne

**isoxsuprine** a *vasodilator* primarily used to increase circulation to the brain and limbs

# K

**kanamycin** an aminoglycoside *antibiotic*

**kaolin** an adsorbent substance and an ingredient of some antidiarrheal drugs

**ketoconazole** an *antifungal*

**ketoprofen** an NSAID *analgesic* used to treat pain, stiffness, and inflammation (especially arthritis)

**ketorolac** an NSAID *analgesic* used to treat pain, stiffness, and inflammation (especially arthritis)

# L

**labetalol** a *beta blocker* used to treat high blood pressure

**lactulose** a *laxative*; also used to treat dementia caused by cirrhosis

**lanolin** a preparation used in the treatment of dry skin

**leucovorin** a substance used to counteract adverse effects of some anticancer drugs

**leuprolide** a *hormone drug* used to treat prostate cancer

**levamisole** an *anticancer drug* and *anthelmintic*

**levobunolol** a *beta blocker* used to treat glaucoma

**levodopa** a drug used to treat parkinsonism

**levorphanol** a narcotic *analgesic* (painkiller)

**levothyroxine** a *hormone drug* used to treat hypothyroidism (underactivity of the thyroid gland)

**lidocaine** a local anesthetic and *antiarrhythmic* used to treat irregular heartbeat

**lincomycin** an *antibiotic*

**lindane** a topical drug used to treat scabies and lice infestations

**liothyronine** a *hormone drug* used to treat hypothyroidism (underactivity of thyroid gland)

**liotrix** a *hormone drug* used to treat hypothyroidism (underactivity of thyroid gland)

**lisinopril** an *ACE inhibitor* used to treat high blood pressure and heart failure

**lithium** a drug used to treat the manic phase of manic-depressive illness

**lomustine** an *anticancer drug*

**loperamide** an *antidiarrheal*

**lorazepam** a *benzodiazepine* used to treat anxiety and insomnia

**lovastatin** a *lipid-lowering drug* used to reduce the level of cholesterol in the blood

**loxapine** an *antipsychotic* used to treat mental disorders

**lypressin** a *hormone drug* used as an antidiuretic

# M

**mafenide** an *antibacterial* used topically to treat serious burns

**magnesium hydroxide** an *antacid* and a *laxative*

**magnesium oxide** an *antacid*

**magnesium salicylate** used as an *anti-inflammatory drug* to treat arthritis

**magnesium sulfate** an *anticonvulsant* primarily used to treat or prevent convulsions associated with some conditions in pregnancy; also used as a *laxative*

**mannitol** a *diuretic* used to treat glaucoma and swelling of the brain

**maprotiline** a tetracyclic *antidepressant*

**mazindol** a *stimulant* used to suppress appetite

**mebendazole** an *anthelmintic* primarily used to treat worm infestations

**mecamylamine** a *sympatholytic* used to treat severe high blood pressure

**mechlorethamine** an *anticancer drug*

**meclizine** an *antiemetic* used to treat nausea and vomiting

**meclocycline** a tetracycline *antibiotic* used topically to treat acne

**meclofenamate** an NSAID *analgesic* used to treat pain, stiffness, and inflammation (especially arthritis)

**medroxyprogesterone** a *hormone drug* used to treat a variety of menstrual disorders and in the treatment of cancers of the kidney and endometrium (lining of the uterus); also used as a long-acting contraceptive

**medrysone** a topical *corticosteroid* used to treat inflammatory conditions of the eye

**mefenamic acid** an NSAID *analgesic* used to treat pain, stiffness, and inflammation (especially arthritis)

**mefloquine** an *antimalarial*

**megestrol** a *hormone drug* used to treat cancers of the breast and endometrium (lining of the uterus)

**melphalan** an *anticancer drug*

**menotropins** a *hormone drug* used to treat infertility

**meperidine** a narcotic *analgesic* (painkiller)

**mephenytoin** an *anticonvulsant* used to treat epilepsy

**mephobarbital** a *barbiturate* used as a *sedative* and to control epileptic seizures

**meprobamate** a *sedative* used to treat anxiety

**mercaptopurine** an *anticancer drug*

**mesalamine** an aspirin derivative used to treat ulcerative colitis (inflammation and ulceration of lining of colon and rectum)

**mesoridazine** an *antipsychotic* used to treat mental disorders

**metaproterenol** a *bronchodilator* used to treat narrowing of airways of the lungs

**metaraminol** a *sympathomimetic* used to treat shock

**methacycline** a tetracycline *antibiotic*

**methadone** a narcotic *analgesic* used to treat heroin addiction and withdrawal symptoms

**methamphetamine** a central nervous system *stimulant* used to treat attention deficit disorder and to suppress appetite

**metharbital** a *barbiturate* used to treat epilepsy

**methazolamide** a weak *diuretic* used to treat glaucoma

**methdilazine** an *antihistamine* primarily used to treat allergies

**methenamine** an *antibacterial* used to treat urinary tract infections

**methicillin** a penicillin *antibiotic*

**methimazole** a drug used to treat hyperthyroidism (overactivity of the thyroid )

**methocarbamol** a *muscle relaxant*

**methotrexate** an *anticancer drug*; also used to treat psoriasis (skin disease) and arthritis

**methoxsalen** a drug used to treat psoriasis (skin disease) and vitiligo (disorder of skin pigmentation)

**methsuximide** an *anticonvulsant* used in the treatment of epilepsy

**methylcellulose** a bulk-forming *laxative*

**methyldopa** a *sympatholytic* primarily used to treat high blood pressure and Raynaud's disease (disorder of the blood vessels)

**methylene blue** used as an antidote for cyanide poisoning

**methylergonovine** a drug used to stimulate contractions of the uterus during labor

**methylformamide** an *anticancer drug*

**methylphenidate** a central nervous system *stimulant* primarily used to treat narcolepsy (sleep disorder) and sometimes used to treat attention deficit disorder

**methylprednisolone** a *corticosteroid* used to treat inflammation

**methyltestosterone** a *hormone drug* used to treat hypogonadism (underactivity of the testes) and impotence caused by hypogonadism

**methyprylon** a *sedative* used to induce sleep

**methysergide** a drug used to prevent migraine headache

**metoclopramide** a drug used to stimulate stomach emptying into the small intestine; also used as an *antiemetic* to treat nausea and vomiting associated with chemotherapy

**metolazone** a weak *diuretic* used to treat glaucoma

**metoprolol** a *beta blocker* primarily used to treat angina, heart attack, and high blood pressure

**metronidazole** an *antibacterial* and an *antiprotozoal*

**metyrosine** a *sympatholytic* primarily used to treat pheochromocytoma (tumor causing excess secretion of the hormones epinephrine and norepinephrine)

**mexiletine** an *antiarrhythmic* used to treat irregular heartbeat

**mezlocillin** a penicillin *antibiotic*

**miconazole** an *antifungal*

**mineral oil** a petroleum derivative used as a *laxative* and a skin softener

**minoxidil** an *antihypertensive*; also used to stimulate hair growth

**misoprostol** a *prostaglandin analogue* used to prevent NSAID–induced ulcers

**mitomycin** an *anticancer drug*

**mitotane** an *anticancer drug*

**mitoxantrone** an *anticancer drug*

**molindone** an *antipsychotic* used to treat acute psychosis

**mometasone furoate** a topical *corticosteroid* used to treat inflammation and allergic skin disorders

**monobenzone** a depigmenting agent used to treat severe vitiligo (disorder of skin pigmentation)

**moricizine** an *antiarrhythmic* used to treat life-threatening irregular heartbeat

**morphine** a narcotic *analgesic* (painkiller)

**moxalactam** a cephalosporin *antibiotic*

**muromonab CD3** an *immunosuppressant* used to prevent rejection of transplanted kidney

# N

**nabilone** an *antiemetic* used to treat nausea and vomiting

**nadolol** a *beta blocker* primarily used to treat angina and high blood pressure

**nafcillin** a penicillin *antibiotic*

**naftifine** an *antifungal*

**nalbuphine** a narcotic *analgesic* (painkiller)

**nalidixic acid** an *antibacterial* used to treat urinary tract infections

**naloxone** used as an antidote for narcotic drug poisoning

**naltrexone** a drug used to treat narcotic drug addiction

**nandrolone** an *anabolic steroid* used to treat some types of anemias

**naphazoline** a *decongestant*

**naproxen** an NSAID *analgesic* used to treat pain, stiffness, and inflammation (especially arthritis)

**natamycin** an *antifungal*

**neomycin** an aminoglycoside *antibiotic*

**neostigmine** a drug used to treat myasthenia gravis (muscle disorder)

**netilmicin** an aminoglycoside *antibiotic*

**niacin** a *lipid-lowering drug* used to reduce the level of fatty substances in the blood

**niacinamide** a *lipid-lowering drug* used to reduce the level of fatty substances in the blood

**nicardipine** a *calcium channel blocker* primarily used to treat high blood pressure and angina

**niclosamide** an *anthelmintic* used to treat worm infestations

**nifedipine** a *calcium channel blocker* primarily used to treat angina; in the sustained-release form used to treat high blood pressure

**nifurtimox** an *antiprotozoal*

**nimodipine** a *calcium channel blocker* used to treat spasm after bleeding from an aneurysm (ballooning of an artery) in the brain, and for migraine headache; also used investigationally in the treatment of stroke

**nitrofurantoin** an *antibacterial* used to treat urinary tract infections

**nitrofurazone** an *antibacterial* used topically in the treatment of burns

**nitroglycerin** a *nitrate* used to relieve pain caused by angina and congestive heart failure

**nizatidine** an *H₂ blocker* used to treat peptic ulcers

**nonoxynol 9** a spermicide used as a contraceptive

**norepinephrine** a *neurotransmitter* (chemical messenger produced in the body) and hormone used to treat shock

**norethindrone** a *hormone drug* used in oral contraceptives

**norfloxacin** an *antibacterial* used to treat urinary tract infections

**norgestrel** a *hormone drug* used in oral contraceptives

**nortriptyline** a tricyclic *antidepressant*

**nystatin** an *antifungal*

# O

**octoxynol** a spermicide used as a contraceptive

**octreotide acetate** a derivative of a *hormone drug* used to treat the diarrhea associated with some types of tumors

**olsalazine** a drug used to treat inflammatory bowel disease

**omeprazole** a *proton pump inhibitor* used to treat peptic ulcers

**oxacillin** a penicillin *antibiotic*

**oxazepam** a *benzodiazepine* primarily used to treat anxiety and insomnia

**oxiconazole nitrate** an *antifungal*

**oxtriphylline** a *bronchodilator* primarily used to treat asthma

**oxybutynin** an *anticholinergic antispasmodic* used to treat urinary incontinence (involuntary urination)

**oxycodone** a narcotic *analgesic* (painkiller)

**oxymetazoline** a *decongestant*

**oxymetholone** an *anabolic steroid* used to treat some types of anemia

**oxymorphone** a narcotic *analgesic* (painkiller)

**oxyphencyclimine** an *anticholinergic antispasmodic* used to treat peptic ulcers

**oxytetracycline** a tetracycline *antibiotic*

**oxytocin** a *hormone drug* used to induce labor and to control bleeding after childbirth

# P

**pancreatin** a preparation containing pancreatic enzymes, used in pancreatic deficiency

**pancrelipase** a preparation containing pancreatic enzymes, used in pancreatic deficiency

**papaverine** a *vasodilator* primarily used to treat circulatory problems

**para-aminobenzoic acid** a *sunscreen*

**paramethadione** an *anticonvulsant* used to treat epilepsy

**paramethasone** a *corticosteroid* used to treat inflammatory or allergic conditions

**paregoric** a narcotic *antidiarrheal*

**paromomycin** an aminoglycoside *antibiotic*; an *anthelmintic* used to treat worm infestation; an *antiprotozoal*

**pemoline** a central nervous system *stimulant* sometimes used to treat attention deficit disorders

**penbutolol** a *beta blocker* used to treat high blood pressure

**penicillamine** an *antirheumatic* used to treat rheumatoid arthritis; also used to treat metal poisoning and a form of cirrhosis

**penicillin G** a penicillin *antibiotic*

**penicillin G benzathine** a penicillin *antibiotic*

**penicillin V** a penicillin *antibiotic*

**pentaerythritol tetranitrate** a *vasodilator* used to treat angina

**pentamidine** an *antiprotozoal* used to treat pneumonia caused by the organism *Pneumocystis carinii*

**pentazocine** a narcotic *analgesic* (painkiller)

**pentobarbital** a *barbiturate* used to treat insomnia

**pergolide** a *dopamine-boosting drug* used to treat parkinsonism and to regulate ovarian function and breast milk secretion

**permethrin** a drug used to treat head-lice infestation

**perphenazine** an *antipsychotic* used to treat mental disorders; an *antiemetic* used to treat nausea and vomiting

**petrolatum** a petroleum derivative used to soften skin

**phenazopyridine** an *analgesic* used to treat pain caused by urinary tract infection

**phendimetrazine** a central nervous system *stimulant* used to suppress the appetite

**phenelzine** an MAO inhibitor *antidepressant*

**phenindamine** an *antihistamine* primarily used to treat allergies

**phenobarbital** a *barbiturate* used to treat epilepsy and anxiety

**phenoxybenzamine** a *sympatholytic* used to treat pheochromocytoma (tumor causing excess secretion of hormones that stimulate heart rate and blood pressure)

**phentermine** a *stimulant* used to suppress appetite

**phentolamine** a *sympatholytic* used to treat pheochromocytoma (tumor causing excess secretion of hormones that stimulate heart rate and blood pressure)

**phenylbutazone** an NSAID *analgesic* used to treat pain, stiffness, and inflammation (especially arthritis)

**phenylephrine** a *decongestant*

**phenylpropanolamine** a *decongestant*; also used to suppress appetite

**phenytoin** an *anticonvulsant* used to treat epilepsy

**physostigmine** a *miotic* used to treat glaucoma

**pilocarpine** a *miotic* used to treat glaucoma

**pindolol** a *beta blocker* used to treat high blood pressure

**piperacillin** a penicillin *antibiotic*

**piperazine** an *anthelmintic* used to treat worm infestations

**pirbuterol acetate** a *bronchodilator* used to treat narrowing of airways of the lungs

**piroxicam** an NSAID *analgesic* used to treat pain, stiffness, and inflammation (especially arthritis)

**plicamycin** an *anticancer drug*; also used to treat high levels of calcium in the blood

**podophyllin** a topical drug used to treat genital warts

**polycarbophil** a bulk-forming *laxative*

**polymyxin B** an *antibacterial* used to treat skin infections

**polythiazide** a *diuretic* used to treat high blood pressure

**potassium iodide** an *expectorant* (promotes coughing up of mucus); also used to treat hyperthyroidism (overactivity of the thyroid gland)

**povidine-iodine** a topical *antiseptic* (prevents infection)

**pralidoxime** an antidote to poisoning by some pesticides

**pramoxine** a topical *anesthetic* (causes loss of sensation)

**prazepam** a *benzodiazepine* primarily used to treat anxiety

**praziquantel** an *anthelmintic* used to treat worm infestation

**prazosin** a *sympatholytic* used to treat high blood pressure

**prednisolone** a *corticosteroid* used to treat inflammation and symptoms of a variety of disorders (including skin disorders and eye irritations and ulceration of the colon)

**prednisone** a *corticosteroid* primarily used to treat inflammatory bowel disease and rheumatoid arthritis (inflammatory disorders)

**primaquine** an *antimalarial*

**probenecid** a drug used to reduce uric acid levels that occur with gout; also used to enhance levels of penicillin and cephalosporin antibiotics

**probucol** a *lipid-lowering drug* used to reduce the level of fatty substances in the blood

**procainamide** an *antiarrhythmic* used to treat irregular heartbeat

**procarbazine** an *anticancer drug*

**prochlorperazine** an *antiemetic* used to treat nausea and vomiting; an *antipsychotic* used to treat mental disorders

**procyclidine** an *anticholinergic* used to treat parkinsonism

**promazine** an *antipsychotic* used to treat psychoses

**promethazine** an *antihistamine* primarily used to treat allergy; an *antiemetic* used to treat nausea and vomiting

**propafenone** an *antiarrhythmic* used to treat irregular heartbeat

**propantheline** an *anticholinergic antispasmodic* used to treat peptic ulcers

**propoxyphene** a narcotic *analgesic* (painkiller)

**propranolol** a *beta blocker* used to treat angina, heart attack, and high blood pressure; used to prevent migraine headache

**propylhexedrine** a *decongestant*

**propylthiouracil** a drug used to treat hyperthyroidism (overactive thyroid gland)

**protriptyline** a tricyclic *antidepressant*

**pseudoephedrine** a *decongestant*

**psyllium** a bulk-forming *laxative*

**pyrantel** an *anthelmintic* used to treat worm infestations

**pyrazinamide** an *antibacterial* used to treat tuberculosis

**pyrethrins** a drug used to treat lice infestation

**pyridostigmine** a drug used to treat myasthenia gravis (muscle disorder)

**pyrilamine** an *antihistamine* primarily used to treat allergies

**pyrimethamine** an *antimalarial* (combined with sulfadoxine)

# Q

**quazepam** a *benzodiazepine* used to treat insomnia

**quinacrine** an *antiprotozoal* used to treat giardiasis

**quinestrol** a *hormone drug* used to treat symptoms of the menopause

**quinethazone** a *diuretic* primarily used to treat high blood pressure

**quinidine** an *antiarrhythmic* used to treat irregular heartbeat

**quinine** an *antimalarial*; also used to treat nighttime cramping of the legs

# R

**ranitidine** an $H_2$ *blocker* used to treat peptic ulcers

**ribavirin** an *antiviral* used to treat viral infections of the respiratory tract in high-risk infants

**rifampin** an *antibacterial* used to treat tuberculosis

**ritodrine** a drug used to prevent uterine contractions that could result in premature labor

# S

**salicylic acid** a drug used to treat acne, warts, and other skin disorders

**salsalate** an NSAID *analgesic* used to treat pain, stiffness, and inflammation (especially arthritis)

**scopolamine** an *anticholinergic antispasmodic* used to prevent motion sickness

**secobarbital** a *barbiturate* primarily used to induce sleep

**selegiline** a drug used to treat parkinsonism

**selenium sulfide** an agent included in dandruff shampoos

**semustine** an *anticancer drug*

**silver nitrate** a chemical used topically to prevent gonorrheal eye infections in newborns; also used to cauterize tissue

**silver sulfadiazine** an *antibacterial* used to treat burns

**sodium bicarbonate** an *antacid*

**sodium iodide** a drug used to treat hypothyroidism (underactive thryroid gland) and some cancers of the thyroid gland

**sodium nitroprusside** a *vasodilator* used to treat high blood pressure in emergencies

**sodium salicylate** an NSAID *analgesic* used to treat pain, stiffness, and inflammation (especially arthritis)

**sodium thiosulfate** an *antidote* for cyanide poisoning

**spectinomycin** an *antibiotic* used to treat penicillin-resistant gonorrhea

**spironolactone** a *diuretic* used to treat overproduction of the hormone aldosterone and in combination with a thiazide diuretic to treat high blood pressure or edema

**stanozolol** an *anabolic steroid* used to reduce the frequency and severity of angioedema (an allergic reaction)

**stibocaptate** an *anthelmintic* used to treat worm infestations

**stibogluconate** an *antiprotozoal*

**streptokinase** a *thrombolytic* used to dissolve blood clots

**streptomycin** an *antibiotic*

**streptozocin** an *anticancer drug*

**sucralfate** a *mucosal protector* used to treat peptic ulcers

**sulconazole nitrate** an *antifungal* primarily used to treat superficial skin infections

**sulfacetamide** an *antibacterial* used to treat vaginal infections and superficial eye infections

**sulfadiazine** an *antibacterial*

**sulfadoxine** an *antimalarial* (combined with pyrimethamine)

**sulfamethizole** an *antibacterial*

**sulfamethoxazole** an *antibacterial* used to treat urinary tract infections

**sulfamethoxazole/ trimethoprim** an *antibacterial* commonly used to treat urinary tract infections

**sulfasalazine** an *anti-inflammatory drug* used in the treatment of inflammatory bowel disease

**sulfinpyrazone** a drug that promotes urinary excretion of uric acid to prevent gout attacks

**sulfisoxazole** an *antibacterial* used to treat eye infections

**sulindac** an NSAID *analgesic* used to treat pain, stiffness, and inflammation (especially arthritis)

**suramin** an *antiprotozoal* used to treat sleeping sickness

# T

**tamoxifen** an *anticancer drug*

**temazepam** a *benzodiazepine* used to treat anxiety

**terazosin** a *sympatholytic* used to treat high blood pressure

**terbutaline** a *bronchodilator* used to treat narrowing of airways in the lungs

**terconazole** an *antifungal*

**terfenadine** a nonsedating *antihistamine* primarily used to treat seasonal respiratory allergies

**testolactone** an *anticancer drug*

**testosterone** a *hormone drug* used to promote male sexual characteristics when testicular function is deficient or absent

**tetracaine** a local and topical *anesthetic* (causes loss of sensation)

**tetracycline** a tetracycline *antibiotic*

**theophylline** a *bronchodilator* used to treat narrowing of airways in the lungs

**thiethylperazine** an *antiemetic* used to treat nausea and vomiting

**thioguanine** an *anticancer drug*

**thioridazine** an *antipsychotic* primarily used to treat schizophrenia

**thiotepa** an *anticancer drug*

**thiothixene** an *antipsychotic* used to treat psychoses

**ticarcillin** a penicillin *antibiotic*

**ticlopidine** an investigational *antiplatelet* being tested in the treatment of stroke

**timolol** a *beta blocker* used to treat heart attacks and high blood pressure; also used to treat glaucoma

**tobramycin** an aminoglycoside *antibiotic*

**tocainide** an *antiarrhythmic* used to treat life-threatening irregular heartbeat

**tolazamide** a *sulfonylurea drug* used to treat diabetes mellitus

**tolbutamide** a *sulfonylurea drug* used to treat diabetes mellitus

**tolmetin** an NSAID *analgesic* used to treat pain, stiffness, and inflammation (especially arthritis)

**tolnaftate** an *antifungal*

**trazodone** an *antidepressant*

**tretinoin** a derivative of vitamin A used to treat acne

**triacetin** an *antifungal*

**triamcinolone** a *corticosteroid* used to treat inflammatory disorders

**triamterene** a *diuretic* primarily used in combination with a thiazide diuretic to treat high blood pressure and edema

**triazolam** a *benzodiazepine* primarily used to treat anxiety

**trichlormethiazide** a *diuretic* used to treat high blood pressure and edema and to prevent some types of kidney stones

**trientine** a drug that removes excess copper in the treatment of Wilson's disease

**trifluoperazine** an *antipsychotic* used to treat mental disorders

**triflupromazine** an *antipsychotic* used to treat mental disorders; an *antiemetic* used to treat nausea and vomiting

**trifluridine** an *antiviral* used to treat herpesvirus infections of the eye

**trihexyphenidyl** an *anticholinergic* used to treat parkinsonism

**trilostane** a drug used in the treatment of Cushing's syndrome (overactivity of the adrenal glands)

**trimeprazine** an *antihistamine* used to treat itching

**trimethadione** an *anticonvulsant* used to treat epilepsy

**trimethaphan** a *sympatholytic* used to reduce blood pressure in emergencies

**trimethobenzamide** an *antiemetic* used to treat nausea and vomiting

**trimethoprim** an *antibacterial* used to treat urinary tract infections

**trimipramine** a tricyclic *antidepressant*

**trioxsalen** a drug used to treat vitiligo (disorder of skin pigmentation)

**tripelennamine** an *antihistamine* primarily used to treat seasonal allergies

**triprolidine** an *antihistamine* primarily used to treat seasonal allergies

**tropicamide** a *mydriatic* used to dilate the pupil

**trypsin** a naturally occurring enzyme used to treat indigestion

# U

**urea** a natural substance included in remedies for dry skin

**urofollitropin** a *hormone drug* used to induce ovulation (to treat infertility)

**urokinase** a *thrombolytic* used to dissolve blood clots

**ursodiol** a drug used to dissolve gallstones

# V

**valproic acid** an *anticonvulsant* primarily used to treat epilepsy

**vancomycin** an *antibiotic*

**vasopressin** a *hormone drug* used to treat diabetes insipidus

**verapamil** a *calcium channel blocker* used to treat angina, irregular heartbeat, and high blood pressure; also used to prevent migraine headache

**vidarabine** an *antiviral* used to treat herpesvirus infections

**vinblastine** an *anticancer drug*

**vincristine** an *anticancer drug*

**vindesine** an *anticancer drug*

# W

**warfarin** an *anticoagulant* primarily used to prevent blood clots

**witch hazel** a soothing *astringent*

# X

**xylometazoline** a *decongestant*

# Z

**zidovudine** an *antiviral* used in the treatment of AIDS

**zinc oxide** a soothing agent used in skin preparations and sunscreens

**zinc sulfate** an *astringent*

# INDEX

Page numbers in *italics* refer to illustrations and captions. See also the DRUG GLOSSARY on pages 134 to 141.

drug interactions 23, 36-37, 48, 52, 55, 58
   case history 59
drug overdoses  see overdoses
drugs
   absorption and metabolism of 36-37, 42-43
   abuse of 25, 26-27, 68
   actions of 30-37
   administration of 38-41, 43
   advertising of 20
   alternatives to 18
   breast-feeding and 47, 55, 66
   costs of 9, 18, 20
   design and development of 16-17, 19-20
   disposal of 62-63
   distribution of, in body 42, 43
   excretion of 42, 43
   history of 10-17
   labeling of 25, 28, 36, 51, 61
   monitoring treatment with 56-57
   naming of 28
   nonmedicinal use of 24, 26-27
   poisoning by 132-133
   pregnancy and 32, 47, 55, 64-65
   questions to ask about 52, 55
   tailor-made 14-15
   targeting of 39
   safety in use of 49, 122
   side effects of 32-35, 54-59
   storage of 60-61, 63
   trials and testing of 15, 19, 21
drug tolerance 68, 69
   case history 45
drug withdrawal 69-70, 83, 89
   case history 71
dyskinesia 35

**E**

ear disorders, drugs for 103, 117, *126*
ear drops 41, *126*
edema 11, 35
Ehrlich, Paul 13
elixirs 10, 40
emollients *118*, *127*
emulsions 40
enemas *125*
enzyme blockers *31*
epilepsy, drugs for *79*, 81
   case history 80
epinephrine 73, 109
ergonovine 13
ergotamine 13, 82
ergot drugs 13
erythropoietin 16
estrogen 108, 110-111
   side effects of 35
expectorants 95, 123
eye disorders, drugs for 103, 116-117, *126*
eye drops 41, *116*, *126*
   disposal of 63
   in medical travel kit 73

**F**

factor VIII 16, 31
FDA (Food and Drug Administration) 121
   drug approval by 19, 20, *126*
   drug classification and monitoring by 24-25, 122
   drug labeling and 25, 28
   generic drugs and 29
   orphan drugs and 21
fetus, drug effects on 32, 64-65
first-pass effect 43
flatulence, drugs for 124
fluconazole 107

fluoride *126*, 128, 131
fluoxetine 82
folic acid 130
Food and Drug Administration  see FDA
foods, drug interactions with 36, *36*, 52, 55, 58
FSH (follicle-stimulating hormone) 110-111
fungicidal drugs 72, 107, 116, *118*, 127

**G**

G6PD (glucose-6-phosphate dehydrogenase) deficiency *44*
GABA (gamma-aminobutyric acid) 78, 79, 81
gallstones 86
gastric acid secretion *85*
gastroenteritis 84
generic drugs 28-29, 121
genetic engineering 16-17
Gerhardt, Charles 12
glaucoma, drugs for 116
glycerin suppositories 87, *125*
goiter, ancient remedy for 10
gold compounds 99
   side effects of 57
gout, drugs for 101
growth disorders, drugs for *109*
growth hormone 16, *109*
gynecomastia 35

**H**

H₂ (histamine) blockers 15, *85*
haloperidol, side effects of 35
hay fever 96
headache 34
heart and circulation, drugs for 88-93
hemorrhoids, drugs for 86, *127*
hepatitis B vaccine 16
heroin 25, *27*, 70
herpesvirus infections 105, 117
hirsutism 35
histamine 15, 96, 97
histamine (H₂) blockers 15, *85*
hives 34
hormone disorders, drugs for 31, 108-109
hormone drugs 31, 108-111
   for cancer 113
   side effects of 35, 110
hydrocortisone *118*, *127*
hyperlipidemia, drugs for 90
hypertension
   case history 93
   drugs for 89, 90, 91
   monitoring treatment of 56
hypnotics 81
hypoglycemic drugs 58

**I**

ibuprofen 65, 123
   side effects of 84
immunization 14
immunosuppressants 87, 99
implants *39*, 110
indigestion remedies  see antacids
infections, drugs for 102-107, 116-117
infestations, drugs for 106-107
inflammation, drugs for 98-101, 116, 117
inflammatory bowel disease 87
inhalers and inhalations 38, 41, *94-95*, 96
injections, types of *38*
insect repellants 73
insulin 16, 31, 108

interactions of drugs  see drug interactions
interferons 16, 113, 115
interleukin-2 16
intestinal disorders, drugs for 86-87
iodine 10, 65, 128, 131
ipecac 48, 133
iron 36, 37, 58, 128, 131
isosorbide dinitrate 45
isotretinoin 119
   pregnancy and 65, 67
   treatment with, case history 67

**J**

Jenner, Edward 11, 14

**L**

lactation disorders, drugs for *109*
laxatives 73, 87, 125
levodopa 83
LH (luteinizing hormone) 110-111
lice, drugs for 107
Lind, James 11
lindane 107
liniments 40
lipid-lowering drugs 31, 90
lithium 65, 77, 81
liver, drug breakdown in 43
lobeline 124
loop diuretics 90
loperamide 72, 86, 125
lotions 40
lovastatin 90
LSD (lysergic acid diethylamide) 25, *27*

**M**

magnesium 128, 131
malaria, drugs for 10, *44*, 73, 106
male pill 111
manic-depressive illness 77
MAO (monoamine oxidase) inhibitor antidepressants 79, 81, 82
   drug interactions of *36*, 37, 58
marijuana 25, *26*, 70
mast cell stabilizers 95
mebendazole 107
medical travel kit 72-73
medication organizers 50, 60
medicine cabinet 61
mefloquine 106
meperidine 37, 58, 100
mercury drugs 11
methotrexate 99, 113, *118*
methylcellulose 86, 125
methylphenidate 27, 82
metoclopramide 78, 82
metronidazole 37, 103, 106
migraine, drugs for 27, 82
minerals 31, 37, 128, 131
minipill (progestin-only pill) *49*, 110, 111
minipump *39*
minoxidil, side effects of 35
miotics 116
misoprostol *84*
mixtures 40
moisturizers 127
monoamine oxidase inhibitors  see MAO inhibitor antidepressants
monoclonal antibodies 39, *39*
morphine 11, 25, *27*, 100, *101*
   dependence on 69
   side effects of 34
   withdrawal from 69, 70
motion-sickness remedies 72, 82
mouth-to-mouth resuscitation 132
mouthwashes *126*

mucolytics 95, 123
mucosal protectors *84*
mupirocin 118
muscle relaxants 99
mydriatics 117

**N**

naloxone 37
narcotic analgesics 24, 25, 100, *101*
   drug interactions of 58
   side effects of 34, 55
narcotic antidiarrheals 86
nausea 34, *78*, *115*
   drugs for 78, 82, 124-125
nebulizers 95
needles 62, 73
nervous system, drugs and 76-83
neuroleptics 77
neurotransmitters 31, *36*, 77, 78, 79
   epilepsy and 81
   gastric acid secretion and 85
   Parkinson's disease and 83
niacin 129
nicotine 25, 27
   dependence on *68*
   withdrawal from 70
   see also smoking
nitrates 45, 88
nitroglycerin 43, 63
   side effects of 34
   treatment with, case history 45
nonnarcotic analgesics 100, 101
nonprescription drugs 121-127
   interactions with prescription drugs 48, 55, 58
nonsteroidal anti-inflammatory drugs  see NSAIDs
norepinephrine 30, 78, 79, 109
   beta blockers and 14, 77, 89
NSAIDs (nonsteroidal anti-inflammatory drugs) 26, 98-99, 100, 101
   drug interactions of 58
   pregnancy and 65
   side effects of 55, 84, 101

**O**

ointments 40
omeprazole *85*
opioids *101*
opium 10, 11
oral contraceptives 29, *51*, 110-111
   drug interactions of 58
   pregnancy and 65
   side effects of 33, 35
oral rehydration preparations 72, 125
orphan drugs 21
osmotic agents 116
osteoarthritis, NSAIDs and 98
osteoporosis 108
   corticosteroids and 34
OTC (over-the-counter) medications 23, 25, 121-131
   interactions with prescription drugs 36, 48, 55, 58
overdoses
   avoiding accidental 49
   case history 59
   emergency treatment for 48, 132-133

**P**

pain 69, *100*
painkillers  see analgesics
pantothenic acid 129
para-aminobenzoic acid *103*, *127*, 130
Paracelsus, Philippus 10-11
parallel track drug treatment 20

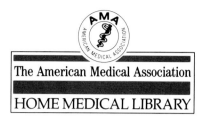

The American Medical Association

HOME MEDICAL LIBRARY

# A HEALTHY DIGESTION

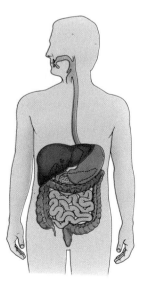

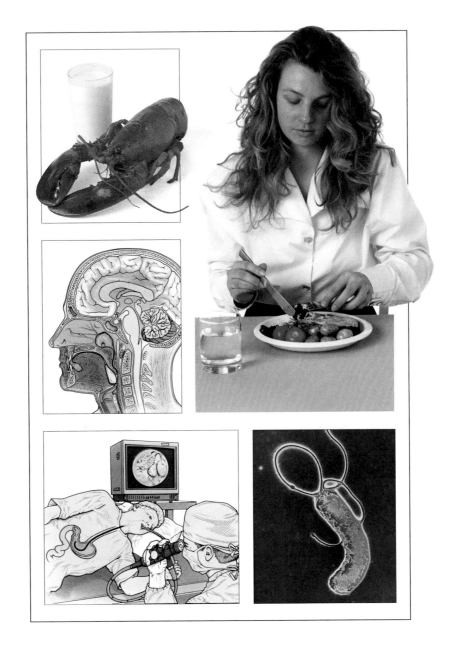

# FOREWORD

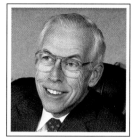

Good digestion is vitally important to your sense of well-being and the quality of your life. That's why it is so important to encourage a healthy digestion by eating a variety of nutritious foods. However, to get the maximum benefit from the foods you eat, your digestive system must break them down and then absorb their nutrients. Any malfunction of the digestive system affects its ability to perform these tasks efficiently.

Digestive disorders are common. They range from minor problems, such as indigestion and constipation, to serious, life-threatening emergencies, such as intestinal obstruction. Many disorders respond to improvements in diet. For example, eating more high-fiber foods, such as whole grains and fruits and vegetables, can help relieve constipation. A high-fiber diet can actually reduce your risk of such serious disorders as diverticulitis. Doctors suspect that even cancers of the digestive system can be prevented by a healthy diet.

Your life-style can also have many serious, long-term effects on your digestive system. Smokers have a higher incidence of peptic ulcers, Crohn's disease, and cancer of the esophagus than do nonsmokers. Stress can bring on digestive tract symptoms and can worsen any digestive system disorders you already have. Modifying such life-style factors now can help prevent digestive system problems in the future.

To maintain the health of your digestive system throughout your life, you need to understand how it works and what you can do to keep it working properly. You also need to know what can go wrong. This volume of the American Medical Association Home Medical Library presents the facts and explains how you can preserve one of your most precious assets – a healthy digestion.

*James S. Todd MD*

**JAMES S. TODD, MD**
Executive Vice President
American Medical Association

# CONTENTS

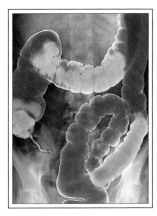

# CHAPTER ONE

# NOURISHMENT FOR LIFE

ALL LIVING ORGANISMS need water, raw materials, and energy to grow and reproduce. Plants obtain their raw materials from soil and water and their energy from sunlight. Animals and humans must fulfill their nutritional needs by eating plant and/or animal material. Most types of food enter your mouth in large pieces that must be broken down. The smaller pieces, consisting of simple molecules, can then more easily be absorbed by and distributed throughout your body. Your cells use these molecules of food to produce energy and materials essential for survival. This process of breaking down food into a usable form is called digestion.

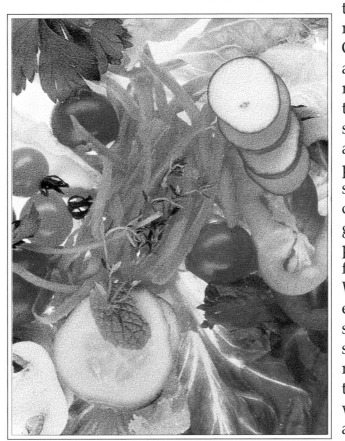

The human digestive system can accommodate many different types of diets. Throughout the world, people depend on very dissimilar types of diets to supply the nutrients and energy they need. In Asia, the diet consists predominantly of rice. Eskimos living near the polar ice cap consume mainly fish and seal meat. The Masai tribe of East Africa has traditionally subsisted on the meat and blood of cattle. These diets may not seem completely balanced, but the digestive system can adapt to them all. By adding foods such as vegetables and fruits to the staple items, these diets can become balanced.

That means they can be modified so they contain enough, but not too much, of all the essential nutrients, including vitamins, minerals, proteins, carbohydrates, and fats. Your digestive system can continue working even when damaged by injury or disease or when weakened immediately after surgery. The digestive system can also tolerate a remarkable amount of stress and abuse. Many people eat irregular, hurried meals that often have low nutritional value. Our diets often lack adequate fiber and may contain potentially harmful substances, such as alcohol. Some people cannot tolerate strong spices, which can irritate the digestive tract. Other people eat spicy foods every day. While some of us eventually develop serious digestive system disorders, most of us go through our lives without developing any serious gastrointestinal disease.

The first section in this chapter compares the human digestive system to those of animals. The section about your dietary needs analyzes the components of what we eat and describes the variety of foods in which they are found. Finally, the section about appetite and hunger describes how different parts of your body interact to signal the need for food and explains individual differences in appetite and hunger.

# THE HUMAN DIGESTIVE SYSTEM

Digestion is the process by which your body converts food into energy and materials for growth and repair. Digestion is one of your body's most important biological processes, and the digestive system makes up about half of the body's total number of internal organs. The digestive system is able to reduce a wide range of complex plant and animal food sources to their basic chemical units. The body absorbs and stores these units and eventually uses them either as fuel or as building blocks for the repair, maintenance, and growth of body tissues. All higher animals have digestive systems that are similar to ours. This sophisticated system has evolved over millions of years to make the most efficient use possible of the food available. A healthy digestive system extracts the nutrients contained in food and eliminates waste from the body.

## FOOD SOURCES AND TYPES OF DIGESTION

People and higher animals need the same basic nutrients – proteins for growth, fats and carbohydrates for energy, essential minerals such as iron (the key ingredient of the red blood cell pig-

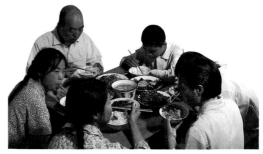

**Primitive diets**
*Humans have always been omnivores (plant and meat eaters). In primitive cultures, people ate fruits, nuts, berries, roots, grains, fish, and any meat they could obtain. Because much of their food was uncooked and often tough, the jaw muscles of primitive peoples were much stronger and their jaws much bigger than ours.*

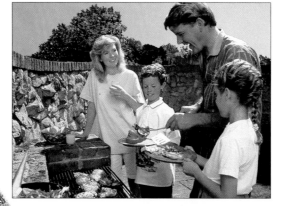

**Diverse eating habits**
*Different cultures have widely contrasting diets and methods of food preparation. But in most cultures, a meal is often a social occasion, shared with family or friends.*

**Human teeth**
*Like the mouths of all omni-*
*vores (plant and meat eaters),*
*the human mouth has several*
*different types of teeth, each*
*adapted for a different func-*
*tion. Sharp incisors are used*
*for cutting; pointed canines are*
*used for tearing; and flat,*
*ridged premolars and molars*
*are used for grinding, crush-*
*ing, and chewing.*

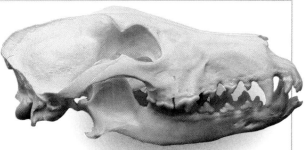

**Teeth of carnivores**
*Carnivores, such as dogs, have large canines (sharp,*
*pointed teeth) for tearing and chopping up meat*
*and powerful jaw muscles for crushing bones.*

Canines

Incisors

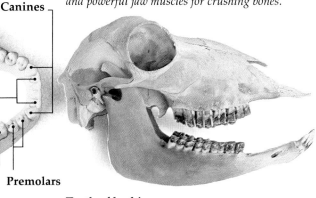

Premolars

Molars

**Teeth of herbivores**
*Herbivores, such as sheep, have small front teeth*
*for clipping through grass and large, flat molars*
*for grinding the grass into a form from which*
*nutrients can be absorbed and used.*

ment hemoglobin), and vitamins (chemical compounds that the body needs but cannot manufacture). The sources from which these nutrients are obtained can vary significantly depending on the way in which an animal has evolved. Humans and animals that have similar digestive systems, such as pigs, are omnivores – they are able to eat and digest a diet of both plant material and meat. An omnivorous diet offers maximum flexibility; if one type of food, such as meat, becomes scarce, the omnivore can switch to another, such as vegetables or fruit.

## Specialized digestive systems

Animals such as lions and tigers, which live on a diet of meat alone, are carnivores. They cannot digest most plant material. Herbivores, such as sheep and cows, can extract energy and nutrients only from plant sources. Herbivores cannot digest meat. Omnivores, carnivores, and herbivores can be distinguished by differences in their teeth, which are specialized in a variety of ways to allow the most efficient mechanical breakdown of their respective types of food.

LACTOSE INTOLERANCE
All infants are born with the enzyme needed to digest lactose (milk sugar). But 60 percent of the world's population lacks this enzyme in adulthood. Members of certain cultures, such as the Semite, Asian, African, Eskimo, and American Indian cultures, lose the enzyme after being weaned from breast milk. The enzyme remains in population groups descended from cultures that continued to consume dairy products in adulthood.

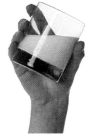

**Symptoms of lactose intolerance**
*Many African and Indian adults cannot tolerate*
*lactose. If they drink milk, they may experience*
*excess gas formation, cramping pains, and*
*sometimes diarrhea. By contrast, most Northern*
*Europeans, as well as people in certain African*
*tribes, have no trouble digesting milk – only*
*10 percent are deficient in the needed enzyme.*

# TYPES OF DIGESTIVE SYSTEMS

All animals – even the most simple ones – have some type of digestive system. All animals must break down their food into smaller units that can be used to produce energy or to synthesize essential materials. The structure of an animal's digestive system depends on the complexity of its diet and on its own complexity as a living organism.

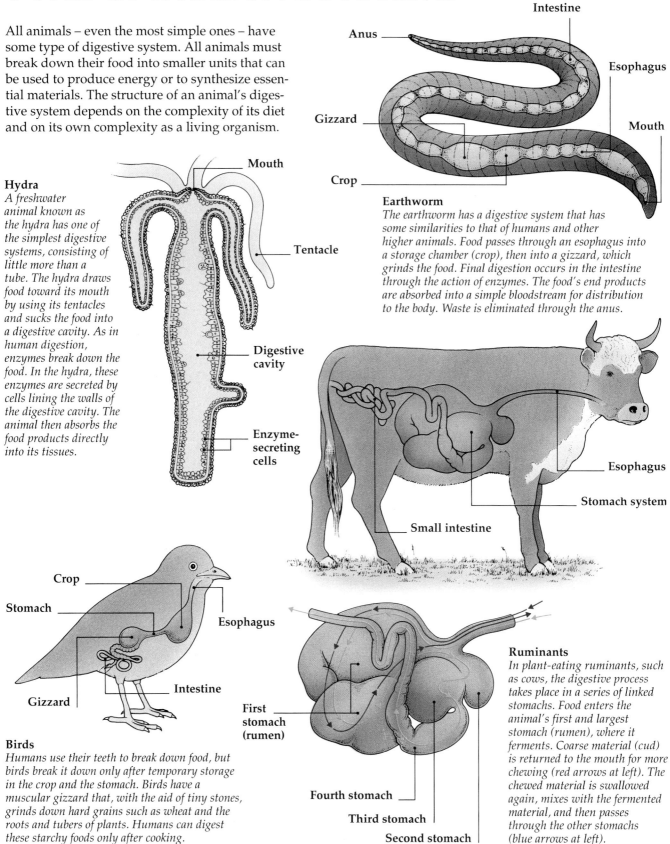

**Earthworm**
*The earthworm has a digestive system that has some similarities to that of humans and other higher animals. Food passes through an esophagus into a storage chamber (crop), then into a gizzard, which grinds the food. Final digestion occurs in the intestine through the action of enzymes. The food's end products are absorbed into a simple bloodstream for distribution to the body. Waste is eliminated through the anus.*

**Hydra**
*A freshwater animal known as the hydra has one of the simplest digestive systems, consisting of little more than a tube. The hydra draws food toward its mouth by using its tentacles and sucks the food into a digestive cavity. As in human digestion, enzymes break down the food. In the hydra, these enzymes are secreted by cells lining the walls of the digestive cavity. The animal then absorbs the food products directly into its tissues.*

**Ruminants**
*In plant-eating ruminants, such as cows, the digestive process takes place in a series of linked stomachs. Food enters the animal's first and largest stomach (rumen), where it ferments. Coarse material (cud) is returned to the mouth for more chewing (red arrows at left). The chewed material is swallowed again, mixes with the fermented material, and then passes through the other stomachs (blue arrows at left).*

**Birds**
*Humans use their teeth to break down food, but birds break it down only after temporary storage in the crop and the stomach. Birds have a muscular gizzard that, with the aid of tiny stones, grinds down hard grains such as wheat and the roots and tubers of plants. Humans can digest these starchy foods only after cooking.*

**Human digestion**
*The organs of the human digestive system –
the esophagus, stomach, pancreas, intestines,
liver, gallbladder, and anus – are common to
all advanced animals. Food enters the mouth
and is propelled through the digestive tract by
waves of muscular contraction. During the
digestive process, substances such as enzymes
(produced by the salivary glands, stomach,
pancreas, and small intestine), hydrochloric
acid (produced by the stomach), and bile salts
(produced by the liver) break down the food
into chemical components that the body can
use. Waste is eliminated through the anus.*

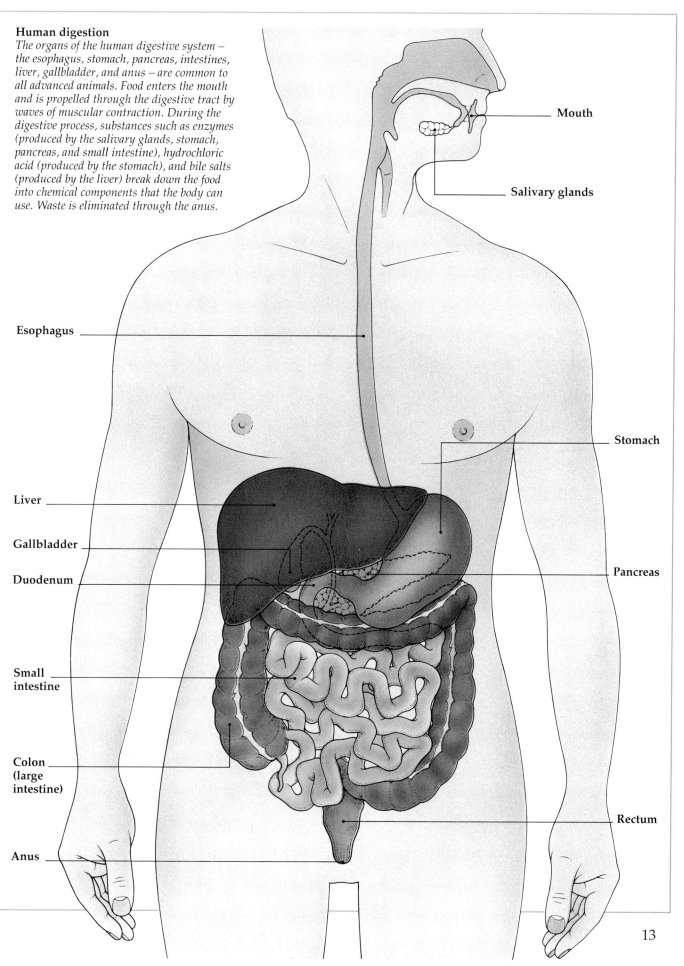

Mouth

Salivary glands

Esophagus

Stomach

Liver

Gallbladder

Pancreas

Duodenum

Small
intestine

Colon
(large
intestine)

Rectum

Anus

# YOUR NUTRITIONAL NEEDS

## VITAMIN SUPPLEMENTS

A person who eats a diet that includes ample protein sources, plenty of fresh fruit and vegetables, and whole grains should not become vitamin deficient. If you eat a balanced diet, vitamin supplements probably will not be beneficial. But vitamin supplements are sometimes necessary for:

◆ Pregnant or breast-feeding women, older people, and infants

◆ People with digestive disorders that impair vitamin and mineral absorption

◆ People whose diets lack a full range of nutrients, such as people living on very low incomes or alcoholics

◆ People taking certain medications, such as oral contraceptives, certain antibacterial drugs (sulfa drugs), or the antituberculosis drug isoniazid

◆ People on restricted-calorie diets

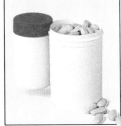

Our species has eaten the same wide variety of foods for millions of years, and our digestive system has become finely tuned to process these foods. Like animals, we need certain dietary components to stay alive and remain healthy. Along with nutrients and water, your diet should include foods that contain certain minerals and 23 additional chemical compounds. These compounds include nine essential amino acids (the basic building blocks for the composition of protein), one fatty acid (linoleic acid, essential for the composition of certain hormones), and 13 vitamins.

## MINERALS

Seventeen minerals are essential for optimal health. They include the major minerals calcium, phosphorus, magnesium, potassium, sodium, chlorine, and sulfur, which the body needs in large quantities, and the trace elements cobalt, chromium, copper, fluorine, iodine, iron, manganese, molybdenum, selenium, and zinc. A balanced diet will provide you with abundant amounts of most of these minerals. The only mineral deficiencies that are relatively common in the US are deficiencies of iron and calcium.

**Fad diets and vitamin deficiencies**
*Some weight-reducing diets that rely on a single food or food group have been advertised as quick ways to lose weight. Such faddish food regimens have included the grapefruit diet, the low-carbohydrate diet, and the liquid-protein diet. These diets can be unhealthy because they lack many essential vitamins, minerals, and other nutrients. The best way to lose weight and keep it off is to eat foods from all food groups and to exercise regularly.*

## VITAMINS

Vitamins are important for your body's internal metabolism. But your body can manufacture only a few of these vital chemicals. If your skin is exposed to adequate sunlight, your cells can make vitamin D. Vitamin K and biotin are produced in small amounts by intestinal bacteria. Your body can produce niacin from the amino acid tryptophan. Your body cannot manufacture vitamins A, C, E, or any of the B vitamins, other than niacin. These vitamins must be absorbed from the food you eat. People living in areas where exposure to sunlight is limited need extra dietary sources of vitamin D. A person also needs additional dietary sources of vitamin K if prolonged use of antibiotics lowers the number of intestinal bacteria that produce the vitamin.

# YOUR BODY'S NEED FOR WATER

Water is your body's most important nutrient. Without it, you could not survive for more than about 5 days. Water is also the most abundant substance in your body, representing about two thirds of body weight. In temperate climates, the minimum daily water requirement is about four 8-ounce glasses. Ideally, you should drink as many as eight 8-ounce glasses of water every day. You may need to drink even more water if you live in a hot climate, if you do heavy manual work, or if you exercise regularly.

## WATER CONTENT OF FOODS

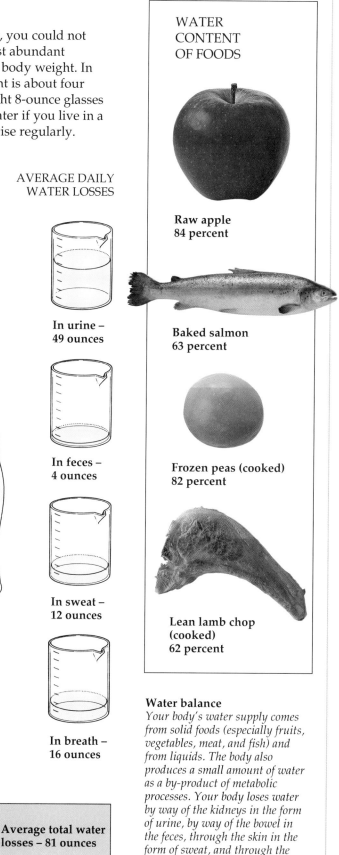

**Raw apple**
84 percent

**Baked salmon**
63 percent

**Frozen peas (cooked)**
82 percent

**Lean lamb chop (cooked)**
62 percent

AVERAGE DAILY
WATER INTAKE

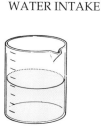

**From liquids –
42 ounces**

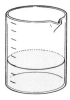

**From solid
foods –
30 ounces**

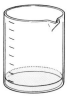

**From water produced
by metabolism –
9 ounces**

AVERAGE DAILY
WATER LOSSES

**In urine –
49 ounces**

**In feces –
4 ounces**

**In sweat –
12 ounces**

**In breath –
16 ounces**

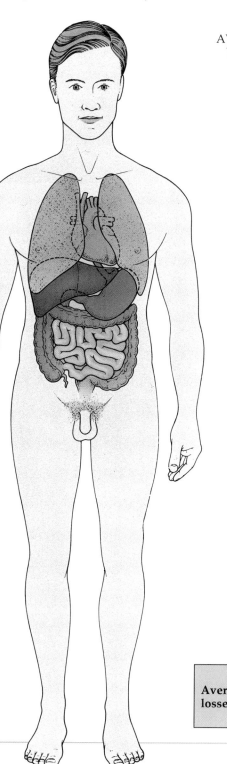

| Average total water intake – 81 ounces |
| --- |

| Average total water losses – 81 ounces |
| --- |

**Water balance**
*Your body's water supply comes from solid foods (especially fruits, vegetables, meat, and fish) and from liquids. The body also produces a small amount of water as a by-product of metabolic processes. Your body loses water by way of the kidneys in the form of urine, by way of the bowel in the feces, through the skin in the form of sweat, and through the lungs as vapor.*

# HOW IMPORTANT IS PROTEIN?

Protein deficiency is rare in the US, except in low-income groups (especially among children). Most people eat more protein than they need. Today, doctors are less concerned about the protein content of a person's diet than about the amount of fiber, vitamins, and minerals it provides. Studies have shown that vegetarians who eat dairy products and eggs are as healthy as people who eat lean meat. Meat is a good source of protein, and the iron in meat is better absorbed than the iron in vegetables. But meat can contain high amounts of cholesterol and saturated fats that have been linked to heart disease and cancer. So the protein content of a food, although important, is of less concern than the food's total nutritional value.

## HOW DOES YOUR BODY USE PROTEINS?

Your body constantly makes new proteins so it can grow and repair its tissues. Protein forms your muscles, blood, skin, organs, hair, and nails. Proteins are large, complex molecules formed from different combinations of 20 basic units called amino acids. Your body can make 11 of these acids from simple substances present in the body, but the other nine – called the essential amino acids – must be obtained from your diet.

**Protein in plants**
*Most staple carbohydrate sources (such as wheat, rice, beans, and nuts) contain protein. But proteins from plant sources provide only some of the essential amino acids. They are known as incomplete proteins. Amino acids that are deficient in one plant food are often present in another. So plant foods must be combined (as in the illustrations below) to provide the complete range of essential amino acids.*

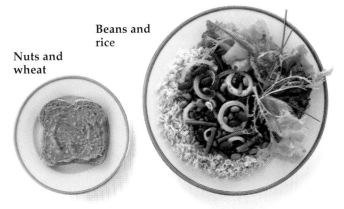

**Beans and rice**

**Nuts and wheat**

**Animal protein sources**
*Animal proteins, such as meat, fish, poultry, or dairy products, contain all nine essential amino acids. They are complete proteins. But meat, especially red meat, and high-fat dairy products, such as ice cream, also contain saturated fats and can raise your blood cholesterol level. Eat small quantities of lean meat, poultry, and fish, and low-fat dairy products, such as skimmed milk.*

**Poultry**

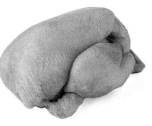

**Fish**

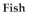

**Food protein breakdown**
*Proteins contained in food consist of long chains of amino acids. Your digestive tract breaks down these chains in stages into individual amino acids.*

**Food proteins**

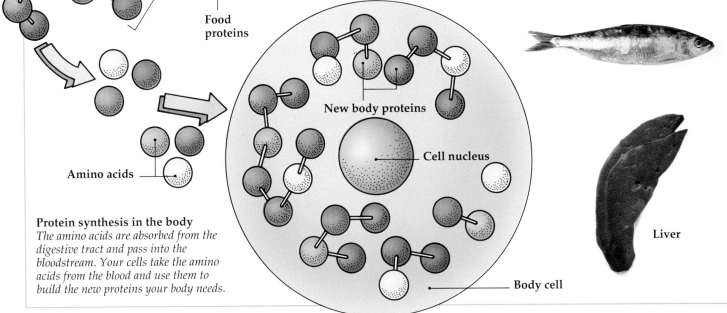

**New body proteins**

**Cell nucleus**

**Amino acids**

**Protein synthesis in the body**
*The amino acids are absorbed from the digestive tract and pass into the bloodstream. Your cells take the amino acids from the blood and use them to build the new proteins your body needs.*

**Body cell**

**Liver**

# WHERE DO WE GET PROTEIN?

## The Mediterranean diet
*People living in the Mediterranean region get their proteins from a wide range of sources, including fish, shellfish, poultry, veal, beef, and pork. This protein often accompanies carbohydrates, such as pasta, made from wheat. Olive oil is used in cooking in place of animal fats, so the Mediterranean diet contains less saturated fat (although as much total fat) than the American diet.*

**Marinara sauce** containing shrimp, tomatoes, and onions is a good source of protein and carbohydrates.

**Pasta** is an incomplete source of protein and must be eaten with another protein source, such as cheese, to provide all essential nutrients.

**Beef** is an excellent source of complete protein, but unless it is lean, it can contain high amounts of saturated fat and cholesterol.

## The American diet
*The American diet relies on a variety of protein sources, including beef, milk, poultry, fish, eggs, cheese, and beans. These protein sources are supplemented by carbohydrates, such as bread and potatoes, and by vegetables and fruits. Because some of these protein sources contain high amounts of saturated fat and cholesterol, many Americans are switching to leaner cuts of meat and low-fat dairy products.*

**Potatoes and vegetables** supply little protein but are excellent sources of energy, vitamins, and minerals.

**Shrimp, pork, chicken, and eggs** are all good sources of complete protein, although they can also be high in fat.

## The Asian diet
*The Asian diet contains a wide range of protein sources. Fish, shellfish, poultry, pork, and beef are all eaten in smaller quantities than in the American diet. Asians get most of their calories from carbohydrates, such as rice and noodles. They also eat large amounts of fresh vegetables, such as cabbage, spinach, green beans, and bean sprouts, and many of their meals are stir-fried. The fat content of the Asian diet is about half that of the American diet.*

**Rice** is an incomplete source of protein and must be combined with another protein source, such as beans, to provide all essential nutrients.

# ENERGY

Your total calorie requirement includes not only the calories you need to keep your body functioning at rest but also those you need for growth, repair, and physical activity. Carbohydrates and fats are your body's main sources of energy. When deprived of adequate carbohydrates and fats, your body can also break down proteins into glucose to produce energy. But carbohydrates are a better energy source when they are part of a balanced diet. You should try to obtain 55 to 60 percent of your total calorie intake from carbohydrates.

## Types of carbohydrates

The carbohydrates in foods fall into three categories: sugars, starches, and a group that includes cellulose (undigestible fiber). All sugars and starches are not equal nutritionally. Ordinary table sugar (sucrose), whether eaten as pure sugar or used as an additive in such foods as pastry or breakfast cereal, provides what nutritionists call "empty calories." Although table sugar contains many calories, it provides few of the nutrients your body needs. Most of your carbohydrate intake should be eaten in the form of complex carbohydrates including starches and cellulose. Whole-grain bread, potatoes, rice, whole-wheat pasta, dried peas and beans, fruits, and vegetables are all good sources of complex carbohydrates. Try to eat carbohydrates in unrefined forms, such as bread made from whole-wheat flour, rather than in refined forms, such as bread made from white flour.

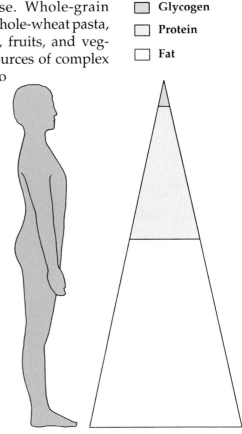

☐ Glycogen
☐ Protein
☐ Fat

**Your body's storage of energy**
*The body stores most excess energy as fat. An average-sized adult has almost 150,000 calories stored as fat, compared with 24,000 calories stored as protein and 300 calories stored as glycogen (the form in which glucose is stored in the body).*

## NUTRITIOUS CARBOHYDRATE SOURCES

Some carbohydrate sources are more "nutrient-dense" than others. This means that, calorie for calorie, they contain more essential nutrients than less nutrient-dense foods. Nutrient-dense foods include whole-grain breads and pasta, potatoes, oranges, and beans. Foods such as cakes and pies contain large amounts of fat and sugar but few nutrients.

## WARNING

The average American diet contains a high proportion of fat – much more than you need for good health. A high-fat diet contributes to obesity, a major risk factor for cardiovascular disease. Fats should constitute no more than 30 percent of your calorie intake. By contrast, a typical US diet supplies 38 percent of its calories in the form of fat. Most of the fat you eat should be unsaturated, such as that found in fish and vegetable oils.

# FIBER

Dietary fiber consists of the parts of plant foods that we cannot digest. Fiber is divided into two types – soluble and insoluble – based on its capacity to dissolve in water. Both types of fiber add bulk to feces and help them retain water, so they are larger, softer, and easier to expel. Fiber helps to prevent constipation and reduces the risk of hemorrhoids. Because soft, bulky feces pass through the intestines more quickly, the bowel lining is exposed to dietary waste toxins for a shorter period of time, which may reduce the risk of bowel cancer. A diet high in fiber also slows down the absorption of sugars from the intestine, resulting in lower blood sugar levels. Control of blood sugar levels is important for diabetics and may also be a way nondiabetics can sustain their energy levels.

SOURCES OF SOLUBLE FIBER

SOURCES OF INSOLUBLE FIBER

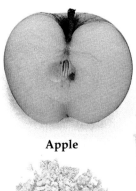

**Apple**

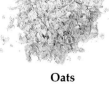

**Oats**

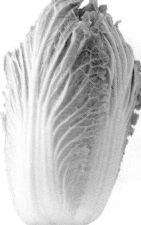

**Cabbage**

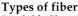

**Celery**

**Types of fiber**
*Insoluble fibers give shape and rigidity to the cell walls of plants (see right) – the stringy filaments in celery are an example. Soluble fiber is found in beans and in the saps and juices of plant foods. Soluble fiber seems to lower blood cholesterol levels, possibly by reducing the amounts of cholesterol absorbed into the bloodstream.*

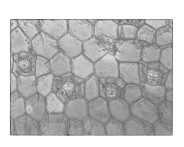

# ASK YOUR DOCTOR
## DIGESTIVE PROBLEMS

Q **My doctor says I have diverticular disease and need to eat more fiber. What is diverticular disease and how did I get it?**

A Diverticular disease is a disorder of the colon caused in part by chronic constipation. Straining to pass small, hard stools raises the pressure in the colon and causes small pouches in its lining to protrude through the outer muscles that surround it. These pouches, called diverticula, may become inflamed or may bleed. Eating more fiber will soften your feces and increase their bulk, so you don't have to strain so hard to pass them.

Q **I have been told to eat more fiber to relieve my constipation. But since I started eating high-bran cereal for breakfast, I have had a lot of gas. Is this normal?**

A Yes. Many people experience more gas when they first increase the amount of fiber they eat. To relieve this problem, add fiber to your diet gradually. Your intestines will eventually adjust to the extra fiber, and the amount of gas will decline in a few weeks.

Q **I have a sweet tooth. How bad are foods such as cake, chocolate, and candy for my health?**

A Sweets are not bad if you eat them infrequently. But these foods do not provide many of the nutrients you need. Their high sugar content contributes to tooth decay, obesity, and increased blood levels of a type of fat that the body uses to form cholesterol. A high consumption of sugar can actually be dangerous for diabetics or for people with hypoglycemia (low blood sugar).

# APPETITE AND HUNGER

Appetite is the pleasant anticipation you feel before eating a meal. Hunger is the less pleasant feeling you have when your body needs food. Appetite combines with hunger to ensure that you eat regularly. But you should eat the right amounts of a wide range of healthy foods. Most people's bodies have an efficient, built-in system that monitors the amount of food they eat. Some active people, such as athletes, can eat much more food than others before their bodies start to store energy as fat. These people burn more calories than less active people. Each individual achieves his or her own body's balance. Most adults stay within a range of weight that varies only slightly.

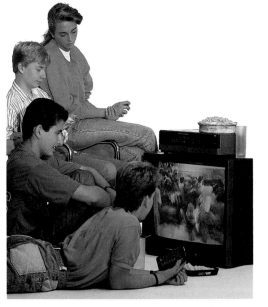

**Breakfast starts your day right**
*Whether or not you eat breakfast affects your appetite throughout the day. Research shows that people who start their day with breakfast consume fewer total calories during the day than do people who skip breakfast. Avoid high-fat breakfast foods, such as eggs, bacon, sausage, and butter. Instead, choose whole-grain breads and cereals, low-fat milk or yogurt, and fruit or fruit juice.*

**Exercise and appetite**
*When you are inactive for a long time you expend little energy but may feel hungry and nibble on snacks. But going for a long walk or a run can actually suppress your appetite and make you feel less hungry.*

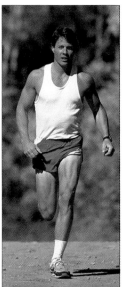

## PREVENTING OBESITY

Most people adjust their eating habits and many exercise more frequently if they begin to gain weight. For example, if you overeat while you are on vacation or during the holidays, you may compensate by eating a little less than usual until

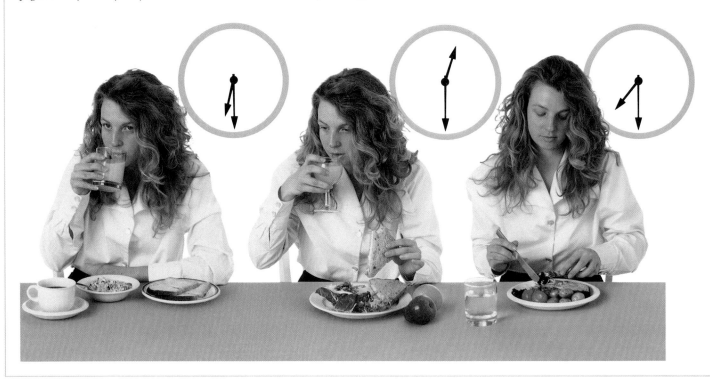

you return to your normal weight. Some people do not change their eating habits and become increasingly overweight if they do not work off the extra calories.

## Overweight children

The factors that contribute to obesity in childhood are complex. Obesity can be an inherited characteristic. For example, a child of overweight parents who is adopted by a family of normal weight is more likely to become an overweight adult than are the family's natural children. But learned behavior also plays a role. For example, if your family has a snack and a drink before going to bed each night, you will probably develop the habit of doing so yourself, even if you are not hungry. Most overweight children are members of overweight families. But overeating is only a part of the problem. One of the most important contributing factors to obesity – even in children – is inactivity. Regular, vigorous exercise can help a child expend the energy needed to offset his or her food intake. Parents should include their children in family activities that provide exercise, such as biking, walking, or sports. Obesity in childhood often leads to obesity in adulthood, which is a risk factor for cardiovascular disease.

## IMPROVING YOUR EATING HABITS

A person who develops eating habits during childhood that lead to excess weight will find it difficult to adjust his or her eating habits during adulthood. If you are overweight, exercise regularly and improve your eating habits so that you can balance the amount of food you eat with the amount your body needs. The following tips can help you:

◆ Eat regularly but eat more at breakfast and lunch than at dinner. Avoid large meals just before bedtime. This pattern of eating will distribute your calorie intake more evenly throughout the day.

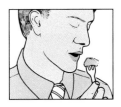

◆ If you have a weight problem and feel hungry between meals, snack on fruit and raw vegetables rather than on candy or potato chips, which have many calories but little nutritional value.

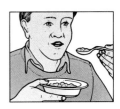

◆ Eat foods low in fat and sugar and high in fiber. Foods such as brown rice provide much of the energy your body needs and contain the fiber that helps your digestive system work efficiently.

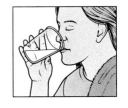

◆ Feeling thirsty? Refresh yourself with water, fruit juice, or skimmed milk rather than with soda pop. Skimmed milk contains essential vitamins and minerals but is not high in calories.

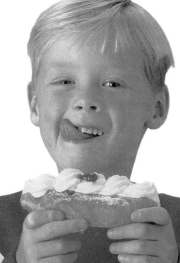

**Teaching healthy eating habits**
*Unhealthy eating habits develop early in life. Parents need to help their children learn healthy eating habits by providing an apple (right) rather than sweets (left) when their children ask for a snack.*

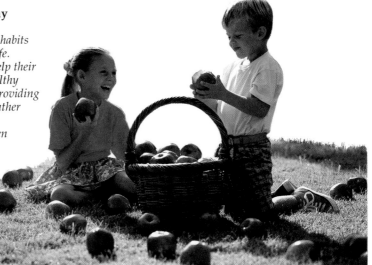

# MECHANISMS OF APPETITE AND HUNGER

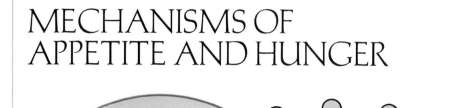

**Limbic system**

**Hypothalamus**

**Vagus nerve**

The control mechanisms for appetite and hunger are located in the part of your brain called the hypothalamus, which becomes stimulated when your blood sugar level is low. The hunger you feel before a meal is usually anticipatory hunger. For example, if you are accustomed to having a meal at noon, you may begin to feel hungry as that time approaches. If you are too busy to eat, these sensations wear off, and a few hours later you may not feel hungry at all. But by that evening, when your next mealtime approaches, you will probably feel very hungry. Appetite and hunger are often increased by certain sensory triggers, such as the sight of a set table or the sight and smell of food.

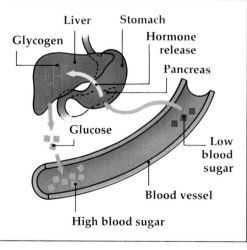

**Low blood sugar level**
*When your body needs food, the level of sugar in your blood falls. This low blood sugar level triggers the release of a hormone from the pancreas. This hormone acts on glycogen (stored sugar) in the liver and divides it into glucose molecules. These molecules pass back into the bloodstream to boost your blood sugar level temporarily, until more glucose is provided by food.*

Liver    Stomach

Glycogen

**Hormone release**

**Pancreas**

**Glucose**

**Low blood sugar**

**Blood vessel**

**High blood sugar**

**Sending the hunger message**
*When the hypothalamus is stimulated by a low blood sugar level, nerve impulses pass along the vagus nerve to the stomach.*

**Registering satisfaction of hunger**
*The brain's limbic system, which regulates automatic body functions and emotions, contains satiety centers that register the satisfaction of hunger. These centers turn off the sensations that signal the need for food. This action takes place long before the food and drink have been digested or absorbed.*

**How the stomach responds**
*In the stomach, nerve impulses trigger the release of digestive juices containing acid, enzymes such as pepsin, and hormones such as gastrin. All are important in the digestive process. These nerve impulses indirectly cause the muscular wall of the stomach to contract, provoking hunger pangs. At this stage, you may feel the growling that often accompanies hunger as air and fluid pass through the intestines. All of these physical triggers signal the need for food.*

Stomach

**Branches of vagus nerve**

**Feeling full**
*Fullness registers immediately in the brain. Physical triggers, such as stomach distention, also indicate satiety. This is why bulky foods with a low-calorie content fill you up quickly and help you lose weight more efficiently.*

## ASK YOUR DOCTOR
## APPETITE AND HUNGER

**Q** **I have heard about people on hunger strikes who have stayed alive for months. How long can people survive without eating?**

**A** If a person has access to water, he or she can stay alive until the body's energy stores are used up. Most energy is stored as fat. When fat stores have been used up, the body begins to use its own stored proteins, found mainly in muscle. Eventually, the heart muscle becomes damaged, leading to death. The length of time this process takes depends on the person's metabolic rate and on the amount of stored fat he or she had at the beginning of the fast.

**Q** **When I am very hungry before a meal, and I eat until I feel satisfied, my stomach becomes huge and feels hard and uncomfortable. Is this normal?**

**A** You may be eating too quickly and swallowing too much air as you eat. Even if you feel very hungry, slow down when eating your meal. You will enjoy your food much more and feel better afterward.

**Q** **I read in a magazine that people tend to crave foods containing elements that they lack. Is this theory true?**

**A** No, although craving sometimes occurs in people with iron deficiency anemia and in pregnant women. Some people have an appetite disorder called pica, in which they crave substances that have no nutritional value, such as dirt or clay. Pica, which can signal iron deficiency, can also lead some people to compulsively eat certain foods.

# CHAPTER TWO

# THE DIGESTION MACHINE

YOUR DIGESTIVE SYSTEM is a highly sophisticated "food factory" that converts the food you eat into valuable substances your cells can use as fuel, construction materials, or agents for biochemical processes. Food contains nutrients, such as complex carbohydrates, proteins, and fats, that your digestive system breaks down into smaller components so they can be absorbed more easily. These components include simple sugars (monosaccharides), protein elements (amino acids), and fatty acids. Vitamins, minerals, and water are absorbed without having to be broken down. These remarkable processes occur inside your digestive tract, which extends from the mouth, down the esophagus, through the stomach and intestines, to the anus. Enzymes secreted by the salivary glands in your mouth, glands in the lining of your stomach and intestines, and your pancreas all work together to transform food into energy for your body's use. The digestion of fats requires a special function that your liver performs. Fats cannot be digested unless a kind of emulsifying agent – a "detergent" – modifies them. This agent is bile, formed in the liver, stored and concentrated in the gallbladder, and released into the intestines when the stomach contents enter the intes-

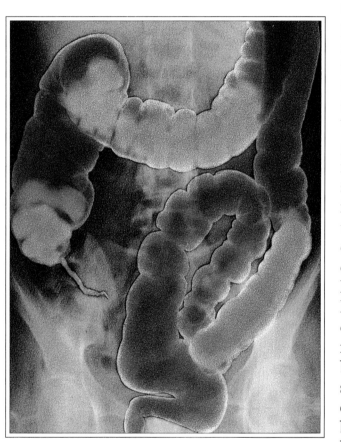

tines. Digested fats then pass into the lymphatic system, which transfers them to the bloodstream. Once digested, most nutrients are absorbed by the lining of your digestive tract. A massive network of blood and lymph vessels supplies the walls of the entire digestive tract. The bloodstream transports the nutrients to the liver for processing. Most of the blood drained from the intestines passes through the liver, which stores many nutrients and processes them even more. From the liver the blood carries nutrients to cells throughout the body. When you drink a glass of water, almost all of it is absorbed in the small intestine. By the time the waste products of the digestive process have reached the lower part of the colon and rectum, most of the water has been reabsorbed into the bloodstream. The solid residue is then evacuated from your body as feces.

Your digestive tract is a largely impenetrable passage through your body. It consists of a single tube that runs from your mouth to your anus that offers no access to the inside of your body except by absorption. Objects ingested accidentally can pass safely through the tract without entering your body. Millions of potentially harmful organisms can exist inside your digestive tract without posing a threat to your general health.

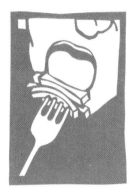

# THE MOUTH AND ESOPHAGUS

THE DIGESTIVE PROCESS begins as soon as you put food in your mouth. Your teeth grind the food and your tongue mixes it with saliva secreted by the salivary glands. Each lump of processed food, called a bolus, then travels down the esophagus, a muscular tube that links your mouth to your stomach.

Your teeth, tongue, and saliva work together to move food around your mouth, reducing it to a soft lump known as a bolus. Your tongue also has taste receptors that, along with smell receptors in the nose, enable you to appreciate food and detect contamination or spoilage.

## THE FUNCTION OF SALIVA

Saliva, a liquid produced by the salivary glands in your mouth, performs several different functions. As you chew, saliva helps form food into a bolus that your

## SALIVARY GLANDS

Your mouth contains three pairs of salivary glands: the parotid, submandibular, and sublingual glands. Numerous, small accessory salivary glands lie beneath the mucous membrane that lines your mouth.

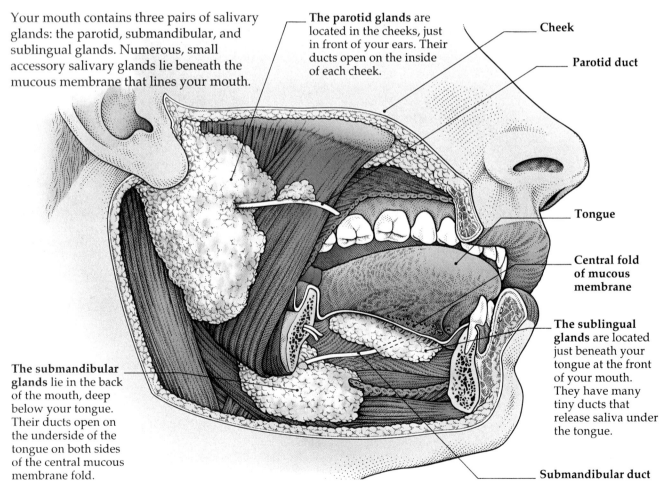

**The parotid glands** are located in the cheeks, just in front of your ears. Their ducts open on the inside of each cheek.

**Cheek**

**Parotid duct**

**Tongue**

**Central fold of mucous membrane**

**The sublingual glands** are located just beneath your tongue at the front of your mouth. They have many tiny ducts that release saliva under the tongue.

**The submandibular glands** lie in the back of the mouth, deep below your tongue. Their ducts open on the underside of the tongue on both sides of the central mucous membrane fold.

**Submandibular duct**

tongue can shift around your mouth for chewing on one side and then the other. Saliva also makes swallowing easier by lubricating both the bolus and the walls of the throat and esophagus. Saliva also dissolves certain molecular particles in food that stimulate the taste buds. Finally, saliva helps clean your mouth and teeth by washing away food debris.

The secretion of saliva by the salivary glands is a reflex action controlled by the autonomic nervous system. Salivation is usually stimulated by the presence of food in the mouth, but it can also occur at the sight, the smell, or even the thought of food. The salivary glands produce about 3 pints of saliva every day.

## Digestive action
Saliva contains a digestive enzyme called amylase, which breaks down starches into the sugar maltose. You can experience this process by holding a piece of bread or potato in your mouth. After a while you will notice a sweet flavor as the starch releases maltose.

## THE ESOPHAGUS

The esophagus is a muscular tube about 10 inches long that extends from the throat through the neck and chest, behind the windpipe (trachea), through the diaphragm, to the stomach. It serves as the passageway for the transfer of swallowed food and liquids from the mouth to the stomach. The upper 1 or 2 inches of the esophagus are usually completely closed. They open only when you swallow. The muscles at the back of your throat that you use to swallow are partially under voluntary control. But once food enters your esophagus, it is automatically propelled into your stomach by the muscles in the esophagus. The lower end of the esophagus, which opens when food approaches, is controlled by a muscle that prevents regurgitation of the stomach contents. The lowest part of the esophagus lies below the diaphragm.

## ATRESIA OF THE ESOPHAGUS

Atresia of the esophagus is a rare and severe birth defect present in about one baby in 3,500. A short segment of the esophagus fails to develop and the upper part ends in a closed-end pouch. The affected baby cannot swallow. Food is simply regurgitated back into the mouth. The upper or the lower segment of the esophagus (more commonly the lower one) may also be abnormally connected to the windpipe (trachea). Babies with a connection between the upper part of the esophagus and the trachea may suck milk into the trachea and lungs, causing severe coughing and breathing difficulties. Immediate surgery is necessary to save the child's life.

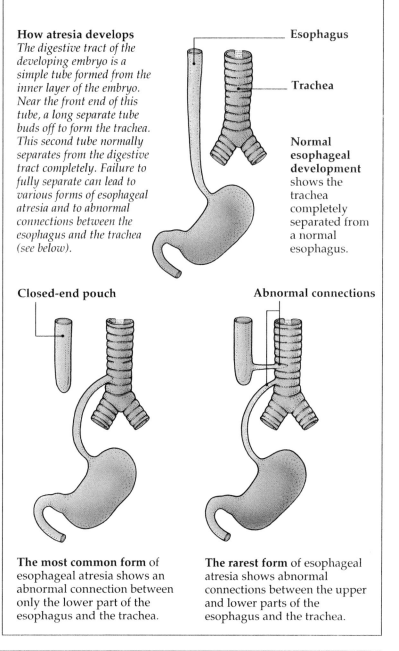

**How atresia develops**
*The digestive tract of the developing embryo is a simple tube formed from the inner layer of the embryo. Near the front end of this tube, a long separate tube buds off to form the trachea. This second tube normally separates from the digestive tract completely. Failure to fully separate can lead to various forms of esophageal atresia and to abnormal connections between the esophagus and the trachea (see below).*

Esophagus

Trachea

**Normal esophageal development** shows the trachea completely separated from a normal esophagus.

**Closed-end pouch**

**Abnormal connections**

**The most common form** of esophageal atresia shows an abnormal connection between only the lower part of the esophagus and the trachea.

**The rarest form** of esophageal atresia shows abnormal connections between the upper and lower parts of the esophagus and the trachea.

# HOW IS FOOD SWALLOWED?

The act of swallowing takes only a few seconds, but it is a complicated process. Partly under the control of the conscious brain (voluntary) and partly an automatic reflex (involuntary), swallowing requires accurate coordination of all body parts involved. Swallowing occurs in three stages: the first in the mouth (the oral stage), the second in the throat or pharynx (the pharyngeal stage), and the third in the esophagus (the esophageal stage).

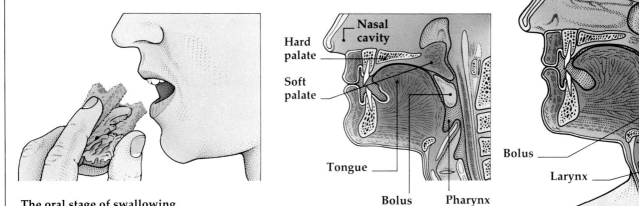

**The oral stage of swallowing**
*Once food has been formed into a bolus, the tongue pushes it to the back of the mouth. The tip of the tongue presses against the hard palate just behind the upper teeth, and the body of the tongue progressively presses backward, forcing the bolus to the back of the mouth and into the throat. At the same time, the soft palate rises and presses firmly against the back wall of the throat, sealing off the nasal cavity so that the bolus cannot move upward. While these activities are mainly voluntary, they are usually performed almost unconsciously.*

## HOW IS BREATHING AFFECTED BY SWALLOWING?

The throat (pharynx) serves as a passageway for both air and food. As food leaves the pharynx, it could enter the trachea instead of the esophagus. To prevent this from happening, the brain stem temporarily inhibits breathing when you swallow and triggers a series of actions to seal off the entrance to the trachea. If food does enter the trachea, the cough reflex is triggered. This reflex immediately returns the food to the mouth to prevent choking.

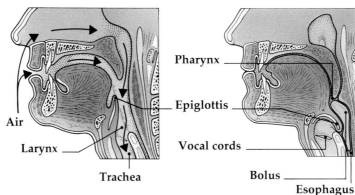

**Breathing**
*During breathing, the space between the vocal cords (the glottis) within the voice box (larynx) is relaxed and open. Air passes through the pharynx into the trachea, not into the esophagus.*

**Swallowing**
*During swallowing, the glottis presses tightly shut. As the bolus passes through the throat into the esophagus, a thin layer of cartilage called the epiglottis tilts down, and the larynx rises. These actions seal off the trachea.*

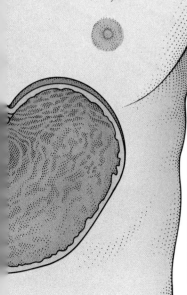

Pharynx

**The pharyngeal stage of swallowing**
*The second stage of swallowing is involuntary. Once the bolus enters the throat (pharynx), it presses against the pharyngeal wall, which contains many nerve endings that are sensitive to pressure. These nerves send messages to the brain stem, which regulates swallowing. Signals from the brain stimulate muscular contraction of the walls of the throat. Brain signals also trigger a sequence of events that prevents food from entering the trachea instead of the esophagus (box at lower left).*

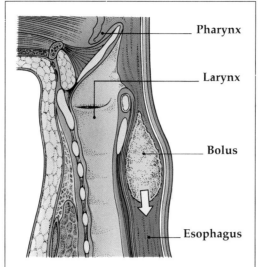

Pharynx

Larynx

Bolus

Esophagus

**The esophageal stage of swallowing**
*The third, esophageal stage of swallowing starts with the relaxation of the upper end of the esophagus so the bolus can pass into it unrestricted. This action, also under the control of the brain stem, takes place immediately after the muscles of the throat contract. As soon as the bolus has passed through the upper end of the esophagus, the larynx relaxes and breathing resumes.*

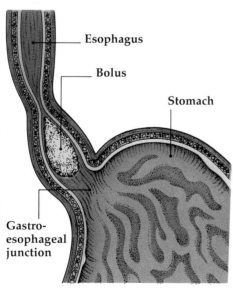

Esophagus

Bolus

Stomach

Gastro-esophageal junction

*The bolus then passes down the length of the esophagus, moved by muscular contractions known as peristalsis (at right). Cells in the lining of the esophagus secrete mucus to reduce friction between the bolus and the esophageal lining. As the bolus moves down the esophagus, muscles at the junction of the esophagus and the stomach relax to allow the bolus to enter the stomach.*

# PERISTALSIS

Once a bolus passes through the upper end of the esophagus, the muscles of the esophagus behind it contract, while the muscles in front of it relax. This pattern of progressive contraction and relaxation moves along the full length of the esophagus, propelling the food to the stomach. These waves of muscular contraction are known as peristaltic waves. Gravity also helps food pass down the esophagus, but peristalsis is so forceful that it would convey food to the stomach even if you were standing on your head.

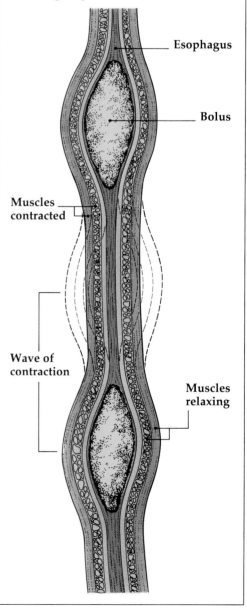

Esophagus

Bolus

Muscles contracted

Wave of contraction

Muscles relaxing

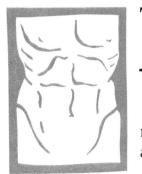

# THE ABDOMINAL CAVITY

Y OUR ABDOMEN extends between your rib cage and your pubic
bone. The abdominal cavity contains most of the organs of
the digestive and urinary systems as well as the internal
reproductive organs. All of these organs lie inside the peritoneum,
a protective membrane that lines the abdominal cavity.

## LOCATIONS OF THE ABDOMINAL ORGANS

**Liver**
The liver is located in the upper right side of the abdomen, just beneath the diaphragm.

**Gallbladder**
The gallbladder is a small, pear-shaped sac located under the liver, to which it is connected by fibrous tissue.

**Small intestine**
Extending from the bottom of the stomach, the small intestine fills most of the center of the abdominal cavity.

**Colon**
The colon (large intestine) has four sections: ascending, transverse, descending, and sigmoid. It starts in the lower right portion of the abdominal cavity, extends up to an area below the liver, and runs across the top of the abdomen. It then turns down the left side of the abdomen to the rectum.

**Pelvic cavity**
The lower part of the abdomen is called the pelvic cavity. It contains the bladder, the rectum, and the internal reproductive organs.

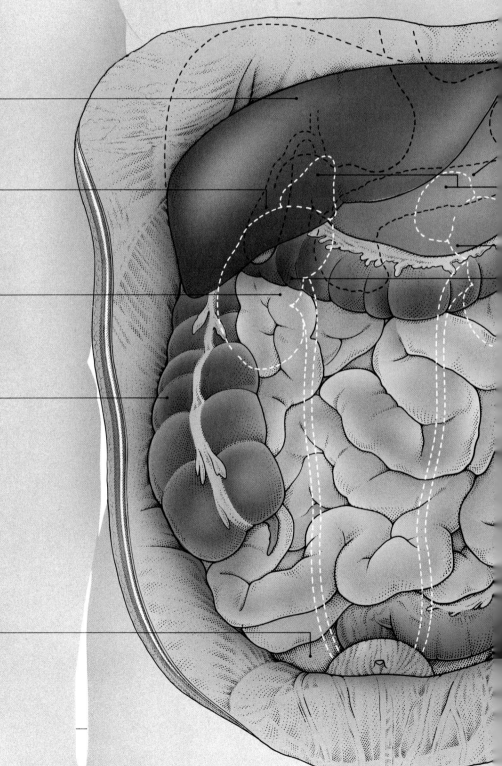

**Stomach**
The stomach sits in the upper left corner of the abdomen, under the diaphragm.

The abdominal organs are held in place and separated by the peritoneum, a thin, translucent membrane. The peritoneum supports the abdominal organs, produces a lubricating fluid so the organs can glide smoothly over each other, and protects against infection. In some areas of the abdomen, the peritoneum becomes multi-layered, forming membranes called the omentum and mesentery.

**Pancreas**
The pancreas lies across the back of the abdomen, behind the stomach.

**Spleen**
The spleen is located in the upper left portion of the abdomen, behind the stomach and lower ribs.

**Adrenal glands**
The two adrenal glands sit on top of each kidney.

**Kidneys**
The kidneys lie behind the peritoneum in the upper abdominal cavity. One kidney sits behind the duodenum (first part of the small intestine) on the right side. The other sits behind the pancreas on the left side.

**Peritoneum**

## OMENTUM

The greater omentum is a double-layered fatty membrane that hangs over the small intestine like an apron. It plays a very specific role in fighting infection because it can move and adhere to an infected area and prevent the infection from spreading to other parts of the abdominal cavity. In obese people, the omentum serves as a reservoir for large quantities of fat. The lesser omentum suspends the stomach and a portion of the duodenum beneath the liver.

## MESENTERY

The mesentery is a double-layered sheet of peritoneum that encloses the small intestine. The mesentery attaches the small intestine to the back of the abdominal wall and ensures that it is securely folded. The arteries, veins, nerves, and lymphatic vessels that supply the small intestine and ascending and descending parts of the colon all lie inside the mesentery. A short part of the mesentery suspends the transverse colon from the back of the abdominal wall.

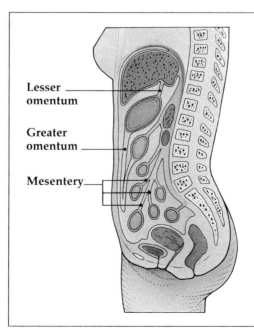

**Lesser omentum**

**Greater omentum**

**Mesentery**

**STRUCTURE OF THE PERITONEUM**

The peritoneum is the membrane that lines the wall of the abdominal cavity. It supplies blood vessels, lymph vessels, and nerves to the organs in the abdominal cavity. Some of these organs are not only covered by peritoneum but also completely surrounded by it. Such multilayered membranes help anchor the organs securely to the abdominal wall.

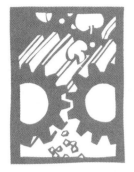

# THE STOMACH

**Y**OUR STOMACH IS A HOLLOW, muscular sac that forms the widest part of the digestive tract. Food enters your stomach by way of the esophagus and exits into the duodenum (the first part of the small intestine). The stomach has two principal jobs: it processes the food you eat and stores it. The stomach gradually releases the processed food into the intestines. Without your stomach's storage capabilities, you would need to eat much more frequently.

The stomach stores food and converts it into units small enough to be acted on by the enzymes in the small intestine. It accomplishes this breakdown by mechanically churning the food so it mixes with gastric juice produced by the stomach's cells. This juice contains digestive enzymes, acid that activates the enzymes and breaks down some foods, and gastrin, a hormone that increases the stomach's muscular activity and stimulates acid production.

## STOMACH ACTIVITY

The wall of the stomach consists of layers of muscle that allow it to churn and mix food. These muscles also enable the stomach to expand and contract. The stomach can contract to hold only about one tenth of a pint but the volume may quickly increase to as much as 3 pints. When you swallow food, your stomach relaxes in anticipation. This relaxation is controlled by the swallowing center in the brain. Wavelike contractions (peristalsis) constantly keep the stomach moving. These waves can occur at a rate of about three per minute.

Powerful contractions of the esophagus force food toward the entrance to the stomach, called the gastroesophageal junction, which opens to allow the food into the

**Muscular structure of the stomach**
*The stomach consists of layers of muscle that rhythmically contract to promote digestion. At the entrance to the stomach, the muscle at the gastroesophageal junction opens and closes to control the passage of food from the esophagus. At the stomach's exit, the pyloric sphincter opens and closes to allow food to pass into the duodenum.*

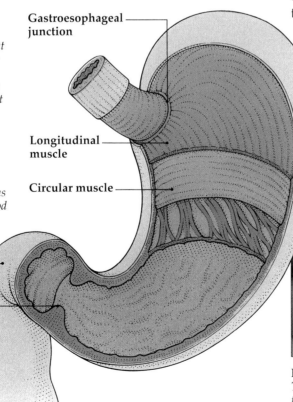

Gastroesophageal junction

Longitudinal muscle

Circular muscle

Duodenum

Pyloric sphincter

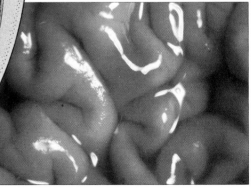

**How does your stomach expand?**
*The inside of your stomach forms folds called rugae that allow it to expand to hold large quantities of food. As the stomach expands, the rugae smooth out.*

stomach. In the stomach, food becomes partially digested, and the products are forced toward the strong ring of muscle at the entrance to the duodenum, called the pyloric sphincter. When the stomach contents have been reduced to a fluid called chyme, which has the consistency of thick cream, the pyloric sphincter allows small quantities to pass into the duodenum. The pyloric sphincter relaxes to accept food of the right consistency, but any lumps of food that strike the pyloric region stimulate the sphincter to close. This action prevents overly large pieces from passing into the small intestine. Such pieces return to the stomach to be broken down further by mechanical digestion and stomach acid.

## Nervous system control of the stomach

The part of the nervous system that regulates automatic body function, called the autonomic nervous system, governs the force of contraction of the stomach wall muscles and the rate at which the stomach empties. The stomach's main link to the brain is the vagus nerve. Shortly before and during a meal, the vagus nerve releases the chemical acetylcholine, which stimulates the production of stomach acid and increases peristalsis, causing the stomach wall muscles to contract more forcibly. Acetylcholine also keeps the pyloric sphincter closed until food has been sufficiently mixed.

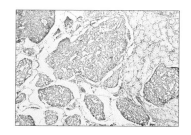
## HOW DOES FOOD MOVE THROUGH THE STOMACH?

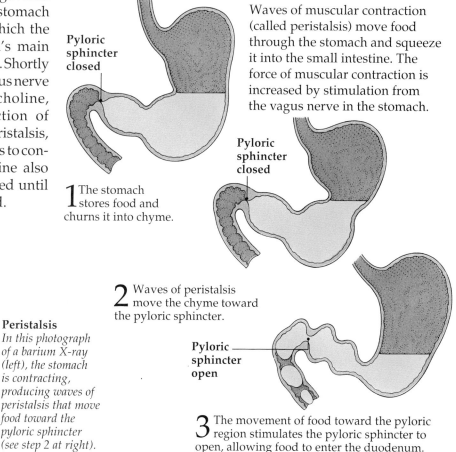

Waves of muscular contraction (called peristalsis) move food through the stomach and squeeze it into the small intestine. The force of muscular contraction is increased by stimulation from the vagus nerve in the stomach.

**Pyloric sphincter closed**

1 The stomach stores food and churns it into chyme.

**Pyloric sphincter closed**

2 Waves of peristalsis move the chyme toward the pyloric sphincter.

**Pyloric sphincter open**

3 The movement of food toward the pyloric region stimulates the pyloric sphincter to open, allowing food to enter the duodenum.

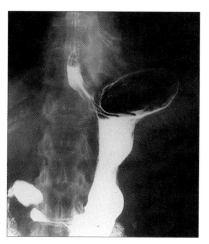

**Peristalsis**
*In this photograph of a barium X-ray (left), the stomach is contracting, producing waves of peristalsis that move food toward the pyloric sphincter (see step 2 at right).*

33

# WHAT HAPPENS IN YOUR STOMACH?

Your stomach homogenizes food by mechanical activity and acid breakdown. It also starts the process of protein digestion. This remarkable organ stores the food you eat, disinfects it, turns it into a semifluid mixture (chyme), and delivers it at regular intervals into the small intestine for further processing. Very few nutrients pass directly from the stomach into your bloodstream because most of the digested material in the stomach consists of chemical molecules that are too large to pass through the stomach wall. Alcohol is one of the few substances that can pass directly from the stomach into the bloodstream.

**Mucus-secreting cells**

**Cells of the stomach glands**

**The stomach lining**
*The stomach lining contains many specialized cells that perform a range of functions.*

### Lipase
*Most fat is digested in the small intestine. But some fat digestion takes place in the stomach, performed by the fat-splitting enzyme lipase. This enzyme is secreted from cells in the stomach glands.*

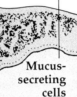

**Lipase**

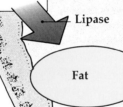

**Fat**

**Fatty acids**

### CELLS OF THE STOMACH LINING

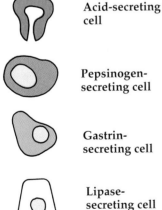

Acid-secreting cell

Pepsinogen-secreting cell

Gastrin-secreting cell

Lipase-secreting cell

Mucus-secreting cell

### Mucus
*The stomach contains cells that secrete mucus. This mucus protects the stomach wall from the corrosive effects of acid and other irritating substances produced in the stomach. Without mucus, the stomach would digest its own wall. Failure of this mucous layer to protect the stomach lining causes the open sores known as ulcers.*

**2** Some cells in the stomach glands secrete pepsinogen, a form of the protein-splitting enzyme pepsin. Hydrochloric acid converts pepsinogen to pepsin, which functions only in acidic conditions.

**3** Pepsin performs the first step in breaking down protein. It splits the proteins in food into smaller units called peptides.

Protein

**1** Cells deep in the stomach glands secrete hydrochloric acid. Hydrochloric acid provides the right environment for stomach enzyme activity. It also kills bacteria and many other microorganisms ingested with food.

## HOW DO STOMACH CELLS INTERACT TO DIGEST PROTEINS?

During the digestion of proteins, several different secretions from cells in the stomach lining interact. The rate of a cell's activity depends on the degree of stimulation it receives from the other elements in the cycle.

**4** The presence of peptides stimulates the release of the hormone gastrin.

Peptides

**5** Endocrine (hormone-secreting) cells in the stomach glands secrete the hormone gastrin into the bloodstream. Gastrin circulates in the bloodstream and returns to the stomach to stimulate the production of more hydrochloric acid. Gastrin also stimulates greater stomach activity and stomach wall movement (called motility).

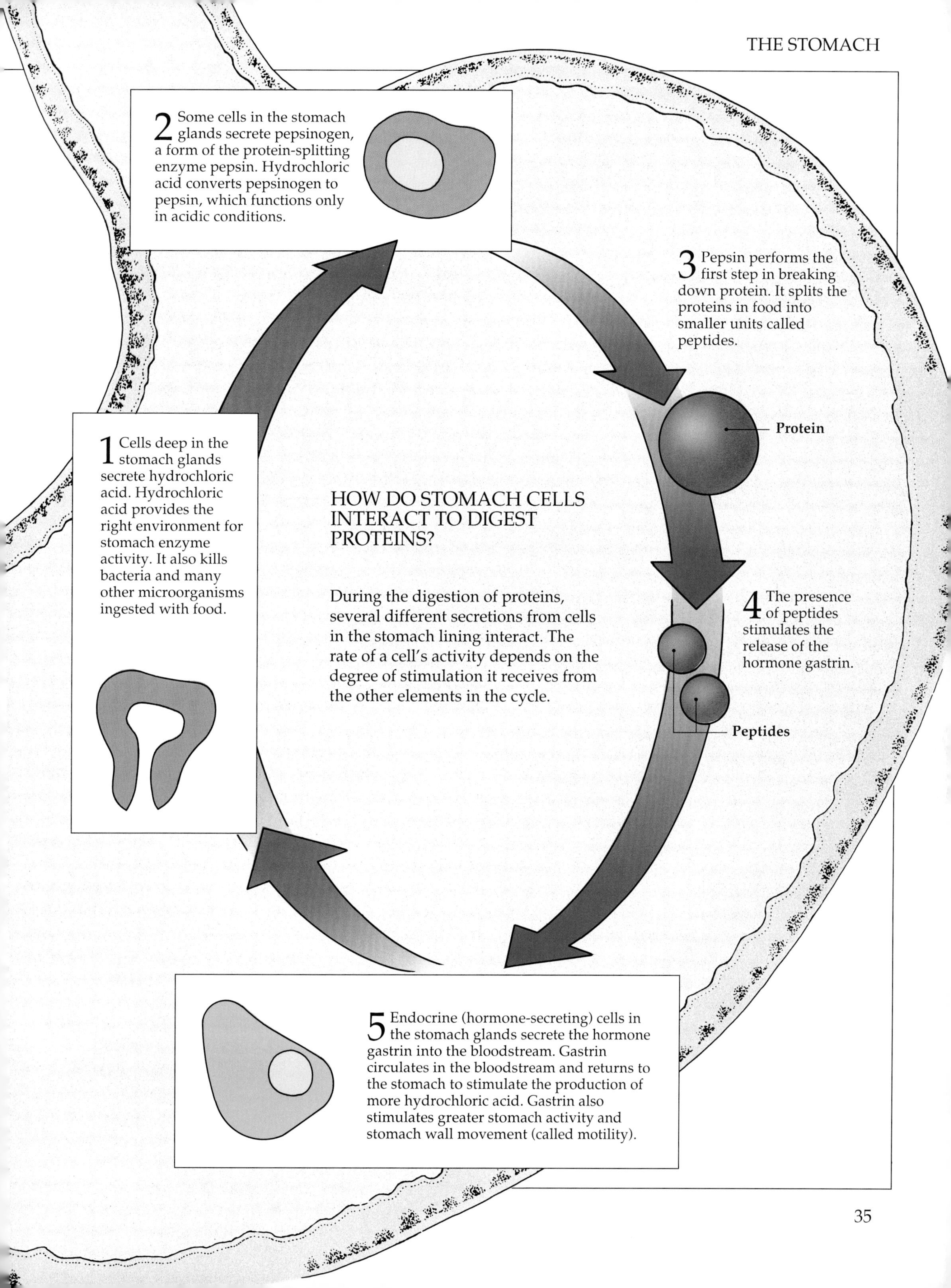

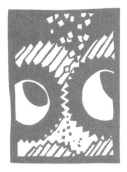

# THE SMALL INTESTINE

THE FOOD YOU EAT passes from your stomach into your small intestine, a coiled tube about 20 feet long. In the small intestine, food is broken down further and nutrients are absorbed. The small intestine joins the stomach at the pyloric sphincter and ends at the first part of the colon, called the cecum.

The small intestine performs two main functions: it completes the chemical breakdown of food and provides a site from which the products of digestion can pass into the bloodstream. The small intestine has an internal structure that allows the absorption of a variety of nutrients from food. The first part of the small intestine is called the duodenum. About 12 inches long, it receives secretions from the pancreas and liver. The second part of the small intestine, the jejunum, extends about 6 feet. Enzymes secreted by the cells that line the jejunum combine with secretions from the duodenum to complete the job of nutrient breakdown. The third part, the ileum, is about 13 feet long. The principal function of the ileum is to absorb nutrients.

**Inside the small intestine**
*The drawing below shows the position of the small intestine in the abdomen. The cross-section (center) shows the four layers that make up the intestinal wall. The inner lining of the small intestine (far right) contains millions of microscopic projections, called villi, that are essential for efficient absorption of nutrients into the bloodstream.*

## INTERNAL STRUCTURE OF THE SMALL INTESTINE

Like the rest of the digestive tract, the small intestine is made up of four layers: the serosa, muscularis, submucosa, and mucosa. The outer layer, called the serosa, is a thin, transparent, protective membrane. The serosa adheres closely to the thick, muscular second layer, called the muscularis. This layer contains a thick, circular inner lining of muscle and a thin, outer lining of longitudinal muscle. The circular muscles mix the creamy fluid called chyme that leaves the stomach and work with the long muscles to move the chyme along by the wavelike movements of peristalsis through the small

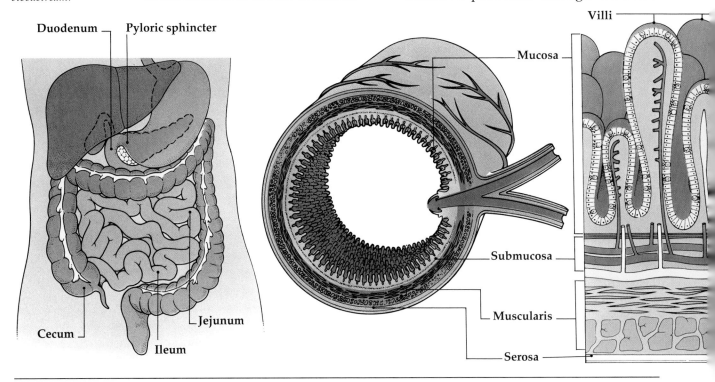

Duodenum · Pyloric sphincter · Villi · Mucosa · Submucosa · Muscularis · Serosa · Cecum · Ileum · Jejunum

intestine. These muscular layers are thickest in the duodenum. In the final few feet of the ileum, the layers of muscle become very thin. Next to the muscularis lies the layer called the submucosa, which contains the blood vessels, lymphatic vessels, and nerves of the small intestine.

## The mucosa

The fourth, innermost layer of the small intestine is the mucosa. This folded layer has millions of fingerlike projections called villi on its surface. Epithelial cells, which cover the surface of the villi, absorb digested nutrients. These cells themselves have projections called microvilli. Together, the mucosal folds, villi, and microvilli increase the surface area of the intestine's lining about 600 times – to an area about the size of a tennis court – for nutrient absorption. Mucosal cells secrete mucus and digestive enzymes. The mucosal layer also contains millions of white blood cells that protect the intestine against infection.

## INTESTINAL MOVEMENT

The small intestine moves in two ways – by segmentation and by peristalsis. In segmentation, the circular muscle of the intestine's muscular coat moves in a series of concentric contractions. An influx of partially digested food from the stomach initiates these movements. Segmentation does not occur at a uniform rate throughout the small intestine. For example, segmentation in the duodenum occurs at a rate of about 12 contractions per minute. The rate in the ileum is only about nine per minute. Peristalsis is the name for the waves of muscular contraction that move the chyme along the intestine. Peristalsis is weaker in the small intestine than in the esophagus and stomach and mainly occurs toward the end of the small intestine.

**Contraction 1**

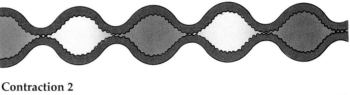

**Contraction 2**

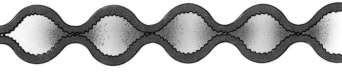

**Contraction 3**

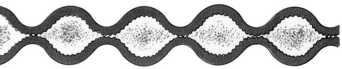

**Segmentation**
*Segmentation is the major contracting activity of the small intestine. Segments of the intestinal wall contract at evenly spaced intervals. Each contraction lasts only a few seconds. As the contracted area relaxes, another set of contractions begins at a point between the previous contractions (see contraction 2 above). This pattern of contractions mixes the chyme up to 12 times per minute, ensuring a thorough blending of the contents with digestive secretions from the intestine, liver, and pancreas.*

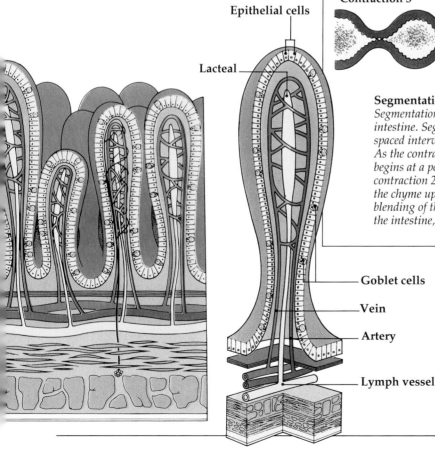

Epithelial cells

Lacteal

Goblet cells

Vein

Artery

Lymph vessel

**Structure of a villus**
*Each villus consists of a central core of muscle and connective tissue, covered by a layer of epithelial cells that absorb nutrients, and special mucus-secreting cells called goblet cells. Inside the muscular core lies a network of delicate blood vessels (capillaries) and a central lymph vessel (lacteal) that joins a network of lymph vessels underlying the villi. The epithelial cells absorb digestive substances that pass into the capillaries or the lacteal.*

# HOW ARE NUTRIENTS BROKEN DOWN AND ABSORBED?

The breakdown of partially digested food from the stomach is completed in the small intestine, aided by secretions from the pancreas, the liver (by way of the gallbladder), and the intestine itself. The nutritional products of digestion then pass into the lymphatic vessels and the bloodstream for distribution to the cells of the body. The enzymes that break down food in the small intestine can function only in alkaline conditions. Food leaving the stomach is highly acidic, so the small intestine must first reduce the acidity of the incoming material. The duodenum secretes the hormone secretin, which reduces the production of stomach acid when food enters the small intestine. Secretin also stimulates alkaline secretions from the pancreas and liver to reduce acidity.

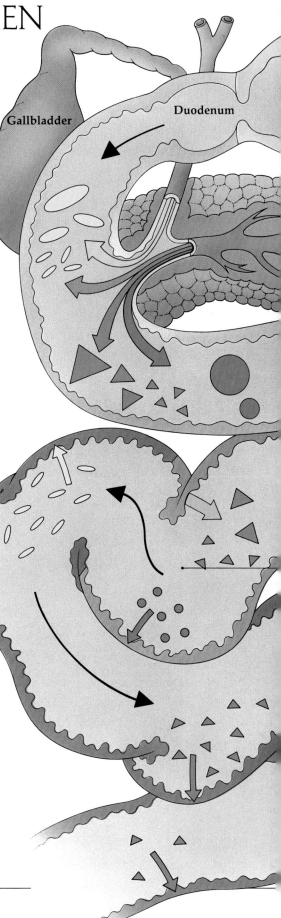

Gallbladder

Duodenum

## Key

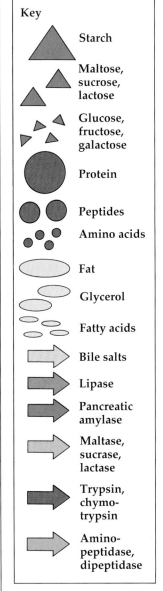

Starch

Maltose, sucrose, lactose

Glucose, fructose, galactose

Protein

Peptides

Amino acids

Fat

Glycerol

Fatty acids

Bile salts

Lipase

Pancreatic amylase

Maltase, sucrase, lactase

Trypsin, chymo-trypsin

Amino-peptidase, dipeptidase

### Breakdown of fat

*Bile, which is produced by the liver and stored in the gallbladder, breaks down fats in the small intestine. Salts contained in the bile break down large fat droplets into many smaller droplets. This action increases the surface area of the droplets and speeds up their digestion by the pancreatic fat-splitting enzyme lipase. Lipase breaks down fats into glycerol (a sugar alcohol) and fatty acids.*

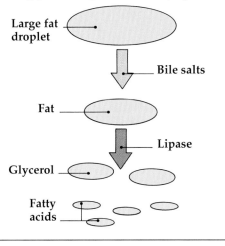

Large fat droplet

Bile salts

Fat

Lipase

Glycerol

Fatty acids

### Absorption of fat

Very little fat appears in the feces because the absorption of the fat we eat is usually rapid and complete. Fat absorption occurs primarily in the jejunum. Tiny fat globules do not pass directly into the bloodstream or liver but pass into the lacteals in the center of the villi (see page 36). These lacteals merge to form large lymphatic channels, which empty into the bloodstream, allowing circulation of fats throughout the body. Most of these fats are transported to the liver for further processing. The rest are deposited in the body as fat.

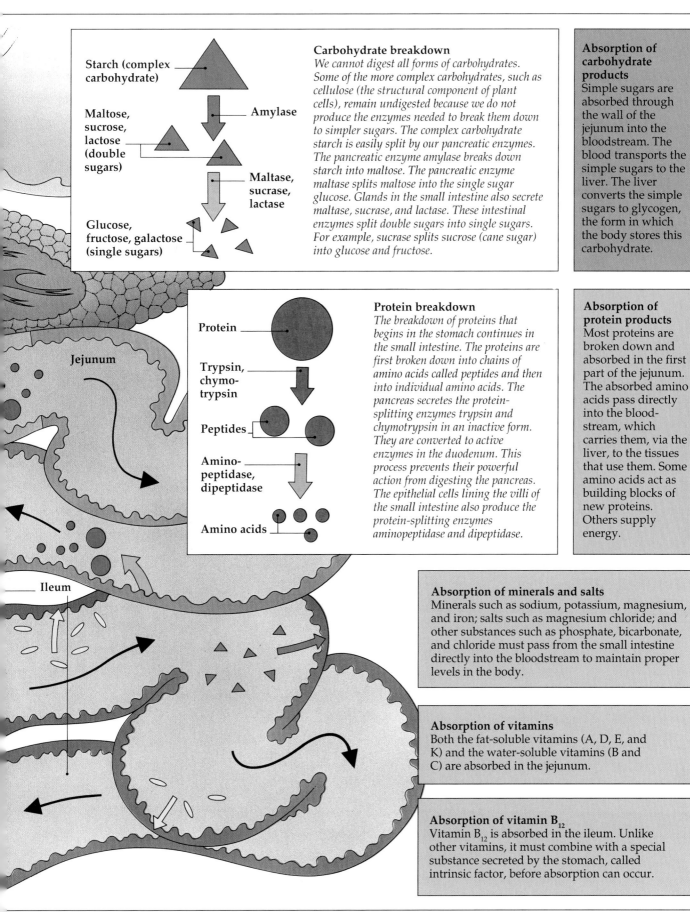

**Starch (complex carbohydrate)**

**Maltose, sucrose, lactose (double sugars)**

Amylase

Maltase, sucrase, lactase

**Glucose, fructose, galactose (single sugars)**

## Carbohydrate breakdown
*We cannot digest all forms of carbohydrates. Some of the more complex carbohydrates, such as cellulose (the structural component of plant cells), remain undigested because we do not produce the enzymes needed to break them down to simpler sugars. The complex carbohydrate starch is easily split by our pancreatic enzymes. The pancreatic enzyme amylase breaks down starch into maltose. The pancreatic enzyme maltase splits maltose into the single sugar glucose. Glands in the small intestine also secrete maltase, sucrase, and lactase. These intestinal enzymes split double sugars into single sugars. For example, sucrase splits sucrose (cane sugar) into glucose and fructose.*

## Absorption of carbohydrate products
Simple sugars are absorbed through the wall of the jejunum into the bloodstream. The blood transports the simple sugars to the liver. The liver converts the simple sugars to glycogen, the form in which the body stores this carbohydrate.

**Jejunum**

**Protein**

Trypsin, chymo-trypsin

**Peptides**

Amino-peptidase, dipeptidase

**Amino acids**

## Protein breakdown
*The breakdown of proteins that begins in the stomach continues in the small intestine. The proteins are first broken down into chains of amino acids called peptides and then into individual amino acids. The pancreas secretes the protein-splitting enzymes trypsin and chymotrypsin in an inactive form. They are converted to active enzymes in the duodenum. This process prevents their powerful action from digesting the pancreas. The epithelial cells lining the villi of the small intestine also produce the protein-splitting enzymes aminopeptidase and dipeptidase.*

## Absorption of protein products
Most proteins are broken down and absorbed in the first part of the jejunum. The absorbed amino acids pass directly into the blood-stream, which carries them, via the liver, to the tissues that use them. Some amino acids act as building blocks of new proteins. Others supply energy.

**Ileum**

## Absorption of minerals and salts
Minerals such as sodium, potassium, magnesium, and iron; salts such as magnesium chloride; and other substances such as phosphate, bicarbonate, and chloride must pass from the small intestine directly into the bloodstream to maintain proper levels in the body.

## Absorption of vitamins
Both the fat-soluble vitamins (A, D, E, and K) and the water-soluble vitamins (B and C) are absorbed in the jejunum.

## Absorption of vitamin B$_{12}$
Vitamin B$_{12}$ is absorbed in the ileum. Unlike other vitamins, it must combine with a special substance secreted by the stomach, called intrinsic factor, before absorption can occur.

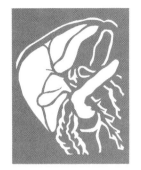

# THE LIVER, PANCREAS, AND GALLBLADDER

T HE FUNCTIONS of your liver, pancreas, and gallbladder are closely linked to those of the digestive tract, but these organs are not actually part of it. In the growing embryo, these structures develop as offshoots of the intestine. Each organ plays a vital role in the digestion of food and in the use of nutrients.

Your liver and pancreas contribute to the digestive process by secreting substances conveyed to the digestive tract by ducts that open into the duodenum. Your gallbladder serves as a storage organ for substances secreted by the liver, concentrating and then releasing them into the duodenum when needed.

## ANATOMY OF THE LIVER

The liver is a spongy, wedge-shaped, reddish brown structure divided into a large right lobe and a smaller left lobe. It lies mainly in the upper right portion of the abdomen, behind the lower ribs and below the diaphragm.

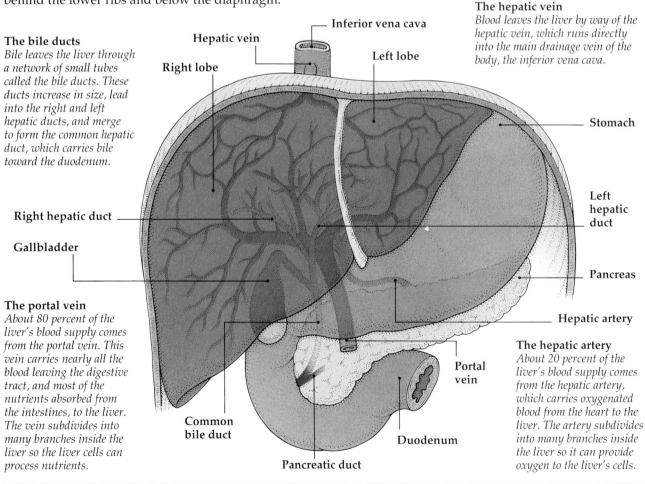

**The bile ducts**
*Bile leaves the liver through a network of small tubes called the bile ducts. These ducts increase in size, lead into the right and left hepatic ducts, and merge to form the common hepatic duct, which carries bile toward the duodenum.*

**The hepatic vein**
*Blood leaves the liver by way of the hepatic vein, which runs directly into the main drainage vein of the body, the inferior vena cava.*

Inferior vena cava

Hepatic vein

Right lobe

Left lobe

Stomach

Right hepatic duct

Gallbladder

Left hepatic duct

Pancreas

**The portal vein**
*About 80 percent of the liver's blood supply comes from the portal vein. This vein carries nearly all the blood leaving the digestive tract, and most of the nutrients absorbed from the intestines, to the liver. The vein subdivides into many branches inside the liver so the liver cells can process nutrients.*

Common bile duct

Pancreatic duct

Portal vein

Duodenum

Hepatic artery

**The hepatic artery**
*About 20 percent of the liver's blood supply comes from the hepatic artery, which carries oxygenated blood from the heart to the liver. The artery subdivides into many branches inside the liver so it can provide oxygen to the liver's cells.*

# LIVER

Weighing about 3 pounds, the liver is the heaviest organ in your body. It is an essential organ because, while a person can function when as much as 90 percent of his or her liver has been removed, a person without a liver cannot survive for more than 1 or 2 days. The liver has numerous functions in the body, aside from its role in the digestive system (see THE LIVER: YOUR BODY'S CHEMICAL FACTORY on page 42). Its only function in digestion is the secretion of bile. The medical term for anything that is related to the liver is "hepatic," which comes from the Greek word "hepar," meaning liver.

# GALLBLADDER

The gallbladder is a pear-shaped, saclike organ located on the underside of the liver. The gallbladder stores and concentrates bile until a hormone from the small intestine stimulates the gallbladder to contract. It then releases the bile into the duodenum. The bile helps to neutralize stomach acid and to emulsify fat.

## Composition of bile

The liver produces up to 2 pints of bile each day. While 97 percent of bile is water, other components include bile salts and pigments from the liver. Bile salts play an important role in the digestion of fat (see HOW ARE NUTRIENTS BROKEN DOWN AND ABSORBED? on page 38). Bile pigments are waste products mainly composed of bilirubin, a yellow substance derived from the pigment of red blood cells after they have been broken down by the spleen. Cholesterol is also secreted into bile. This mechanism is important in controlling blood cholesterol levels. The intestine reabsorbs some bile salts, cholesterol, and most of the water.

## THE BILIARY SYSTEM

The gallbladder is transparent, but concentrated bile gives it a bluish green color (see below). A healthy gallbladder is about 3 inches long and has the capacity to hold about 2 fluid ounces. The wall of the gallbladder is made of fibrous tissue strengthened by smooth muscle and lined with a folded mucous membrane. Bile, the bile ducts, and the gallbladder form the biliary system.

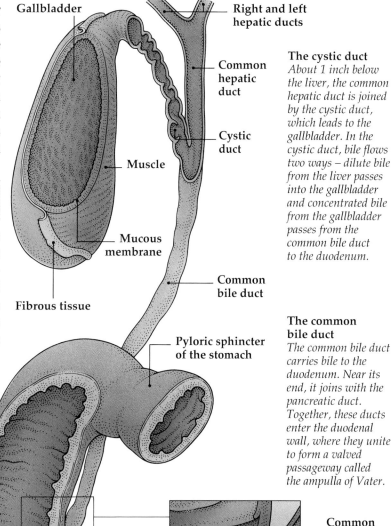

Gallbladder

Right and left hepatic ducts

Common hepatic duct

**The cystic duct**
*About 1 inch below the liver, the common hepatic duct is joined by the cystic duct, which leads to the gallbladder. In the cystic duct, bile flows two ways – dilute bile from the liver passes into the gallbladder and concentrated bile from the gallbladder passes from the common bile duct to the duodenum.*

Cystic duct

Muscle

Mucous membrane

Common bile duct

Fibrous tissue

Pyloric sphincter of the stomach

**The common bile duct**
*The common bile duct carries bile to the duodenum. Near its end, it joins with the pancreatic duct. Together, these ducts enter the duodenal wall, where they unite to form a valved passageway called the ampulla of Vater.*

Common bile duct

Pancreatic duct

Ampulla of Vater

Duodenum

# THE LIVER: YOUR BODY'S CHEMICAL FACTORY

Your liver is composed of millions of cells called hepatocytes. These cells perform more than 500 different functions, including the storage of nutrients; the breakdown of drugs (including alcohol), poisons, and waste products; and many chemical conversions. The liver functions like a factory that filters and processes the chemicals in your body.

## Glucose and other carbohydrates

Hepatocytes remove excess glucose (a sugar) from your blood and convert it to glycogen, which is stored. The cells then convert glycogen back to glucose when blood glucose levels become too low. The liver also converts simple sugars, such as fructose, from the food you eat into glucose. The liver stores only a small amount of glucose as glycogen and converts most of the surplus glucose into fat, which the blood then carries to your body's fat stores.

## Amino acids

Hepatocytes remove amino acids, the breakdown products of the protein you eat, from your blood and use them to make proteins for their own use or for release into the blood. For example, your liver makes blood plasma proteins, such as albumin, which is used to maintain blood volume, and coagulation factors, such as fibrinogen, which is used in blood clotting. A toxic by-product of this protein processing is ammonia, which the liver converts into urea for excretion in urine. Your liver also converts excess amino acids to fats, glucose, or glycogen.

## Fats and cholesterol

Hepatocytes convert the fats you eat into fats that can be stored by your body or used as fuel. Hepatocytes

### LIVER LOBULES

Your liver is made up of thousands of tightly packed, hexagonal units called lobules (below). Lobules are the basic functional units of the liver. Each one consists of layers of cells (called hepatocytes), just one cell thick, that radiate from a central vein.

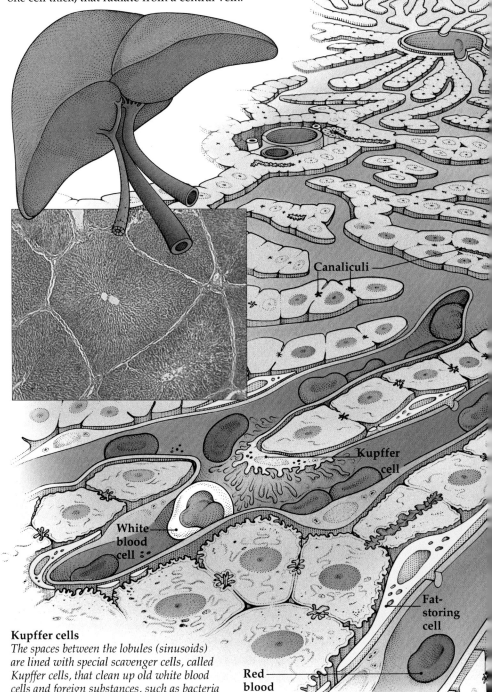

Canaliculi

Kupffer cell

White blood cell

Fat-storing cell

Red blood cell

**Kupffer cells**
*The spaces between the lobules (sinusoids) are lined with special scavenger cells, called Kupffer cells, that clean up old white blood cells and foreign substances, such as bacteria and viruses, from the blood.*

**Bile secretion**

*Hepatocytes manufacture bile and secrete it into tiny channels called bile canaliculi lying between the cells. The canaliculi drain into small bile ducts. These ducts run between the lobules that have end branches of the hepatic portal vein and hepatic artery branches. The bile ducts converge to form the left and right hepatic ducts.*

also play an important role in maintaining your body's cholesterol levels. You obtain a small amount of cholesterol from your diet. But your liver manufactures most of the cholesterol in your body from saturated fats in the food you eat. The more of these saturated fats you eat, the more cholesterol your liver produces. High levels of cholesterol in your blood inhibit the production of cholesterol by the liver. Falling blood cholesterol levels stimulate the liver to produce cholesterol. Hepatocytes also store excess cholesterol and use it to manufacture bile salts.

## Other liver functions

Your liver stores fat-soluble vitamins, some water-soluble B vitamins, and iron. It also breaks down many harmful chemicals, such as alcohol and other drugs, into safer substances. In an embryo, the liver produces red blood cells – a function performed by the bone marrow in an adult.

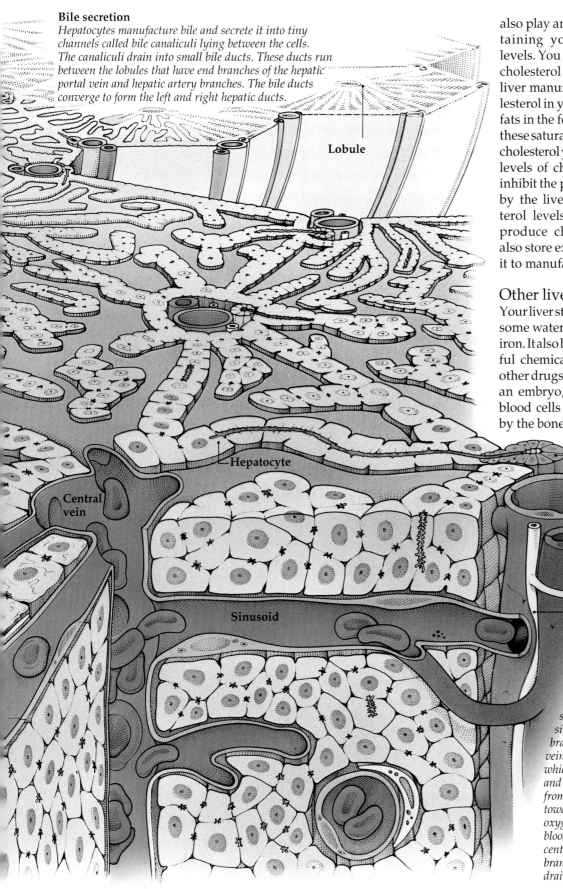

Lobule

Hepatocyte

Central vein

Sinusoid

Bile duct

Branch of portal vein

Branch of hepatic artery

Lymphatic vessel

**Blood flow in the lobules**

*Between the layers of hepatocytes lie blood-filled spaces called sinusoids. The sinusoids are formed by end branches of the hepatic portal vein and the hepatic artery, which run between the lobules and small bile ducts. Blood flows from the outside of the lobule toward its central vein, carrying oxygenated and nutrient-laden blood to the hepatocytes. The central vein of each lobule is a branch of the hepatic vein, which drains blood from the liver.*

# PANCREAS

The pancreas secretes certain substances through its duct. They include digestive enzymes that break down proteins, carbohydrates, and fats as well as sodium bicarbonate, which neutralizes stomach acid (see HOW ARE NUTRIENTS BROKEN DOWN AND ABSORBED? on page 38). All of these substances pass through the pancreatic duct to the duodenum. The pancreas also releases the hormones insulin, glucagon, and somatostatin directly into the bloodstream. Together, these three hormones control blood sugar levels. Control of blood sugar levels is the pancreas' main function.

## Regulating blood sugar levels

The pancreas secretes insulin when blood sugar levels are too high. Insulin moves glucose (a form of sugar) from the blood into muscle, fat, and liver cells, reducing glucose levels in the blood. Insulin also promotes the production and storage of a form of glucose in the liver. The hormone glucagon produces effects that are opposite to those of insulin. Glucagon raises the level of glucose in the blood in two ways. First, it stimulates the release of glucose from the liver. Second, it increases the rate at which the liver makes glucose. The process by which somatostatin controls the level of glucose in the blood is less well understood than are the roles of insulin and glucagon. Somatostatin seems to inhibit the secretion of both insulin and glucagon and prevents the overly rapid absorption of nutrients from the small intestine.

ANATOMY OF THE PANCREAS

The pancreas is a long, tapered organ with a large head and thin tail. The head lies in the curve of the duodenum, the body sits behind the stomach, and the tail ends near the spleen. Almost all of the pancreas is made up of exocrine tissue, which secretes substances by way of a duct. Endocrine tissue, which secretes hormones directly into the bloodstream, is scattered throughout the pancreas. The main pancreatic duct runs through the middle of the pancreas to the duodenum, where it joins the common bile duct and leads to an opening in the duodenum called the ampulla of Vater (see GALLBLADDER on page 41).

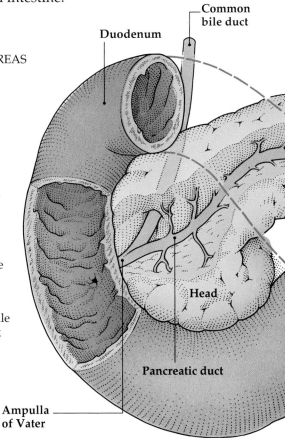

Common bile duct

Duodenum

Head

Pancreatic duct

Ampulla of Vater

---

GILBERT'S SYNDROME

Gilbert's syndrome is a disorder, usually occurring in young adults, in which the yellow pigment bilirubin accumulates in the blood. An early indication is mild jaundice (a yellowish coloring of the skin), which occurs either for no obvious reason or after an attack of viral hepatitis from which recovery was thought to have been complete. Many doctors believe that the syndrome may be inherited. Mild jaundice is often the only sign. Occasionally, an affected person loses his or her appetite and feels pain in the upper part of the abdomen.

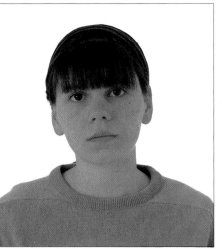

**How does Gilbert's syndrome cause jaundice?**
*Gilbert's syndrome is caused by the deficiency of a certain liver enzyme, glucuronyl transferase, which is needed by the liver to process the yellow pigment bilirubin. In the absence of this enzyme, bilirubin is not as effectively secreted in bile and accumulates in the blood. This accumulation leads to the yellow staining of body tissues called jaundice (shown at left).*

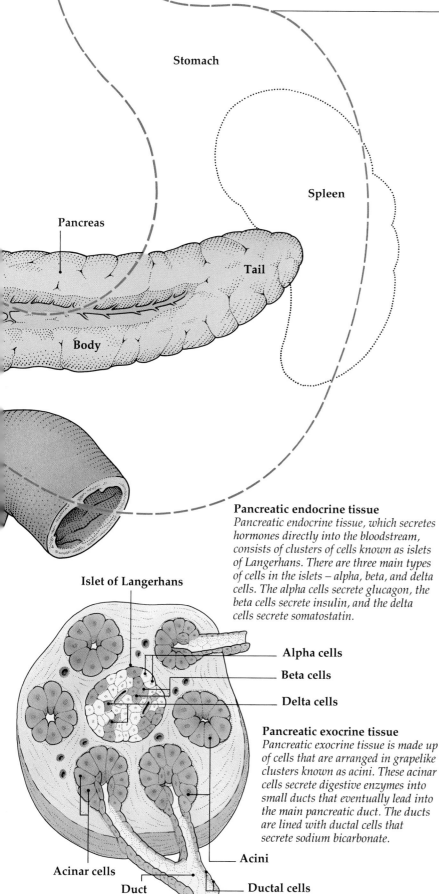

Stomach

Spleen

Pancreas

Tail

Body

**Pancreatic endocrine tissue**
*Pancreatic endocrine tissue, which secretes hormones directly into the bloodstream, consists of clusters of cells known as islets of Langerhans. There are three main types of cells in the islets – alpha, beta, and delta cells. The alpha cells secrete glucagon, the beta cells secrete insulin, and the delta cells secrete somatostatin.*

Islet of Langerhans

Alpha cells

Beta cells

Delta cells

**Pancreatic exocrine tissue**
*Pancreatic exocrine tissue is made up of cells that are arranged in grapelike clusters known as acini. These acinar cells secrete digestive enzymes into small ducts that eventually lead into the main pancreatic duct. The ducts are lined with ductal cells that secrete sodium bicarbonate.*

Acinar cells

Duct

Acini

Ductal cells

## ASK YOUR DOCTOR
## THE LIVER, PANCREAS, AND GALLBLADDER

**Q** I am starting a new job as a hospital orderly. Why have I been advised to be immunized with a hepatitis vaccine?

**A** Hepatitis, inflammation of the liver, can lead to permanent liver damage and even death. It can be caused by several types of viruses, but the one for which a vaccine exists is the hepatitis B virus. Hepatitis B can be transmitted by infected blood and blood products, which you may be handling in the hospital. You should have the vaccinations even though the risk of infection is very low. They are relatively painless and will protect you for life.

**Q** My wife had tests that show she has gallstones. They don't cause her any pain. Her doctor is not recommending any treatment. Should we be concerned?

**A** If your wife has never been troubled by the gallstones, they are probably not worth worrying about. But if she has intermittent abdominal pain on the upper right side, fever, nausea, and vomiting, she may need to have the gallstones or her gallbladder removed.

**Q** A friend told me that I am drinking too heavily and could develop diabetes if I don't reduce my alcohol intake. Is this true?

**A** Yes. Long-term alcohol abuse can cause inflammation of the pancreas (pancreatitis). Several episodes of inflammation can permanently damage your pancreas, ultimately reducing or destroying its insulin-producing cells. This damage leads to diabetes mellitus.

45

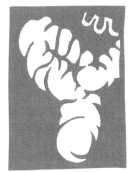

# THE COLON, RECTUM, AND ANAL CANAL

B Y THE TIME FOOD residue enters the final section of the digestive tract, absorption of nutrients, such as glucose and amino acids, into the bloodstream has stopped. The colon (large intestine) gradually converts the waste products of the digestive process into a form suitable for excretion from the body, concentrating and storing the waste before it passes out of the rectum and anal canal as feces.

The principal job of the colon, rectum, and anal canal is the disposal of waste products from the digestive system. About a quart and a half of liquid intestinal contents enter the colon each day, but little of this is food residue. Along with indigestible cellulose and other dietary fiber, the material passing into the colon consists of water, bile pigments, a residue of minerals, billions of bacteria, dead cells shed from the lining of the digestive tract, and secretions of mucus from the lower end of the ileum.

## COLON

The colon secretes no digestive enzymes, although it does produce mucus that may serve as a lubricant to move feces. The colon absorbs water from the fecal matter, changing it from a liquid to a solid form. Absorption is efficient and continuous; the colon normally absorbs about 2 ½ pints of water per day. If the contents of the colon remain there long enough, almost all the water is absorbed, making the feces soft, formed, and solid.

### Bacteria in the colon

Billions of bacteria normally occupy your colon. These bacteria are harmless to your body as long as the intestinal wall remains intact. Certain strains of bacteria synthesize small amounts of vitamins that are later absorbed. Although the amounts of vitamins are small compared with those in the food you eat, these amounts can become important if the vitamins are deficient in your diet. For example, your liver needs vitamin K to synthesize the blood-clotting factor prothrombin. Bacteria in your colon can produce enough vitamin K to compen-

## SECTIONS OF THE COLON

**Ascending and transverse segments**
These sections of the colon are the sites at which water is extracted from fecal matter.

**Descending and sigmoid segments**
Feces are stored in these parts of the colon before defecation.

**Cecum**
The cecum, the first portion of the ascending colon, is a wide, closed-ended pouch that contains the appendix.

**Rectum**
Feces pass into this final section of the colon just before defecation.

**Anal canal**
This passage, which ends at the anus, transports feces out of the body.

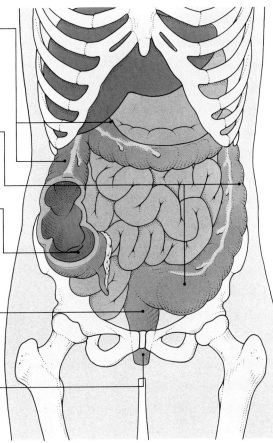

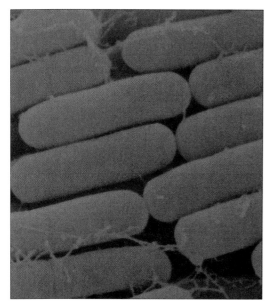

**Escherichia coli bacteria**
*Escherichia coli is the naturally occurring species of bacterium that predominates in the large intestine of humans and animals. It is used in genetic research because its DNA can be manipulated to produce valuable human proteins, such as insulin.*

sate for a lack of leafy green vegetables, which contain vitamin K, in your diet. Bacteria also modify the structure of cholesterol and hormones secreted in bile.

## Intestinal gas

Fermentation of certain foods by intestinal bacteria may produce considerable quantities of gas (flatus). A person produces about a half quart of gas each day. Flatus consists mainly of nitrogen and carbon dioxide, with smaller quantities of methane and hydrogen. These gases are all odorless, but flatus may also contain the odorous gas hydrogen sulfide. Certain foods, such as beans, can increase gas. They contain complex sugars that are not digestible and are fermented by bacteria in the colon. Excess gas probably does not cause most abdominal bloating, which is usually caused by altered bowel muscle function.

### WARNING
Antibiotics taken for many weeks or months may reduce the number and types of bacteria in the colon. This process diminishes bacterial production of some vitamins, leading to vitamin deficiency if your diet does not contain enough of the vitamins. In the ill or elderly, 2 or 3 weeks of antibiotics may reduce the number of bacteria in the colon, permitting the overgrowth of less useful, harmful bacteria and fungi that can cause diarrhea.

## FAMILIAL POLYPOSIS

Familial polyposis is a rare disorder in which small tumors (polyps) grow over the surface of the colon and rectum. The condition is inherited and appears in adolescence. It is detected by diagnostic tests, such as air contrast barium X-rays (see caption on page 119), and endoscopy, an examination that uses a flexible fiberoptic instrument to investigate a body cavity. In almost all cases of familial polyposis, many of the polyps become malignant within about 15 years of onset. Without treatment, most affected people die of cancer before the age of 40.

The most effective treatment is colectomy and ileostomy, a complete surgical removal of the colon and rectum. Surgeons create a permanent opening in the wall of the abdomen through which the lower end of the small intestine can eliminate waste products. An alternative treatment is to remove the colon and link the end of the ileum to the rectum. Any polyps that appear in the rectum are destroyed by burning (diathermy).

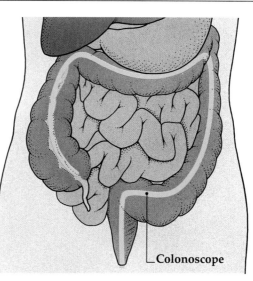

Colonoscope

**Endoscopic investigation**
*To confirm a diagnosis of familial polyposis, a long fiberoptic viewing instrument called a colonoscope is inserted into the large intestine by way of the anus. Doctors can check for the presence of polyps by viewing the channel projected on a monitor. Suspicious polyps can be removed and examined for signs of cancer.*

**Tubular adenomas**
*Two tubular adenomas, or polyps, can be seen as dark growths in the center of the photograph at right of a cross-section of colon. A person with familial polyposis may have thousands of these polyps scattered over the mucosal surface of his or her colon and rectum.*

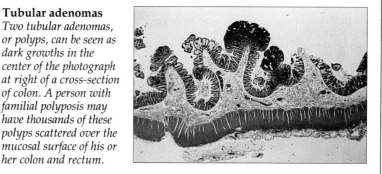

# STOOL FORMATION AND DEFECATION

The colon, like the stomach, serves an important storage function. Just as food stored in the stomach enables us to work for hours without hunger pangs, feces stored in the colon reduce the need to defecate to about one bowel movement a day. To allow enough time for the reabsorption of water from the feces, movement of contents is slower in the colon than in any other part of the digestive tract.

## HOW DOES THE COLON MOVE FECES?

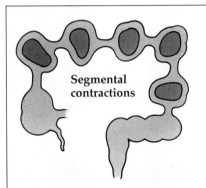

**Segmentation movements**
*The feces are mixed and churned by segmentation movements that occur about once every half hour. Segmentation movements involve no forward movement of contents toward the anus.*

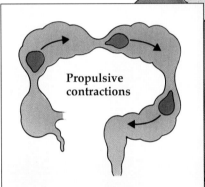

**Propulsive contractions**
*Wavelike propulsive contractions work with segmentation movements to ease the feces toward the rectum. Propulsive contractions occur in the colon about once every 30 minutes.*

**Mass movements**
*After each meal, a mass movement occurs in the descending colon. This movement squeezes part of the feces down into the lower part of the sigmoid colon and rectum.*

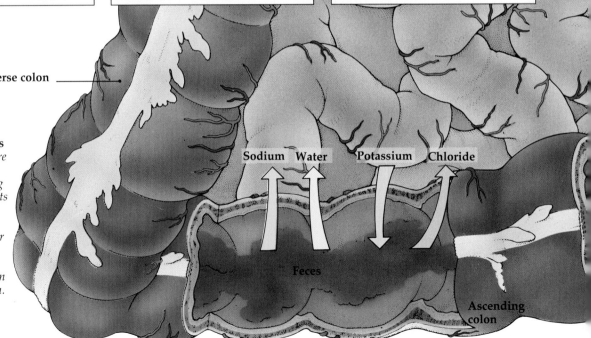

Transverse colon

**Dehydration of feces**
*Sodium and chloride are absorbed from fecal matter in the ascending and transverse segments of the colon. This process creates a need for the removal of water from the feces through the colon wall. Potassium is secreted in this section of the colon.*

Sodium   Water   Potassium   Chloride

Feces

Ascending colon

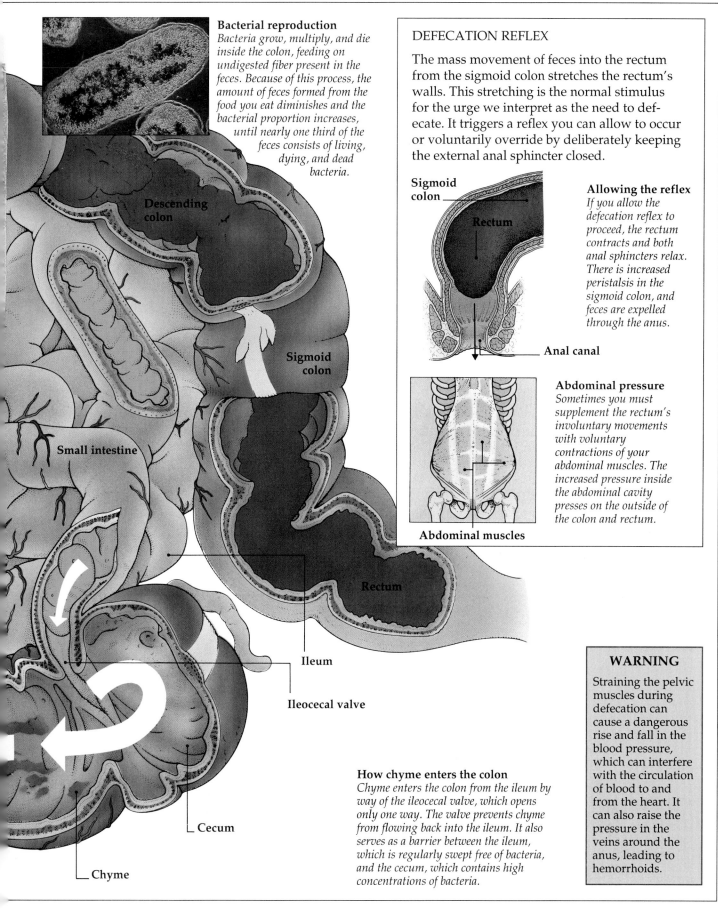

**Bacterial reproduction**
*Bacteria grow, multiply, and die inside the colon, feeding on undigested fiber present in the feces. Because of this process, the amount of feces formed from the food you eat diminishes and the bacterial proportion increases, until nearly one third of the feces consists of living, dying, and dead bacteria.*

Descending colon

Sigmoid colon

Small intestine

Ileum

Ileocecal valve

Rectum

Cecum

Chyme

## DEFECATION REFLEX

The mass movement of feces into the rectum from the sigmoid colon stretches the rectum's walls. This stretching is the normal stimulus for the urge we interpret as the need to defecate. It triggers a reflex you can allow to occur or voluntarily override by deliberately keeping the external anal sphincter closed.

Sigmoid colon

Rectum

Anal canal

**Allowing the reflex**
*If you allow the defecation reflex to proceed, the rectum contracts and both anal sphincters relax. There is increased peristalsis in the sigmoid colon, and feces are expelled through the anus.*

**Abdominal pressure**
*Sometimes you must supplement the rectum's involuntary movements with voluntary contractions of your abdominal muscles. The increased pressure inside the abdominal cavity presses on the outside of the colon and rectum.*

Abdominal muscles

### WARNING
Straining the pelvic muscles during defecation can cause a dangerous rise and fall in the blood pressure, which can interfere with the circulation of blood to and from the heart. It can also raise the pressure in the veins around the anus, leading to hemorrhoids.

**How chyme enters the colon**
*Chyme enters the colon from the ileum by way of the ileocecal valve, which opens only one way. The valve prevents chyme from flowing back into the ileum. It also serves as a barrier between the ileum, which is regularly swept free of bacteria, and the cecum, which contains high concentrations of bacteria.*

# RECTUM AND ANAL CANAL

The rectum is the final portion of the large intestine, located just below the sigmoid colon and directly above the anal canal. It is smooth and curved and lies in front of the sacral part of the spine. Extending about 5 inches, the rectum serves as the temporary storage site for feces just before defecation. It also provides most of the expulsive force during defecation. The rectum can distend widely but is normally empty, with collapsed walls, except just before and during defecation. There is no contracting muscle, or sphincter, between the sigmoid colon and the rectum. But feces are held above the level of the rectum until shortly before defecation.

## The anal canal

The anal canal extends about 1½ inches below the rectum. It is the final part of the digestive tract, extending through the muscular floor of the pelvis. When closed, the final section forms a half-inch-long slit, but it is capable of considerable stretching and is surrounded by strong, circular muscles. The lining of the anal canal is easily damaged by bulky, hardened feces.

The anal canal is lined with a mucous membrane that opens onto the puckered, pigmented skin of the anus. The skin of the anus contains large sebaceous and sweat glands. Large veins lying just under the mucous membrane form the membrane into 10 vertical columns. These columns press together to form an efficient, watertight sealing mechanism.

### CONSTIPATION

Having a regular bowel movement is very important in preventing constipation. If you regularly ignore or suppress the urge to defecate, tension in the walls of the rectum subsides. This means you will not feel the urge again when the next mass of feces moves into the rectum. It is possible but unwise to repeatedly ignore the urge to defecate. Water will continue to be extracted from the bowel contents. The feces then become increasingly dry, hard, and difficult to expel.

## ANATOMY OF THE RECTUM AND ANUS

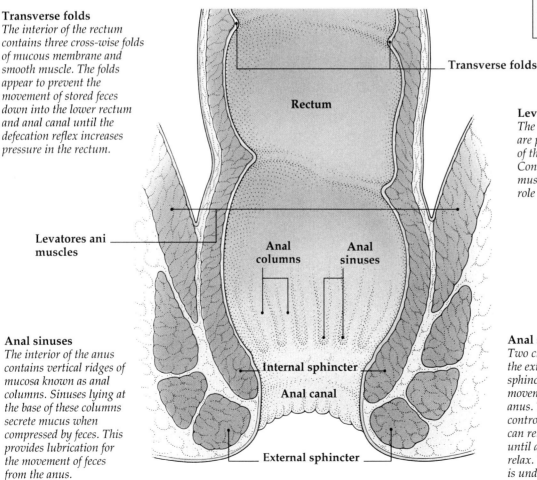

**Transverse folds**
*The interior of the rectum contains three cross-wise folds of mucous membrane and smooth muscle. The folds appear to prevent the movement of stored feces down into the lower rectum and anal canal until the defecation reflex increases pressure in the rectum.*

**Levatores ani muscles**
*The levatores ani muscles are part of the musculature of the pelvic floor. Contractions of these muscles play an important role in the defecation reflex.*

**Anal sinuses**
*The interior of the anus contains vertical ridges of mucosa known as anal columns. Sinuses lying at the base of these columns secrete mucus when compressed by feces. This provides lubrication for the movement of feces from the anus.*

**Anal sphincters**
*Two circular bands of muscle, the external and internal anal sphincters, control the movement of feces from the anus. The involuntarily controlled internal sphincter can retain feces in the rectum until a reflex causes it to relax. The external sphincter is under voluntary control.*

Transverse folds

Rectum

Levatores ani muscles

Anal columns

Anal sinuses

Internal sphincter

Anal canal

External sphincter

# FACTORS THAT CAN ALTER THE STOOLS

Changes in your diet and life-style can cause temporary changes in the character of your stools. These factors also affect the frequency of bowel movements. Occasionally, people become alarmed at the appearance of their stools. Several factors that give stools an unusual appearance are described below. The color and consistency of stools can be an important early indication of certain disorders (see LOWER DIGESTIVE TRACT SYMPTOMS on page 78). Be sure to report to your doctor any persistent and unexplained changes in your stools or defecation habits.

## DIET

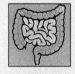

Some foods contain fibrous, insoluble elements that pass though the intestinal tract unchanged. These elements include the seeds of tomatoes, pomegranates, kiwi fruit, and watermelons; apple and tomato skins; and sweet corn husks. Their presence in the stools is a normal part of a healthy diet.

## MEDICAL TESTS

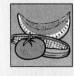

**Barium X-rays**
After having a barium X-ray, you may pass white or very pale stools. This is normal and indicates only that your body is expelling the barium that was introduced or that you swallowed.

**Transit time studies**
Doctors use transit time studies to investigate abnormal bowel movements. Patients swallow colored pellets in water that do not dissolve, and doctors time the passage of the pellets through the digestive tract. Pellets may appear in the stools.

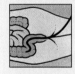

**Endoscopy**
After endoscopy, you may notice a little blood in your stools. This bleeding usually stops shortly after the procedure. If large amounts of blood appear, you should notify your doctor.

## MEDICATIONS

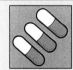

**Antibiotics**
Long-term use of antibiotics can cause diarrhea due to a reduction in the number of bacteria in the colon. This reduction permits the overgrowth of toxin-secreting bacteria or fungi.

**Codeine**
Codeine-containing medications, such as cough medicines and painkillers, often cause constipation. A high-fiber diet, plenty of fluids, and glycerine suppositories can help you overcome this temporary problem.

**Iron and bismuth**
Medications containing the metals iron or bismuth can cause the feces to be black. But dark or black stools passed while not taking these medications may indicate the presence of blood in the stools. If you are in doubt, ask your doctor to check the problem.

# ASK YOUR DOCTOR
## PROBLEMS OF THE LARGE INTESTINE

**Q** My mother has been told that she has a tumor in her rectum and may need to have a permanent colostomy. What does this mean?

**A** A colostomy is an artificial connection between the colon and an opening in the skin of the abdomen that allows the bowel contents to pass into a bag attached to the abdominal wall. Doctors create the opening during an operation called a colectomy, in which they remove the diseased part of the colon or rectum. Removal of the rectum usually means that the colostomy must remain in place permanently.

**Q** Why did the doctor perform a rectal examination after my husband complained of being unable to pass urine properly?

**A** The doctor's examination of the rectum with his or her finger can reveal enlargement of the prostate gland, a common cause of urinary problems in older men. Doctors also perform rectal examinations to detect cancers of the prostate gland and rectum and some colon cancers.

**Q** Recently, my anus has become itchy. It is often painful during or after my bowel movements. My doctor diagnosed hemorrhoids, but how did I get them?

**A** Hemorrhoids are dilated veins that lie close to the surface of the anal canal. If your diet is low in fiber and you are often constipated, the combination of straining to expel a stool and injury from the passage of hard feces can damage these veins. They become itchy, tender, and dilated, and they sometimes bleed.

# CHAPTER THREE

# SYMPTOMS OF DIGESTIVE TROUBLE

DIGESTIVE TRACT SYMPTOMS, such as bloating and heartburn, affect all of us from time to time. Many people experience these symptoms regularly. About 10 percent of the US population have heartburn every day and another 30 percent experience it occasionally. Millions of Americans have indigestion. About half of all Americans develop painful or bleeding hemorrhoids at one time or another; many others have them without feeling any discomfort. Diarrhea and constipation also occasionally trouble otherwise healthy people. Looking for relief from these common problems, Americans spend almost $1 billion every year on nonprescription remedies for digestive tract symptoms. These symptoms do not usually signal a serious disease, although they may be uncomfortable. But sometimes they serve as a warning sign of a serious disorder, so you should not ignore them. You can learn to distinguish between temporary or recurring symptoms that you have experienced for some time and those that are unusual or persistent. Any new, recurring symptom should be investigated by your doctor. Use over-the-counter medications only when you are sure about the nature of your symptoms, and do not take such medications for a long period of time.

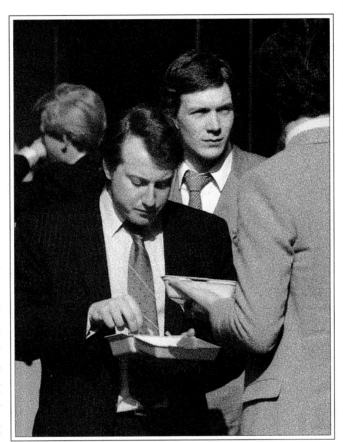

Your life-style can provide clues about the possible cause of a digestive tract symptom. Stress has been linked to a host of symptoms, including a lump in the throat, nausea, bloating, belching, gnawing or cramping pain, stomach growling, flatulence, diarrhea, and constipation. Drinking heavily can cause nausea, vomiting, diarrhea, and indigestion. Long-term alcohol abuse can lead to cirrhosis of the liver, central nervous system disorders, and pancreatic disease. Indigestion and peptic ulcers occur more frequently in smokers than in nonsmokers, as does cancer of the esophagus. Doctors also suspect that many cancers of the digestive tract are linked to diet. For example, cancer of the colon, which kills about 60,000 people in the US every year, may be caused by too little fiber and too much fat in the diet.

This chapter begins with a discussion of the relationship between your life-style choices and the health of your digestive tract. We then explore general digestive tract symptoms and demonstrate how doctors analyze abdominal pain to make a diagnosis. Common symptoms of the upper and lower digestive tracts are described so you can learn to tell the difference between the sensations of normal digestive function and those that may indicate the onset of a serious disorder.

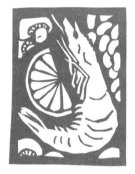

# LIFE-STYLE AND YOUR DIGESTIVE SYSTEM

**Y**OU'VE COME HOME late from work. Just as you sit down to dinner, the phone rings. It's your boss, reminding you about a deadline. Upset, you go back to the table and gulp your food. You have a few glasses of wine and smoke cigarettes to relieve the stress. A pressured life can affect your digestion. And your response to stress can bring on or worsen digestive problems.

Everyone occasionally experiences some event that provokes anxiety. At such times, you might have nausea, vomiting, and diarrhea – the most common gastrointestinal signs of extreme anxiety. These symptoms usually go away when the stressful event passes. But constant stress can have more serious, long-term effects on your digestive system. The heavy use of alcohol and tobacco, often part of an overly stressful life-style, can also impair digestion.

## ALCOHOL

Alcohol can damage the digestive system in two ways. Occasional intoxication brings on the familiar symptoms of nausea, vomiting, and severe indigestion the next morning. These symptoms are the direct result of alcohol's effects on the digestive system. They usually improve within a few hours. Long-term overconsumption of alcohol has more serious consequences (see page 55).

### Alcohol tolerance
Some people can drink more alcohol than others before becoming intoxicated. These people are said to have a higher tolerance to alcohol. The reasons for this disparity are unclear. Alcohol's short-term effects on the brain depend on the quantity consumed and the size of the person consuming it. The smaller the person, the higher the concentration of alcohol in the bloodstream, given the same alcohol intake. Your level of intoxication is no indication of the damage you may be doing to your body. Many people who never seem intoxicated develop serious alcohol-related health problems.

**Diet and cancer**
*The chart below shows that there has been little change in the number of deaths from colon cancer during the past few decades in the US. But the death rate for stomach cancer has decreased substantially. The reasons for this decrease are unknown, but some nutritionists see a link between falling rates of stomach cancer and healthy changes in diet. Stomach cancer is relatively rare in the US today.*

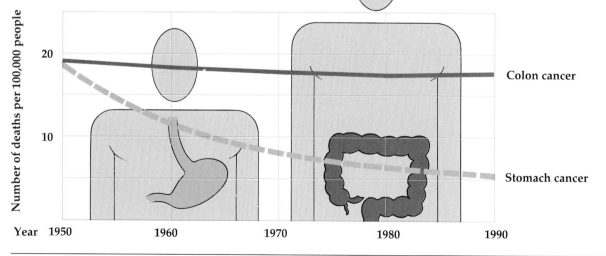

| Number of deaths per 100,000 people | | | | | |
|---|---|---|---|---|---|
| 20 | | | | | Colon cancer |
| 10 | | | | | Stomach cancer |
| Year 1950 | 1960 | 1970 | 1980 | 1990 | |

# ALCOHOL'S LONG-TERM EFFECTS ON YOUR DIGESTIVE SYSTEM

Habitual, heavy drinking adversely affects many parts of your body, including your brain and your heart. Within your digestive system, damage from alcohol can occur in several forms:

**Liver failure**
Prolonged alcohol abuse can cause hepatitis and accumulation of fat in liver cells. This process causes scarring and, eventually, cirrhosis of the liver, which can lead to liver failure and liver cancer. If the liver is affected, appetite may diminish and the abdomen may swell with fluid.

**Skin changes**
Indications that severe alcoholic liver disease has occurred may include skin that is jaundiced (yellow) and more susceptible to bruising. The palms of the hands turn red, and tiny, spiderlike blood vessels appear on the chest and arms.

**Esophageal damage**
Ulcers and/or varicose veins may develop in the esophagus. Varicose, or dilated, veins occur at the base of the esophagus when the liver is not functioning properly. If the veins burst, the resulting hemorrhage can be fatal.

**Stomach damage**
Heavy drinking causes repeated attacks of gastritis, which is inflammation of the stomach lining. Sometimes the stomach lining erodes. Heavy drinking also increases the chance of developing ulcers in the duodenum and stomach.

**Pancreatitis**
Chronic alcohol abuse often causes inflammation of the pancreas (pancreatitis). Pancreatitis causes a deficiency of the fat-splitting enzyme lipase. Lipase deficiency results in excess fat in the feces. Insulin deficiency from an impaired pancreas causes diabetes.

## SMOKING AND YOUR DIGESTIVE SYSTEM

Smoking is harmful to all parts of your body, including the digestive system. When a smoker inhales, swallowed air and smoke can cause or aggravate abdominal distention and belching. Indigestion, diarrhea, and duodenal and stomach ulcers occur more commonly in smokers than in nonsmokers. If a person continues to smoke during treatment for an ulcer, the healing process is prolonged. Ulcers recur more frequently in smokers and relapse occurs sooner after treatment ends.

**Esophageal cancer**
*Cancers of the digestive system, especially of the esophagus and oral cavity, occur more commonly in smokers. The photograph (right) shows a tumor obstructing the esophagus in a person with esophageal cancer.*

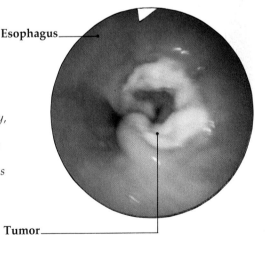

Esophagus

Tumor

# IS YOUR DIGESTIVE SYSTEM AT RISK?

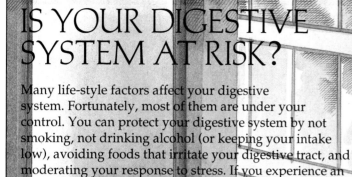

Many life-style factors affect your digestive system. Fortunately, most of them are under your control. You can protect your digestive system by not smoking, not drinking alcohol (or keeping your intake low), avoiding foods that irritate your digestive tract, and moderating your response to stress. If you experience an allergic response to a particular food, try to avoid it.

### Alcohol: long-term effects

*Regular, long-term alcohol consumption damages liver tissues, leading to cirrhosis (scarring that interferes with function). In most cases, cirrhosis eventually results in liver failure or liver cancer. Inflammation of the pancreas (pancreatitis) is also common in habitual drinkers. Pancreatitis prevents secretion of digestive enzymes by the pancreas and may lead to diabetes. Pancreatitis can be fatal.*

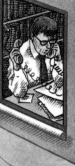

### Stress

*If you are under a lot of stress, you may suffer from nausea, vomiting, and diarrhea. Chronic stress can cause duodenal ulcers and other digestive system disorders.*

### Alcohol: immediate effects

*Drinking can cause nausea, vomiting, diarrhea, and indigestion. Women are more susceptible to the harmful effects of alcohol than are men. Women have less of the enzyme that breaks down alcohol, leading to a higher concentration of alcohol in the bloodstream. People in certain ethnic groups, such as the Chinese, lack this enzyme almost completely. They become intoxicated more easily than other ethnic groups, and the alcohol remains in their bloodstream for a longer time.*

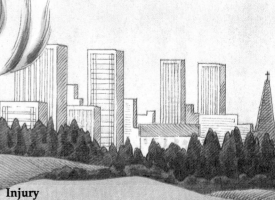

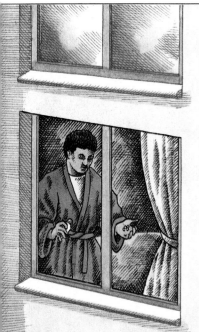

## Drugs

Drugs can affect the digestive system in a variety of ways. For example, antibiotics can cause diarrhea. Painkillers that contain codeine or codeine derivatives can cause constipation.

## Injury

Severe injury, from such emergencies as a major fire or an automobile accident, sometimes results in the development of acute stress ulcers, usually in the stomach. Occasionally, duodenal ulcers develop later. While acute superficial stress ulcers in the stomach tend to heal quickly, duodenal ulcers may not heal for a long time.

## Smoking

Smoking can seriously impair your digestive system. Smokers have a higher incidence of peptic ulcers, the inflammatory bowel condition Crohn's disease, and cancers of the esophagus. The chronic cough that accompanies long-term smoking can weaken the abdominal muscles and aggravate an abdominal hernia.

## Low-fiber diet

A low-fiber diet can lead to constipation. Many people with chronic constipation strain to have a bowel movement and develop or aggravate anal hemorrhoids and abdominal hernias. A diet that is high in refined carbohydrates and low in fiber also increases the risk of diverticular disease (see page 120) in the intestines and may contribute to the formation of cancer in the digestive system.

## STRESS

In a stressful situation, your body reacts by increasing its production of certain hormones, including cortisol and epinephrine. This so-called arousal response produces a more rapid heartbeat, increased blood flow to the muscles, a faster breathing rate, and greater mental alertness. Your body puts itself in a state of maximum readiness to cope with the source of the stress. If you cannot overcome the stressful situation, your body remains physically prepared to escape by running away. This reaction is called the "fight-or-flight" response.

## Normal digestive response

The body's automatic stress responses also affect the digestive tract by inhibiting release of saliva, slowing down the emptying of the stomach into the intestines, and increasing intestinal contractions. In some cases, these effects can produce a dry mouth, nausea, diarrhea, and even vomiting. When the stress is acute, such as in a potentially dangerous situation, these symptoms are fairly common. They usually stop as soon as the source of stress disappears.

## Abnormal digestive response

If your exposure to stress continues for a long time, symptoms can develop in many parts of your body. Long-term effects of stress can manifest themselves in such conditions as a rash or elevated blood pressure. Ongoing stress can cause headaches, backaches, heart palpitations, or panic attacks. Long-term stress can also cause disturbances of the digestive tract. Doctors think that stress may play a part in peptic ulcers and inflammatory bowel disease. Infection or inflammation of the digestive tract may render it more susceptible to the effects of stress (see page 59). But the reason people respond to long-term stress in different ways remains unknown.

## HOW DOES STRESS AFFECT THE DIGESTIVE SYSTEM?

**Psychogenic vomiting**
*Chronic or recurrent vomiting that occurs with no other symptoms is often psychogenic (psychological in origin). The vomiting may be accompanied by anxiety and a history of "nervous stomach" or irritable bowel syndrome.*

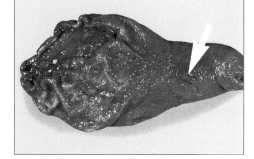

**Peptic ulcers**
*Although no evidence exists that stress causes peptic ulcers, doctors believe stress may aggravate an existing ulcer and cause complications. Perforation occurs when an ulcer penetrates through the wall of the digestive tract (see arrow above).*

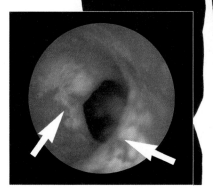

**Inflammatory bowel disease**
*The arrows at right point to ulceration of the colon in inflammatory bowel disease. The cause of inflammatory bowel disease (see INFLAMMATORY BOWEL DISEASE on page 115) remains unknown, but symptoms of the disease often flare up during emotionally stressful events, such as the death of a loved one.*

## Globus hystericus

*Globus hystericus is the constant sensation of having a lump in the throat, with no difficulty in swallowing. It is almost always a symptom of stress and is especially common in people with emotional problems, such as depression and anxiety.*

## Chronic abdominal pain

*Doctors frequently treat people who experience chronic abdominal pain. Most cases are not due to disease but to problems with digestive function.*

## Indigestion

*As many as half of the people seen by a gastroenterologist (a doctor who specializes in disorders of the digestive system) have indigestion but no evidence of disease. Most of these people have irritable bowel syndrome.*

## Irritable bowel syndrome

*Some doctors believe that emotional stress can precipitate irritable bowel syndrome (see* IRRITABLE BOWEL SYNDROME *on page 123). The symptoms of irritable bowel syndrome vary, but in most cases produce intermittent, cramplike abdominal pain, bloating, and irregular bowel habits (diarrhea and/or constipation). These symptoms can also be a normal reaction to a single episode of stress in many people who do not have this condition.*

## PHYSICAL STRESS DISORDERS

Acute peptic ulcers, commonly called stress ulcers, often occur in people suffering from severe injuries, burns, infections, or shock. Erosive gastritis (inflammation and superficial ulceration of the stomach lining) may occur in up to 90 percent of people who are critically ill and receiving intensive care. Most cases of erosive gastritis develop about 24 hours after the physical trauma.

# YOUR DIGESTIVE TRACT'S OWN NERVOUS SYSTEM

In a sense, your digestive tract has its own nervous system, called the enteric nervous system, made up of more than 5 million nerve cells. This nervous system can initiate and transmit signals within the digestive tract independently of the brain. The enteric nervous system determines the pattern of muscular contraction at every point along your digestive tract. Infection or inflammation of the digestive tract may disrupt the workings of this nervous system.

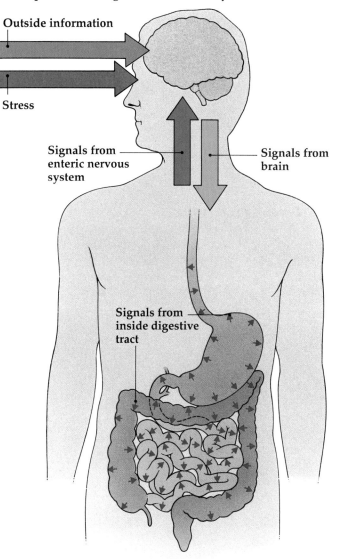

**Outside information**

**Stress**

**Signals from enteric nervous system**

**Signals from brain**

**Signals from inside digestive tract**

## The brain/digestive tract link

*The brain stays informed of what is happening in the digestive tract by way of impulses that pass along branches of the vagus nerve. The brain processes this information, along with information from the outside world, and passes instructions back down the vagus nerve to the enteric nervous system. Stress may cause more frequent or more alarming instructions to pass from the brain to the enteric nervous system, disrupting digestive tract function.*

## DIET

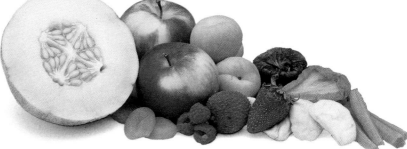

Your digestive system receives and processes the food you eat, absorbs nutrients, and eliminates waste products. Your eating habits – which include not only what you eat but also how much you eat and the way you eat – all affect your digestive system's functions and occasionally produce symptoms. Too much of any food – even healthy foods – can cause digestive problems. For example, beans contain large quantities of certain carbohydrates that are poorly absorbed. These carbohydrates remain largely undigested when they pass into the colon. The residue becomes fermented by bacteria, producing large quantities of gas.

### Food intolerance and allergy

Some people develop unwanted symptoms when they eat foods that most people can easily digest. These people are said to have a food intolerance. For example, some people cannot digest milk because they do not have enough of the enzyme necessary for the digestion of lactose, the main sugar found in milk (see LACTOSE INTOLERANCE on page 11). Other foods that can provoke digestive symptoms include albumin (egg white) and shellfish. Symptoms result from an inability to digest these foods rather than from an allergy. In true food allergy,

substances in food trigger an allergic response from the immune system. Even a trace can cause severe symptoms. Food allergy affects only about 1 percent of children and adults. Food intolerance is more common, affecting about 20 percent of children in the US.

### Inadequate diet

Diets that do not contain enough nutrients, including vitamins and minerals, can cause a variety of disorders throughout the body. For example, anemia can be caused by a lack of folic acid, a vitamin found in leafy green vegetables. Symptoms of anemia include inflammation of the tongue, diarrhea, and mental confusion. Diets that contain inadequate amounts of fiber often lead to constipation because the feces lack bulk. Many minor digestive tract conditions probably result from a lack of dietary fiber. Low-fiber diets can also produce more serious digestive tract problems, including

**Fiber and health**
*Dietary fiber consists of those parts of plant food that cannot be broken down by enzymes in the human digestive system. Fiber is a valuable component of a healthy diet because it helps to maintain bowel function and prevents constipation. Fiber achieves this by absorbing water during digestion, ensuring that the feces are soft and easy to pass. High-fiber foods include most fruits and vegetables and whole-grain breads and cereals.*

**Adverse reactions to food**
*Some people experience adverse reactions to substances in certain foods, such as seafood and milk. They develop characteristic symptoms, such as facial flushing, itching, and swelling of the face and throat, whenever they eat foods containing these substances. Rashes, such as urticaria (which produces the itchy patches shown at right), are also common.*

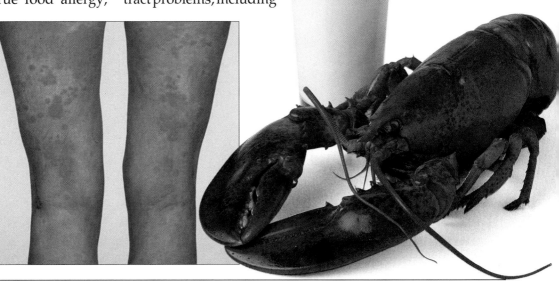

hemorrhoids, hernias, and diverticular disease. These problems are caused or aggravated by the excessive straining required to expel stools. To avoid such problems, you should consume a diet that contains plenty of fiber and eat a wide variety of naturally occurring foods. No strict rules exist about the frequency or size of meals, unless a bowel disease is already present. For a healthy person, the type of food eaten is more important than when it is eaten.

## DRUGS

Almost all drugs have side effects, and many drugs adversely affect the digestive tract. Antibiotics can irritate the lining of the intestine and cause diarrhea, one of the most common side effects of prescribed medications. Nonsteroidal anti-inflammatory drugs (NSAIDs), such as aspirin; potassium supplements; and corticosteroid drugs can irritate the lining of both the stomach and the intestine, producing indigestion, nausea, vomiting, and diarrhea. In severe cases, NSAIDs can cause bleeding from stomach ulcers or erosions, resulting in anemia and even life-threatening bleeding.

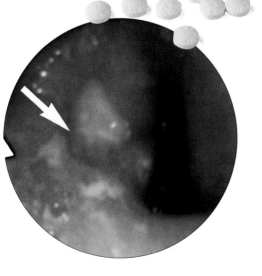

**Ulceration of the digestive tract**
*NSAIDs, such as aspirin, sometimes damage the esophagus or stomach. Such drugs can act on the lining of these organs to produce gastric erosions, ulceration (arrow at left), and bleeding. Ulceration (shown at left) is most common in older people taking NSAIDs because the stomach's protective mechanisms deteriorate gradually with age.*

## ASK YOUR DOCTOR
### INDIGESTION

**Q** **When I finish a meal, I seem to have an uncomfortable feeling of fullness, even though I don't eat very much. What could be wrong?**

**A** You may be eating your food so quickly that you swallow a lot of air with each mouthful, distending your stomach. Rich foods, such as gravy, that have a high fat content delay the movement of food from your stomach into your intestine, which can add to your discomfort. Try to eat slowly, allow yourself to relax after your meal to help you digest it, and avoid high-fat foods.

**Q** **I often have indigestion after meals. My mother says I should adopt a diet of milk and other bland foods. Is this true?**

**A** No. The belief that people with digestive tract disorders should eat only bland foods has long been abandoned. Consume small meals four or five times a day and consult your doctor if your symptoms of indigestion last more than 2 or 3 weeks.

**Q** **I have been under a lot of pressure at work lately. I feel bloated almost immediately after eating and recently have been getting heartburn regularly. Are these symptoms related to stress?**

**A** Possibly. You may be suffering from nervous indigestion, which is a common symptom in people who are under too much stress. Try not to rush when eating so you do not swallow air along with your food. When you feel the heartburn coming on, you can take an antacid, but if your symptoms persist, see your doctor to rule out the possibility of a peptic ulcer.

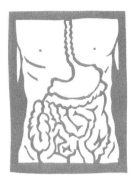

# NONSPECIFIC SYMPTOMS

DIGESTIVE TRACT SYMPTOMS affect almost everyone from time to time. Often, they do not indicate disease and are nothing to worry about. Most clear up on their own. But persistent symptoms, or those for which you cannot establish a cause, may signal a serious illness and should be investigated by your doctor.

Doctors usually label digestive tract symptoms as either specific or nonspecific (general). Specific symptoms can be pinpointed to a certain part of the digestive tract. Nonspecific symptoms, such as weight loss, may not be related to a particular part of the digestive system. Usually, a combination of symptoms alerts a doctor to a particular diagnosis.

## TYPES OF SYMPTOMS

Although nonspecific symptoms of the digestive tract suggest digestive tract disease, they can also indicate a disorder somewhere else in the body. Often, these symptoms do not help doctors locate the specific site of the illness. When making

## ABDOMINAL DISTENTION

Distention (swelling) of the abdomen may arise from a number of factors, but the most common are obesity, fluid, gas, feces, or pregnancy. Your doctor must establish whether you have visible abdominal distention or simply the sensation of distention without swelling. A feeling of distention without visible swelling can be caused by your stomach or colon failing to relax enough to hold their contents.

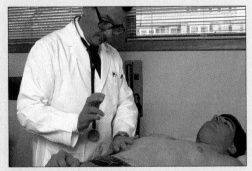

**Percussion of the abdomen**
*A doctor can distinguish fluid in the abdomen from gas by tapping the abdomen. This procedure is called percussion. Fluid gives off a dull sound, and gas produces a drumlike sound.*

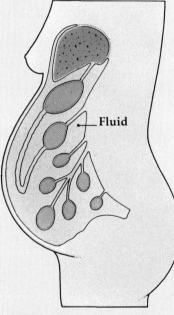

**Fluid**
*The presence of fluid in the abdominal spaces (peritoneal cavity) is called ascites. It is usually a result of severe liver disease, as pictured above, or of a cancer in the abdominal cavity. It can also accompany heart disease or kidney failure.*

**Pregnancy**
*A doctor always considers the possibility of pregnancy in any woman of child-bearing age who experiences abdominal swelling. The woman pictured below is about 5 months pregnant. Her abdomen is becoming enlarged.*

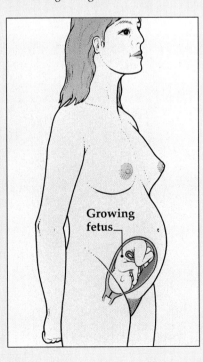

Growing fetus

a diagnosis, doctors note general symptoms along with more specific symptoms, such as pain in a certain location, to try to determine if these symptoms follow a pattern.

## Loss of appetite

Loss of appetite is a nonspecific bodily response to many diseases, from anxiety and depression to viral infections or life-threatening cancers. The importance of the loss of appetite depends on how long it lasts and whether you have any accompanying symptoms or problems.

## Weight loss

If you have a healthy appetite, weight loss is a serious nonspecific symptom. Explanations for weight loss can include an increased demand by your body for energy. This can occur with an overactive thyroid gland. Another cause is malabsorption of food. If weight loss arises from malabsorption of food, feces will be bulky, greasy, and yellow or gray in color and may contain recognizable pieces of food. Weight loss is also a late symptom of many cancers. If you have a poor appetite, weight loss is a natural consequence of inadequate food intake.

## Nausea and vomiting

The feeling of nausea with or without vomiting cannot be used to diagnose a specific disease. These symptoms can have many causes, from disturbed brain function to obstruction of the digestive tract. A single episode of nausea and vomiting can result from acute gastroenteritis (inflammation of the stomach lining), excess alcohol consumption, treatment with anticancer drugs, or stress. Frequent nausea and/or vomiting should be investigated by your doctor.

### TYPES OF ABDOMINAL PAIN

Digestive tract obstruction, or a stone stuck in the bile duct, causes a strong, spasmodic pain. Sudden, severe pain can arise from perforation of the digestive tract wall. Recurrent abdominal pain often signals digestive tract dysfunction that may not be serious. If sudden abdominal pain is caused by a serious digestive tract disorder, symptoms such as fever, vomiting, and distention also usually occur.

**Obesity**
*The body commonly stores excess fat in the abdomen, within the greater omentum (a membrane in front of the intestines). This explains why overweight people often have large abdomens that may look swollen (see illustration below).*

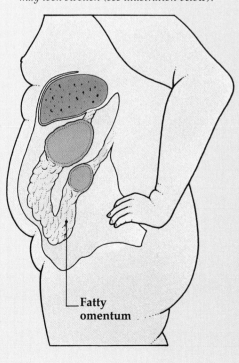

Fatty omentum

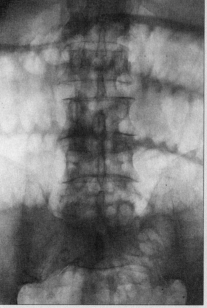

**Gas**
*Gaseous distention of the small intestine (see X-ray above) signals obstruction of the small intestine. A bowel obstruction needs immediate medical intervention. But excess gas usually arises after swallowing air or from bacterial fermentation of food residue in the colon. Belching or passing of gas is normal.*

**Impacted feces**
*Excessive impaction of feces in the rectum and colon produces abdominal distention. Swelling occurs as stool accumulates throughout the intestine (see arrows below).*

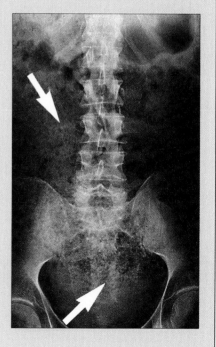

# ABDOMINAL PAIN

Abdominal pain is the term that describes any feeling of discomfort in the abdominal cavity, which extends from the pelvis to the lower border of the ribs. The pain may originate in the skin, muscles, or peritoneum (lining of the abdominal cavity), or from the organs inside the cavity.

## ABDOMINAL REGIONS

For the sake of convenience, doctors usually describe abdominal pain by the site or sites at which it is predominantly felt. For this purpose, they divide the abdomen into seven areas, including four quadrants.

**Right upper quadrant**
*Pain in the right upper quadrant is intense and spasmodic. Pain in this region is commonly caused by an inflamed gallbladder or a trapped gallstone, which also causes nausea, vomiting, and fever. The pain often spreads around the edge of the ribs and toward the center of the abdomen (epigastric area). It then penetrates through to the back.*

**Umbilical area**
*The umbilical area is centered at the navel. Disorders of the small intestine can cause pain in this area.*

**Right lower quadrant**
*The intense, localized pain of the later stage of appendicitis usually occurs in the right lower quadrant. Pain from an irritable colon is comparatively milder and shorter in duration, and relief comes with the passage of gas or stool. In women, pain in both the right and left lower quadrants can occur at the time of ovulation. It can also be caused by diseases of the ovaries or fallopian tubes.*

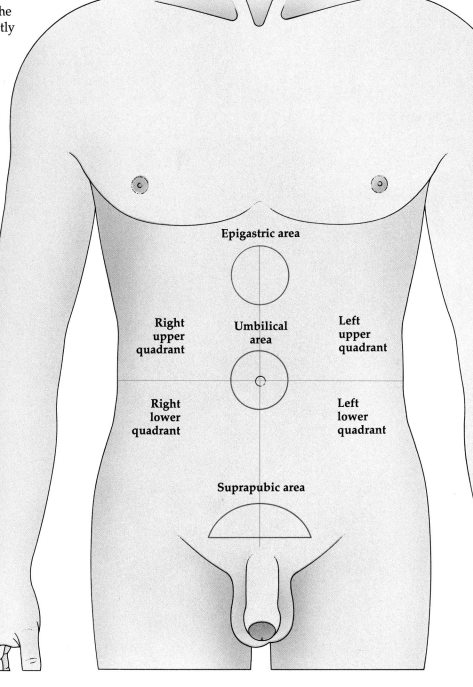

Epigastric area

Right upper quadrant

Umbilical area

Left upper quadrant

Right lower quadrant

Left lower quadrant

Suprapubic area

**Left upper quadrant**
*Pain in the left upper quadrant is uncommon. It may occasionally signal a disorder of the colon.*

**Epigastric area**
*Digestive tract pain in the epigastric area usually arises from stomach acid, causing inflammation or ulceration of the esophagus, stomach, or duodenum. Pain felt at this site also arises from a disorder of the pancreas, such as pancreatitis (inflammation of the pancreas) or cancer.*

**Suprapubic area**
*The suprapubic area is centered in the region around the pubic bone. Pain in the suprapubic area may indicate disorders of the colon but more often results from a lower urinary tract infection.*

**Left lower quadrant**
*Left lower quadrant pain can indicate a disturbance of the descending and sigmoid colons. For example, an irritable colon causes pain relieved by the passage of gas or stool, while diverticulitis produces a more constant pain. Although left lower quadrant pain can indicate serious disease, it more commonly accompanies less serious conditions, such as diverticulosis or irritable colon.*

# RADIATING AND REFERRED PAIN

Pain that originates in specific abdominal locations can spread, or radiate, to other areas of the abdomen. You may even feel it in other areas of your body, some of them far from the source. This phenomenon is known as referred pain. It occurs because sensory nerves from the abdomen also supply certain other areas of the body. Nerve impulses reaching the brain from the abdomen may be misinterpreted as coming from somewhere else.

**Gallbladder pain**
Pain caused by a trapped gallstone or an inflamed gallbladder can radiate to the back between the shoulder blades or to the tip of the right shoulder blade or right shoulder.

**Duodenal ulcer pain**
The pain from a duodenal ulcer may radiate to the middle of the back, particularly if the ulcer has penetrated the back wall of the duodenum and entered the pancreas.

**Pancreatic pain**
The pain of pancreatitis (inflammation of the pancreas) may radiate to the left side, just below the ribs. It may be severe. Pain from pancreatic cancer can be felt in the middle of the back and can even extend up between the shoulder blades.

**Kidney pain**
Pain from an infected kidney or severe, fluctuating pain from a kidney stone passing down one of the two ureters can begin in the outer part of the back above the waist. These types of pain may also be felt in the groin, the tip of the penis, or the scrotum.

**Large bowel pain**
Irritable bowel syndrome, inflammatory bowel disease, and other disorders of the large intestine can cause general lower back pain.

# MONITOR YOUR SYMPTOMS
# RECURRENT ABDOMINAL PAIN

Consult this chart if you have abdominal pain (between the bottom of your ribcage and your groin) that comes and goes but always feels the same. Most cases of recurrent abdominal pain signal long-standing digestive problems. Your doctor may treat these problems with drugs and suggest that you change your eating and bowel habits. Early diagnosis can exclude the slight possibility of serious underlying digestive system or reproductive organ disease.

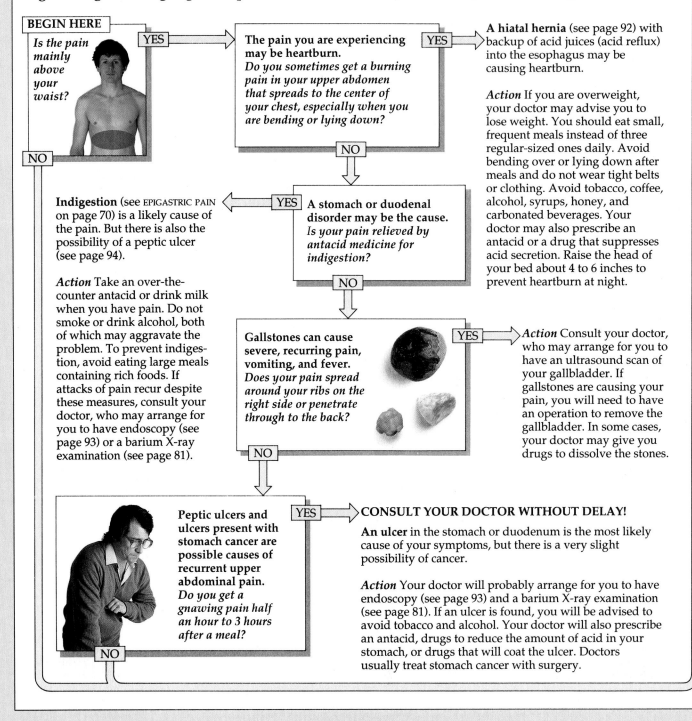

**BEGIN HERE**

*Is the pain mainly above your waist?*

YES

**The pain you are experiencing may be heartburn.**
*Do you sometimes get a burning pain in your upper abdomen that spreads to the center of your chest, especially when you are bending or lying down?*

YES

**A hiatal hernia** (see page 92) with backup of acid juices (acid reflux) into the esophagus may be causing heartburn.

*Action* If you are overweight, your doctor may advise you to lose weight. You should eat small, frequent meals instead of three regular-sized ones daily. Avoid bending over or lying down after meals and do not wear tight belts or clothing. Avoid tobacco, coffee, alcohol, syrups, honey, and carbonated beverages. Your doctor may also prescribe an antacid or a drug that suppresses acid secretion. Raise the head of your bed about 4 to 6 inches to prevent heartburn at night.

NO

**Indigestion** (see EPIGASTRIC PAIN on page 70) is a likely cause of the pain. But there is also the possibility of a peptic ulcer (see page 94).

*Action* Take an over-the-counter antacid or drink milk when you have pain. Do not smoke or drink alcohol, both of which may aggravate the problem. To prevent indigestion, avoid eating large meals containing rich foods. If attacks of pain recur despite these measures, consult your doctor, who may arrange for you to have endoscopy (see page 93) or a barium X-ray examination (see page 81).

YES

**A stomach or duodenal disorder may be the cause.**
*Is your pain relieved by antacid medicine for indigestion?*

NO

**Gallstones can cause severe, recurring pain, vomiting, and fever.**
*Does your pain spread around your ribs on the right side or penetrate through to the back?*

YES

*Action* Consult your doctor, who may arrange for you to have an ultrasound scan of your gallbladder. If gallstones are causing your pain, you will need to have an operation to remove the gallbladder. In some cases, your doctor may give you drugs to dissolve the stones.

NO

**Peptic ulcers and ulcers present with stomach cancer are possible causes of recurrent upper abdominal pain.**
*Do you get a gnawing pain half an hour to 3 hours after a meal?*

YES

**CONSULT YOUR DOCTOR WITHOUT DELAY!**

**An ulcer** in the stomach or duodenum is the most likely cause of your symptoms, but there is a very slight possibility of cancer.

*Action* Your doctor will probably arrange for you to have endoscopy (see page 93) and a barium X-ray examination (see page 81). If an ulcer is found, you will be advised to avoid tobacco and alcohol. Your doctor will also prescribe an antacid, drugs to reduce the amount of acid in your stomach, or drugs that will coat the ulcer. Doctors usually treat stomach cancer with surgery.

NO

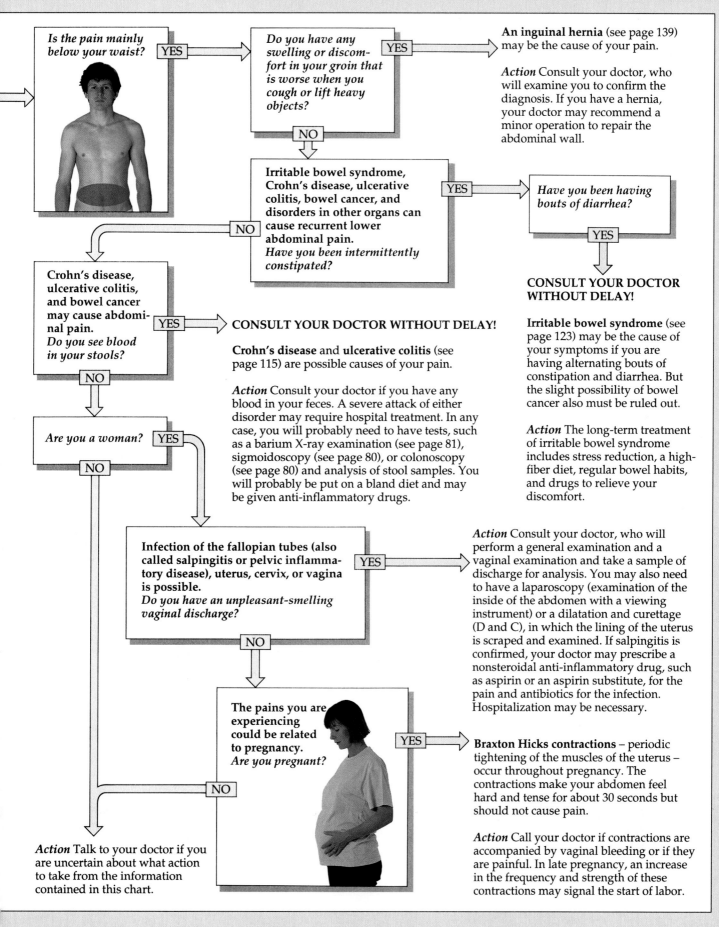

**Is the pain mainly below your waist?** — YES →

**Do you have any swelling or discomfort in your groin that is worse when you cough or lift heavy objects?** — YES →

**An inguinal hernia** (see page 139) may be the cause of your pain.

*Action* Consult your doctor, who will examine you to confirm the diagnosis. If you have a hernia, your doctor may recommend a minor operation to repair the abdominal wall.

— NO ↓

**Irritable bowel syndrome, Crohn's disease, ulcerative colitis, bowel cancer, and disorders in other organs can cause recurrent lower abdominal pain.** *Have you been intermittently constipated?* — YES →

**Have you been having bouts of diarrhea?** — YES ↓

**CONSULT YOUR DOCTOR WITHOUT DELAY!**

**Irritable bowel syndrome** (see page 123) may be the cause of your symptoms if you are having alternating bouts of constipation and diarrhea. But the slight possibility of bowel cancer also must be ruled out.

*Action* The long-term treatment of irritable bowel syndrome includes stress reduction, a high-fiber diet, regular bowel habits, and drugs to relieve your discomfort.

— NO →

**Crohn's disease, ulcerative colitis, and bowel cancer may cause abdominal pain.** *Do you see blood in your stools?* — YES →

**CONSULT YOUR DOCTOR WITHOUT DELAY!**

**Crohn's disease** and **ulcerative colitis** (see page 115) are possible causes of your pain.

*Action* Consult your doctor if you have any blood in your feces. A severe attack of either disorder may require hospital treatment. In any case, you will probably need to have tests, such as a barium X-ray examination (see page 81), sigmoidoscopy (see page 80), or colonoscopy (see page 80) and analysis of stool samples. You will probably be put on a bland diet and may be given anti-inflammatory drugs.

— NO ↓

**Are you a woman?** — YES →

— NO ↓

**Infection of the fallopian tubes (also called salpingitis or pelvic inflammatory disease), uterus, cervix, or vagina is possible.** *Do you have an unpleasant-smelling vaginal discharge?* — YES →

*Action* Consult your doctor, who will perform a general examination and a vaginal examination and take a sample of discharge for analysis. You may also need to have a laparoscopy (examination of the inside of the abdomen with a viewing instrument) or a dilatation and curettage (D and C), in which the lining of the uterus is scraped and examined. If salpingitis is confirmed, your doctor may prescribe a nonsteroidal anti-inflammatory drug, such as aspirin or an aspirin substitute, for the pain and antibiotics for the infection. Hospitalization may be necessary.

— NO ↓

**The pains you are experiencing could be related to pregnancy.** *Are you pregnant?* — YES →

**Braxton Hicks contractions** – periodic tightening of the muscles of the uterus – occur throughout pregnancy. The contractions make your abdomen feel hard and tense for about 30 seconds but should not cause pain.

*Action* Call your doctor if contractions are accompanied by vaginal bleeding or if they are painful. In late pregnancy, an increase in the frequency and strength of these contractions may signal the start of labor.

— NO →

*Action* Talk to your doctor if you are uncertain about what action to take from the information contained in this chart.

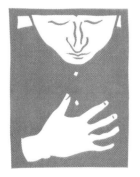

# UPPER DIGESTIVE TRACT SYMPTOMS

YOUR UPPER DIGESTIVE TRACT includes your mouth, esophagus, stomach, and duodenum (the first part of the small intestine). From time to time, everyone experiences some discomfort or isolated symptoms in these areas. Patterns of symptoms often indicate specific disorders, but no clear-cut diagnosis can be made without a careful examination by your doctor.

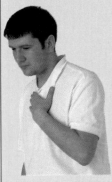

Most symptoms that occur in the upper digestive tract signal minor disorders. For example, painful swallowing often suggests nothing more serious than a sore throat. Other symptoms may be brought on by a temporary case of food poisoning or a viral infection. But some problems indicate a more serious condition. Only by taking a complete history of your symptoms and performing certain tests can your doctor reach a definite diagnosis.

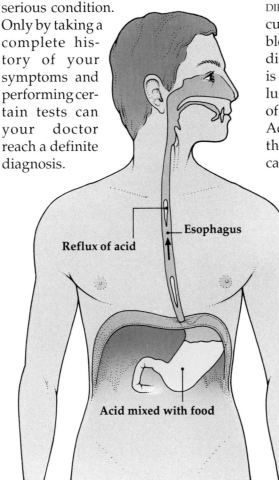

**Reflux of acid**

**Esophagus**

**Acid mixed with food**

## SYMPTOMS IN THE THROAT AND ESOPHAGUS

Many people experience symptoms in the throat and esophagus. You may feel as if food is sticking in either your throat or your chest (see the symptoms chart DIFFICULTY SWALLOWING on page 69). Difficulty swallowing can be caused by a blockage, a throat infection, or a nerve disorder (because the act of swallowing is partially controlled by the brain). A lump in your throat may be a symptom of anxiety. Chest pain can also occur. Acid reflux, the movement of acid from the stomach up into the esophagus, causes pain in the upper part of the abdomen, chest, and throat as the acid bathes the lining of the esophagus. If the reflux is persistent and severe, inflammation of the esophagus can occur. This inflammation can cause a spasm in the muscle of the esophagus, sometimes resulting in the burning sensation known as heartburn.

**Acid reflux**
*Acid reflux can occur even in healthy people if they eat a large meal and lie down immediately after eating. Reflux may be caused by decreased tone (relaxation) of the muscles at the junction of the esophagus and the stomach. If you experience reflux, do not overfill your stomach and avoid syrupy and carbonated drinks.*

# MONITOR YOUR SYMPTOMS
# DIFFICULTY SWALLOWING

Painful or difficult swallowing is usually caused by an infection that produces soreness, swelling, and excess mucus at the back of the throat. Persistent difficult or painful swallowing that is unrelated to a sore throat should be evaluated by your doctor.

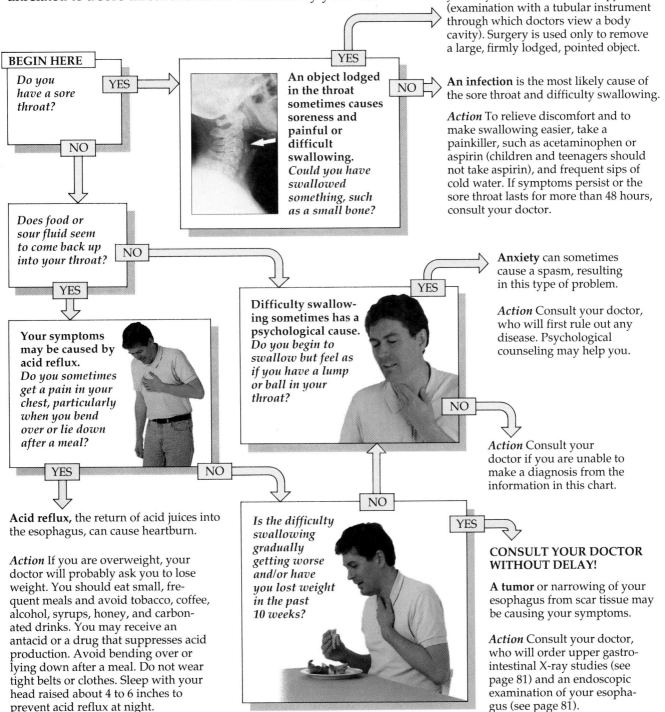

**BEGIN HERE**

*Do you have a sore throat?*

YES →

NO ↓

**An object lodged in the throat sometimes causes soreness and painful or difficult swallowing.** *Could you have swallowed something, such as a small bone?*

YES

NO →

*Action* Consult your doctor, who will examine your throat and possibly remove the object at the same time. If he or she cannot pinpoint the problem, you may need to have endoscopy (examination with a tubular instrument through which doctors view a body cavity). Surgery is used only to remove a large, firmly lodged, pointed object.

**An infection** is the most likely cause of the sore throat and difficulty swallowing.

*Action* To relieve discomfort and to make swallowing easier, take a painkiller, such as acetaminophen or aspirin (children and teenagers should not take aspirin), and frequent sips of cold water. If symptoms persist or the sore throat lasts for more than 48 hours, consult your doctor.

*Does food or sour fluid seem to come back up into your throat?*

NO →

YES ↓

**Difficulty swallowing sometimes has a psychological cause.** *Do you begin to swallow but feel as if you have a lump or ball in your throat?*

YES

NO →

**Anxiety** can sometimes cause a spasm, resulting in this type of problem.

*Action* Consult your doctor, who will first rule out any disease. Psychological counseling may help you.

*Action* Consult your doctor if you are unable to make a diagnosis from the information in this chart.

**Your symptoms may be caused by acid reflux.** *Do you sometimes get a pain in your chest, particularly when you bend over or lie down after a meal?*

YES ↓

NO →

*Is the difficulty swallowing gradually getting worse and/or have you lost weight in the past 10 weeks?*

NO ↑

YES →

**Acid reflux,** the return of acid juices into the esophagus, can cause heartburn.

*Action* If you are overweight, your doctor will probably ask you to lose weight. You should eat small, frequent meals and avoid tobacco, coffee, alcohol, syrups, honey, and carbonated drinks. You may receive an antacid or a drug that suppresses acid production. Avoid bending over or lying down after a meal. Do not wear tight belts or clothes. Sleep with your head raised about 4 to 6 inches to prevent acid reflux at night.

**CONSULT YOUR DOCTOR WITHOUT DELAY!**

**A tumor** or narrowing of your esophagus from scar tissue may be causing your symptoms.

*Action* Consult your doctor, who will order upper gastrointestinal X-ray studies (see page 81) and an endoscopic examination of your esophagus (see page 81).

# EPIGASTRIC PAIN

Pain felt in the center of the highest part of the abdomen is called epigastric pain. Such pain is a common problem that people often describe as indigestion. It may be accompanied by a feeling of nausea or a gnawing, hungry feeling that cannot be traced to a definite location. Epigastric pain can originate in the lower end of the esophagus, stomach, and duodenum and occasionally in the biliary system (the structures that convey bile) and pancreas. Possible causes include peptic esophagitis (inflammation of the esophagus by stomach juices), ulcers of the duodenum and stomach, and pancreatitis. The presence of other symptoms often helps the doctor pinpoint the problem to a particular organ.

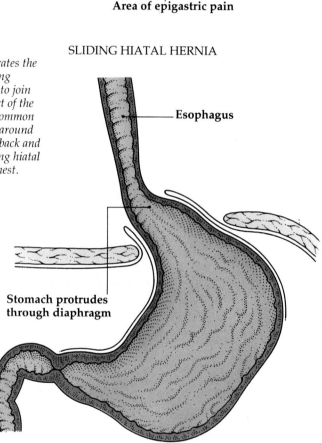

**Area of epigastric pain**

ANATOMY OF
NORMAL STOMACH

**Hiatal hernia**
*The diaphragm is a sheet of muscle that separates the chest from the abdomen. It contains an opening (hiatus) through which the esophagus passes to join the stomach. A hiatal hernia occurs when part of the stomach protrudes through this opening. A common type of hiatal hernia occurs when the muscle around the hiatus allows part of the stomach to slide back and forth between the abdomen and chest. A sliding hiatal hernia produces a burning sensation in the chest.*

SLIDING HIATAL HERNIA

**Esophagus**

Diaphragm

**Stomach protrudes
through diaphragm**

Stomach

**Inflamed pancreas**

**Pain from the pancreas**
*Epigastric pain can originate in the pancreas. A sudden, severe pain accompanied by other symptoms, such as vomiting and abdominal distention, can indicate acute inflammation of the pancreas (pancreatitis, right), which is a medical emergency. Chronic (long-lasting or recurrent) pancreatitis can cause epigastric pain that sometimes spreads to the back. The condition brings on other symptoms, such as pale, fatty stools and increased production of urine, with thirst and weight loss.*

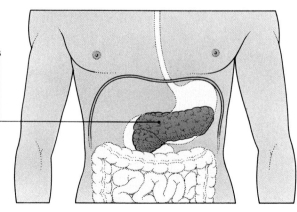

## Peptic ulcers

*Peptic ulcers are open sores in the lining of the digestive tract that can develop when the lining is exposed to acid and the digestive enzyme pepsin. The acid can destroy the lining of the stomach and duodenum. All peptic ulcers produce intermittent epigastric pain that may radiate through to the back.*

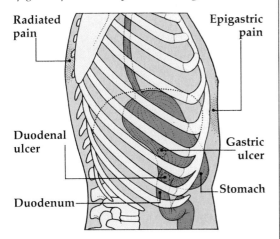

Radiated pain

Epigastric pain

Duodenal ulcer

Gastric ulcer

Duodenum

Stomach

## Stomach cancer

*In rare cases, epigastric pain is caused by stomach cancer, a malignant tumor (see arrow at right) that appears in the lining of the stomach. An ulcerating stomach cancer produces symptoms that are very similar to those caused by a peptic ulcer.*

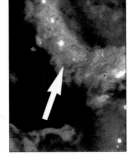

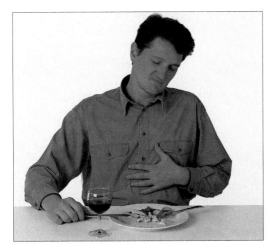

## Indigestion

*Indigestion, or dyspepsia, is characterized by such upper gastrointestinal tract symptoms as belching, bloating, a feeling of fullness, nausea, heartburn, and sometimes vague epigastric pain. Such symptoms without pain are not usually caused by disease.*

# EPIGASTRIC PAIN UNRELATED TO THE DIGESTIVE SYSTEM

Although epigastric pain often arises from a disorder of the upper digestive tract, it may also be a sign of heart disease. Your doctor should always investigate such pain to rule out this possibility.

### Angina

*Angina is chest pain that extends to the arms and may also radiate to the epigastric area (below right). At rest, no pain may be felt. During exercise (below) and stress, especially after a meal, the heart's demand for oxygen increases. If the demand is not fulfilled, pain occurs.*

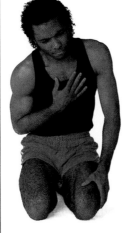

**Area of epigastric pain**

### Coronary thrombosis

*Coronary thrombosis, a blocking of one of the coronary arteries, deprives the heart muscle of oxygen. Such a blockage can be fatal. Its most common symptom is a severe, crushing pain in the chest, which may begin in the epigastric area. The diagram below shows how a blood clot can block an artery. The photograph at right shows the structure of a blood clot.*

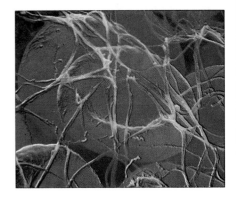

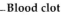

**Blood clot**

# BELCHING

Each time you swallow food, liquids, or saliva, you also swallow air. Belching is the expulsion of this air from your stomach. Belching once or twice soon after a meal is normal. It can be intensified by eating or drinking too quickly, consuming carbonated drinks, or taking antacid drugs. Antacids react with acid in the stomach to form carbon dioxide, which you then expel in a belch. Belching can also result from anxiety, if you swallow excess amounts of air when you are stressed. Belching accompanies indigestion, sometimes producing a recurring cycle of swallowing air, discomfort, belching, relief, and swallowing more air. During pregnancy, belching often accompanies nausea and heartburn. A hormone released during pregnancy relaxes the gastroesophageal junction. This process irritates the esophagus, causing belching and nausea.

**Is belching normal?**
*When you eat, you swallow air along with your food. It is normal for excess air to be expelled by belching. But if you belch frequently, persistently, and loudly, or if the air expelled is foul smelling, you should consult your doctor.*

Gas

**How do you hiccup?**
*When you hiccup, your diaphragm involuntarily contracts, causing an intake of breath that is suddenly checked by the epiglottis (a structure over the opening to your larynx, or voice box). This action produces the characteristic sound of the hiccup as the column of incoming air is suddenly stopped.*

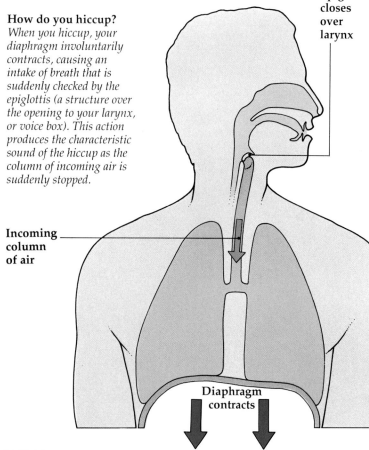

Epiglottis closes over larynx

Incoming column of air

Diaphragm contracts

# HICCUPS

Intermittent, sudden, involuntary contractions of the diaphragm, followed by a rapid closing of the epiglottis over the vocal cords, produces the sound we call hiccups. Hiccups are normal and almost all attacks of hiccups last for only a few minutes. Hiccups can occur when something irritates the diaphragm or the nerves that control it. Many home remedies for hiccups exist, but doctors know of no single effective treatment.

Frequent, persistent hiccups can lead to exhaustion in extreme cases and can result from a disorder of the nervous system or the kidneys. In rare cases, they are caused by irritation of the diaphragm from disorders such as pancreatitis, hepatitis, or inflammation of the esophagus by stomach juices.

# VOMITING

Vomiting is the involuntary, forcible ejection of the stomach contents through the esophagus and mouth. Vomiting is a common symptom that accompanies many minor stomach problems and is not a sign of serious disease unless it is recurrent, prolonged, or accompanied by severe pain, or contains blood (see the symptoms chart VOMITING on page 74). Vomiting can be brought on by high levels of certain substances in the blood (such as hormones during pregnancy and some poisons, bacterial toxins, and drugs) or by increased pressure inside the skull from fluid accumulation in the brain caused by a tumor or inflammation. It can also accompany disturbances of the balance center in the inner ear.

**Causes of fecal vomiting**
*Vomiting of foul-smelling intestinal contents is rare. It is usually caused by a fistula, an abnormal passage between organs of the upper digestive tract and the colon (below).*

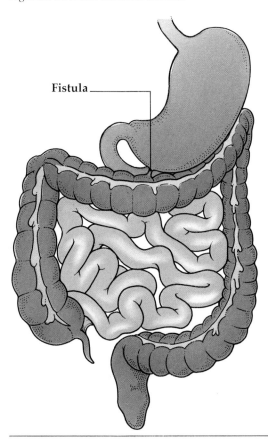

Fistula

**Vomiting caused by pyloric obstruction**
*Pyloric obstruction is blockage of the pylorus, the outlet from the stomach to the duodenum. Causes of pyloric obstruction include scarring from a long-standing ulcer (pyloric stenosis) or, very rarely, a cancer that blocks the outlet (below). The obstruction blocks the passage of stomach secretions and food into the duodenum. It also causes the stomach to expand and involuntary vomiting may occur several hours after eating. People with this condition may vomit an entire day's intake of food in the evening.*

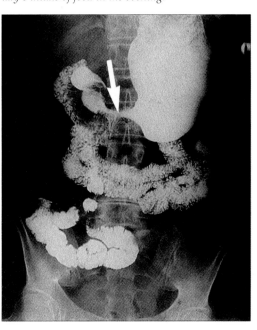

## What can you tell from the appearance of vomit?

It is normal for vomit to contain undigested food and clear, sour acid. The presence of bitter-tasting, green or green-brown bile in the vomit is caused by the return of bile from the duodenum into the stomach.

If your vomit is red or black or resembles coffee grounds, you should seek immediate medical care. These abnormal characteristics indicate the presence of fresh blood or partly digested blood, which may have come from bleeding in the upper gastrointestinal tract. Unusually foul-smelling vomit may indicate the regurgitation of intestinal contents (fecal vomiting). This condition can result from an abnormal channel between the intestinal wall and the stomach or from intestinal obstruction, which forces food back up the esophagus.

**ANTIEMETIC DRUGS**

Doctors sometimes use antiemetic drugs, such as prochlorperazine, to treat nausea and vomiting. The drugs work by suppressing the vomiting reflex at different sites in the brain. Some antiemetic drugs also increase muscle pressure in the lower esophagus and stimulate the muscles in the lower part of the stomach, allowing food to move into the small intestine. If vomiting accompanies vertigo (dizziness), doctors administer drugs that diminish nerve activity from the balance centers of the inner ear and the brain. These drugs also suppress the vomiting center in the brain stem. Antiemetic drugs should not be taken without medical advice, because they may mask a serious underlying disorder. Pregnant women who experience vomiting should use antiemetic drugs only when prescribed.

# MONITOR YOUR SYMPTOMS
# VOMITING

Vomiting occurs when the muscles of the stomach and abdomen suddenly contract and expel the stomach's contents. Vomiting usually signals irritation of the stomach from infection, overindulgence in rich food or alcohol, or the presence of drugs or poisons. It may also be triggered by nerve impulses sent to the brain from the stomach or elsewhere in the body or by toxic substances carried to the brain in the bloodstream. Occasionally, nerve signals that come from the brain, or from the balance mechanism in the inner ear, also induce vomiting. Vomiting that is prolonged or accompanied by severe abdominal pain, intense headache, or eye pain requires immediate medical attention.

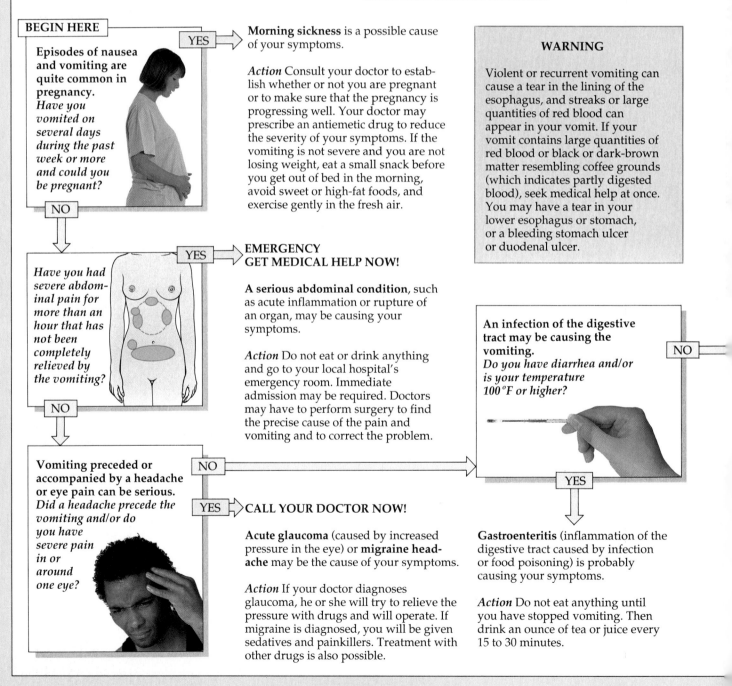

**BEGIN HERE**

**Episodes of nausea and vomiting are quite common in pregnancy.** *Have you vomited on several days during the past week or more and could you be pregnant?*

YES →

**Morning sickness** is a possible cause of your symptoms.

*Action* Consult your doctor to establish whether or not you are pregnant or to make sure that the pregnancy is progressing well. Your doctor may prescribe an antiemetic drug to reduce the severity of your symptoms. If the vomiting is not severe and you are not losing weight, eat a small snack before you get out of bed in the morning, avoid sweet or high-fat foods, and exercise gently in the fresh air.

NO ↓

*Have you had severe abdominal pain for more than an hour that has not been completely relieved by the vomiting?*

YES →

**EMERGENCY
GET MEDICAL HELP NOW!**

**A serious abdominal condition,** such as acute inflammation or rupture of an organ, may be causing your symptoms.

*Action* Do not eat or drink anything and go to your local hospital's emergency room. Immediate admission may be required. Doctors may have to perform surgery to find the precise cause of the pain and vomiting and to correct the problem.

NO ↓

**Vomiting preceded or accompanied by a headache or eye pain can be serious.** *Did a headache precede the vomiting and/or do you have severe pain in or around one eye?*

NO →

YES → **CALL YOUR DOCTOR NOW!**

**Acute glaucoma** (caused by increased pressure in the eye) or **migraine headache** may be the cause of your symptoms.

*Action* If your doctor diagnoses glaucoma, he or she will try to relieve the pressure with drugs and will operate. If migraine is diagnosed, you will be given sedatives and painkillers. Treatment with other drugs is also possible.

**WARNING**

Violent or recurrent vomiting can cause a tear in the lining of the esophagus, and streaks or large quantities of red blood can appear in your vomit. If your vomit contains large quantities of red blood or black or dark-brown matter resembling coffee grounds (which indicates partly digested blood), seek medical help at once. You may have a tear in your lower esophagus or stomach, or a bleeding stomach ulcer or duodenal ulcer.

**An infection of the digestive tract may be causing the vomiting.** *Do you have diarrhea and/or is your temperature 100°F or higher?*

NO →

YES ↓

**Gastroenteritis** (inflammation of the digestive tract caused by infection or food poisoning) is probably causing your symptoms.

*Action* Do not eat anything until you have stopped vomiting. Then drink an ounce of tea or juice every 15 to 30 minutes.

**Overindulgence in food is a possible cause.**
*In the past few hours, have you either overeaten or eaten spicy or rich foods (such as those containing butter or creamy sauces)?*

→ **YES** → **Acute indigestion** can easily occur after such overindulgence.

*Action* Follow the advice on treating vomiting (right). An over-the-counter antacid medication may help. Consult your doctor if you do not feel better within 24 hours.

**NO** ↓

**Drinking large quantities of alcohol in a short time can make you sick.**
*In the past few hours, have you consumed a large amount of alcohol?*

→ **YES** → **Inflammation** of the stomach lining by alcohol is possible.

*Action* Follow the advice on treating vomiting (above right). An over-the-counter antacid medication may help. Consult your doctor if you do not feel better within 24 hours.

**NO** ↓

**Food poisoning from contaminated food, or food to which you are allergic, can cause vomiting.**
*Have you eaten anything that may have gone bad or to which you may be allergic – for example, shellfish?*

→ **YES** → **Food poisoning** can result from food contaminated by bacteria or their toxins. **Food allergy** is a less common problem.

*Action* Follow the advice on treating vomiting (above right) and call your doctor.

**NO** →

**A disorder of the balance mechanism of the inner ear can cause vomiting and dizzy spells.**
*Before you vomited, did you feel dizzy and notice ringing in your ears?*

**YES** → *Action* Consult your doctor, who may recommend rest and prescribe antiemetic drugs. If your symptoms persist, you may have an inner-ear disorder, which requires testing.

**NO** →

**A disorder of the liver or gallstones may be the underlying cause of your vomiting.**
*Do the whites of your eyes or does your skin look yellow?*

**NO** / **YES**

**YES** ↓ **Jaundice** indicates a liver or gallbladder disorder.

*Action* Consult your doctor, who may order blood tests and possibly an ultrasound scan or a computed tomography (CT) scan. Treatment will depend on the underlying disorder.

**NO** ↓

**Certain medications can cause vomiting as a side effect.**
*Are you taking any medication?*

**YES** ↓ *Action* Discuss the problem with your doctor.

**NO** → *Action* Consult your doctor if you are unable to make a diagnosis from the information in this chart.

**TREATMENT FOR VOMITING**

If you have been vomiting and you suspect no serious cause, try the following self-help measures:
◆ Do not eat solid food for several hours after you have stopped vomiting.
◆ Drink clear (nonalcoholic) fluids in small sips at 15- to 30-minute intervals, once the nausea and vomiting subside.
◆ Do not smoke.
◆ Do not take aspirin.

If you vomit repeatedly for more than 6 hours or if other symptoms develop, call your doctor.

**WARNING**

If you are taking oral contraceptive pills and experience vomiting, your protection against conception may be reduced. Continue to take your pills as usual but use another form of contraception until you start a new cycle of pills.

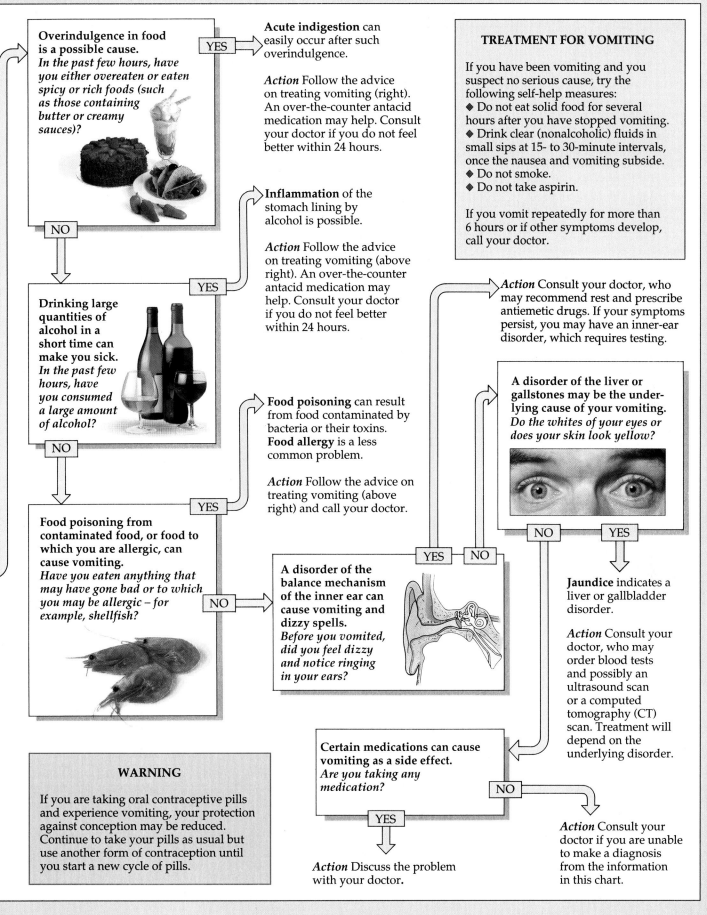

75

## THE VOMITING REFLEX

Vomiting occurs when the vomiting center in the brain is activated. This activation may be triggered by information coming from the brain, the bloodstream, or the digestive tract or by disturbances of the balancing mechanism in the inner ear. Once the vomiting center is activated, a precise sequence of events leads to the eventual propulsion of the stomach's contents through the mouth. Doctors call this sequence the vomiting reflex.

**1** The vomiting center in the brain stem is activated by the stimuli listed above. The vomiting center then sends nerve impulses toward the stomach and abdomen.

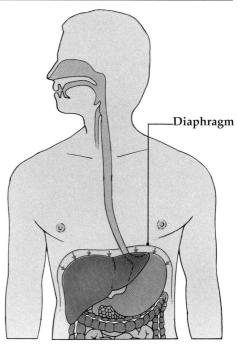

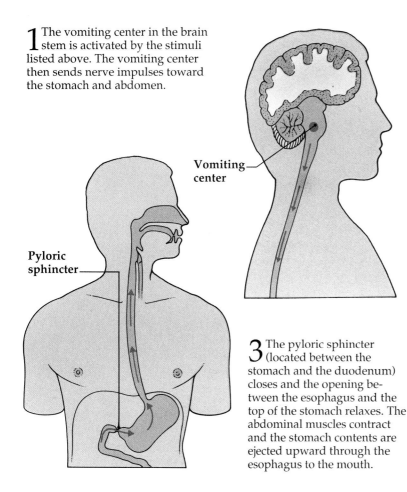

Vomiting center

Pyloric sphincter

**2** The nerve impulses cause the diaphragm to press down into the abdomen and stimulate the stomach wall to contract.

Diaphragm

**3** The pyloric sphincter (located between the stomach and the duodenum) closes and the opening between the esophagus and the top of the stomach relaxes. The abdominal muscles contract and the stomach contents are ejected upward through the esophagus to the mouth.

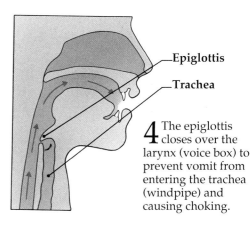

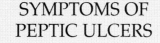

Epiglottis

Trachea

**4** The epiglottis closes over the larynx (voice box) to prevent vomit from entering the trachea (windpipe) and causing choking.

## SYMPTOMS OF PEPTIC ULCERS

Although some people with peptic ulcers have no symptoms, ulcers of both the stomach and duodenum often produce pain in the upper part of the abdomen (see EPIGASTRIC PAIN on page 70). The characteristics of the pain can help doctors distinguish one type of ulcer from the other. Stomach ulcers may cause pain soon after eating. Duodenal ulcers do not usually cause pain until 2 to 3 hours after eating. Vomiting, eating, or taking antacids usually relieves both types of ulcer pain temporarily. The pain of a duodenal ulcer often occurs between 1 and 3 AM, the only time the stomach secretes acid that is not neutralized by eating food. People with duodenal ulcers rarely lose weight unless they have pyloric stenosis (see page 73) and vomit frequently. Other symptoms that can accompany both types of ulcers include nausea, vomiting, and blood in the stools.

# CASE HISTORY
# FATIGUE AND PALLOR

**B**ETTY, WHO HAS SEVERE ARTHRITIS, **had become increasingly tired over the last few months. Her friends told her she looked pale. She noticed she was becoming breathless during even the slightest exertion and became worried about her ability to continue taking care of herself. She decided to see her doctor.**

**PERSONAL DETAILS**
**Name** Betty Griffith
**Age** 73
**Occupation** Retired attorney
**Family** Betty has lived alone since her husband died 2 years ago. She has had problems with her arthritis, but she is determined not to lose her independence.

## MEDICAL BACKGROUND
For several months Betty has been taking two or three aspirin four times a day to relieve the pain caused by the osteoarthritis that affects her hip, knees, and thumbs.

## THE CONSULTATION
Noticing how pale she looks, Betty's doctor asks her about the type of painkiller she has been using for her arthritis and discovers she has been taking a large quantity of aspirin. Betty says she has slight indigestion but she has never worried about it. During further questioning, she tells her doctor that the color of her stools has changed to black. She has never vomited blood. Examination of her abdomen reveals no abnormality.

## THE DOCTOR'S IMPRESSION
The doctor suspects that Betty is anemic from bleeding in her digestive tract. This suspicion is strengthened by her excessive use of aspirin, her obvious pallor, and the occurrence of black stools. Her breathlessness probably signals a failure of her depleted red blood cells to carry sufficient oxygen. The doctor obtains samples of her stools and blood and examines them.

**Gastroscopy**
*To confirm Betty's condition, the doctor visually examines the inside of her stomach with a fiberoptic endoscope (right). The instrument reveals multiple gastric erosions (above).*

## THE DIAGNOSIS
The blood test confirms that Betty is anemic. The test for blood in her stool sample is positive, confirming that she is losing blood from her digestive tract. The doctor believes that Betty's anemia is caused by GASTRIC EROSIONS resulting from her excessive aspirin intake. A gastric erosion is a superficial injury to the mucosa (innermost layer) of the stomach wall. These erosions can bleed slowly and persistently and often cause anemia. They can also bleed suddenly and heavily, causing a medical emergency.

## TREATMENT
Betty's doctor prescribes iron supplements to reverse her anemia. He recommends that she take acetaminophen for her arthritis pain because it is less likely to cause gastrointestinal bleeding. He also prescribes antacids and some ulcer-healing drugs. These medications help Betty's gastric erosions heal in a few days. Betty switches to acetaminophen, which relieves her arthritis pain as effectively as aspirin. The iron supplements restore Betty's vigor, and she resumes her daily activities with increased energy.

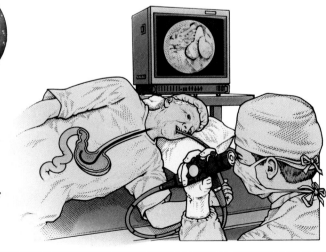

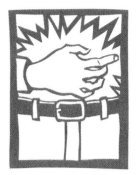

# LOWER DIGESTIVE TRACT SYMPTOMS

THE LOWER DIGESTIVE TRACT consists of the colon, rectum, and anal canal. The principal symptom produced by disorders of the lower digestive tract is a change in bowel habits, such as the development of diarrhea or constipation. Visible changes in the appearance of the feces may accompany many of these disorders.

Feces sometimes change in color, odor, consistency, or content. Dramatic changes may result from a harmless condition, but they sometimes indicate a serious digestive tract disorder. Talk to your doctor about any change in bowel habit or in the appearance of your feces that lasts for longer than a week.

## REPLACING LOST BODY FLUIDS

If you have watery diarrhea, you can rapidly become dehydrated. Children and older people are especially at risk. Call your doctor and replace lost body fluids by drinking at least 2 to 3 pints of rehydration solution every day until your diarrhea stops. If dehydration is severe, your doctor may administer fluids intravenously.

### WARNING

If you are taking oral contraceptive pills and have had diarrhea for more than 24 hours, your protection against conception may be reduced. Diarrhea can prevent your oral contraceptive from being absorbed through your intestines. To ensure that you are protected against conception, you should use an additional method of contraception for the remainder of your current menstrual cycle.

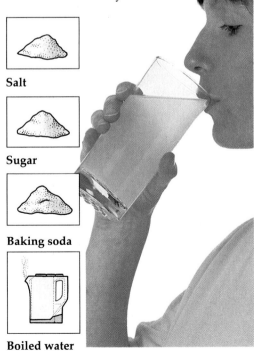

**Salt**

**Sugar**

**Baking soda**

**Boiled water**

## DIARRHEA

Doctors define diarrhea as the passing of loose and frequent bowel movements, but this definition requires further explanation. The sudden occurrence of profuse, watery stools and a frequent, urgent need to defecate is undoubtedly diarrhea. But the point at which normal stools become diarrhea is subject to individual interpretation. Most doctors agree that more than three soft or loose stools in a day constitute diarrhea.

### The influence of your diet

In part, the food you eat determines the volume and consistency of your feces and the frequency of your bowel movements. Most people regard one bowel movement a day as normal. But high-fiber diets can produce soft stools up to three times a day. People who consume large quantities of fiber may have even more frequent bowel movements.

Most diarrhea results from infection and lasts no more than 48 hours. Special treatment is rarely needed. You should report persistent or recurrent diarrhea to your doctor.

**Rehydration solutions**
*Rehydration preparations that contain potassium chloride are available from your pharmacist. You can make your own rehydration solution by mixing ½ teaspoon of salt, 2 teaspoons of sugar, and ½ teaspoon of baking soda into 1 pint of boiled water (left). Let the mixture cool before drinking.*

## Types of diarrhea

Diarrhea can contain excess water, or blood, pus, mucus, or fat. Watery diarrhea tends to be profuse and lasts for only a day or two. The most common cause of watery diarrhea is food poisoning, although it can also be caused by anxiety, food intolerance or allergy, and drug toxicity. Some rare tumors also cause profuse watery diarrhea. Bloody diarrhea, which often contains mucus or pus, can be caused by inflammation and ulceration of the digestive tract. If it lasts for only a short time, infection is usually the cause. If bloody diarrhea continues for more than a few days, it is more likely to be a result of inflammatory bowel disease (see page 115). Pus contained in diarrhea comes from areas of infection in the intestinal wall, such as infection of ulcers that develop during episodes of severe inflammatory bowel disease. Mucus in the diarrhea may be caused by irritable bowel syndrome (see page 123), inflammatory bowel disease, intestinal polyps, or cancer of the colon. Bulky, greasy, yellow stools signal an inability to absorb fat and other nutrients in the small intestine. Factors that can produce such stools include stomach or intestinal surgery, disease of the pancreatic or biliary tract (made up of the ducts that convey bile), and intestinal disorders.

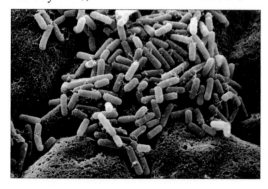

**Travelers' diarrhea**
*When traveling, you may be at increased risk of diarrhea from certain types of viruses, bacteria, or parasites in contaminated food and water. The bacterium* Escherichia coli *(above, magnified 850 times) inhabits your digestive tract harmlessly. But in some parts of the world you may be exposed to strains of* E. coli *that are unfamiliar to your digestive tract.*

## WHAT CAUSES DIARRHEA?

When your digestive tract is functioning normally, the colon absorbs water from the liquid food residue it processes to produce semisolid feces. Diarrhea occurs when the inflamed lining of the small intestine cannot absorb the intestinal contents (as when you eat spoiled food) and secretes large quantities of salts and water into the digestive tract. Diarrhea can also occur when digestive tract contractions increase in frequency and force.

**Increased contractions**
*When digestive tract contractions increase, liquid and semiliquid food residue passes through the colon quickly.*

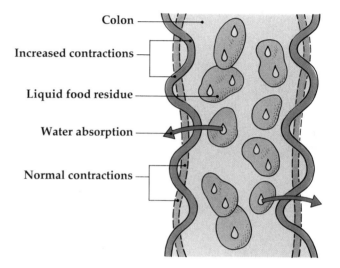

**Excess water loss**
*If the small intestine deposits excess amounts of water into food residue, the colon cannot absorb enough water to form semisolid feces. Sometimes the colon secretes additional water into the stools.*

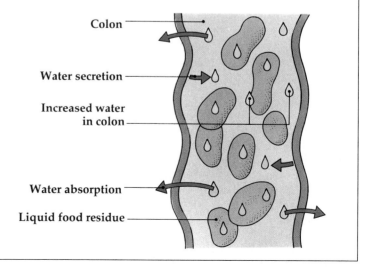

# HOW DO DOCTORS INVESTIGATE BLOOD IN THE STOOLS?

Blood in the stools signals a disorder somewhere in the digestive system. The blood may be visible on the surface of the feces or may be mixed in with the feces. It can also be separate from the feces, appearing either bright red or black. People may pass normal-looking stools that contain blood. Doctors perform a fecal occult (hidden) blood test to confirm the presence of blood. Other tests might be performed to determine the cause. The arrows in the chart below show the sequence of investigation your doctor might follow to reach a diagnosis.

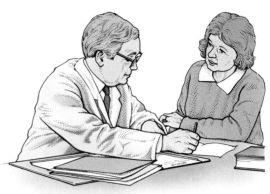

**Consulting your doctor**
*Determining the cause of internal bleeding may require many tests, including endoscopy, X-rays, and ultrasound. Your doctor will first gather clues to the diagnosis by taking a thorough, detailed medical history.*

## IF THE FECES APPEAR NORMAL

### Fecal occult blood test
*A test of the feces for occult (hidden) blood is a routine part of an examination for anyone over 50. The test is also done for anyone with iron-deficiency anemia. A sample of feces is placed on a chemical strip. A substance dropped on the white strip turns blue if blood is present.*

## IF THE FECAL BLOOD IS BLACK

### Testing for internal bleeding
*Visible black (partly digested) blood in the stools suggests bleeding from a place in the upper digestive tract or from as far down as the ascending colon. If blood loss is rapid, the stool appears inky black and blood pressure can fall, leading to shock. This condition requires immediate diagnosis and treatment.*

## IF THE FECAL BLOOD IS BRIGHT RED

### Proctoscopy and sigmoidoscopy
*Bright red blood usually originates near the anus. Your doctor may locate the bleeding site with a proctoscope, a rigid cylindrical tube that is inserted into the rectum, or with a flexible sigmoidoscope to view the rectum and sigmoid colon.*

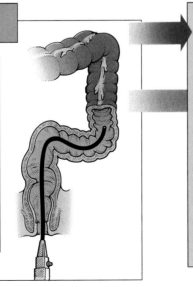

### Colonoscopy
*Doctors perform colonoscopy with a flexible, fiberoptic instrument called a colonoscope. (Fiberoptics permit the transmission of images through solid plastic or glass tubes.) You may be lightly anesthetized. The colonoscope is passed through the anus to the cecum. The doctor withdraws the instrument slowly, examining the inside of the colon. Biopsy samples may be taken, or polyps removed, with instruments passed through the colonoscope.*

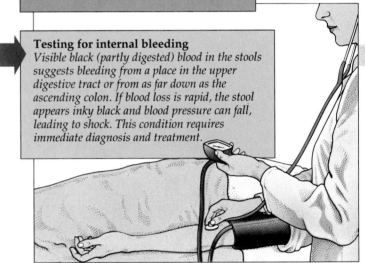

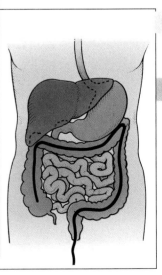

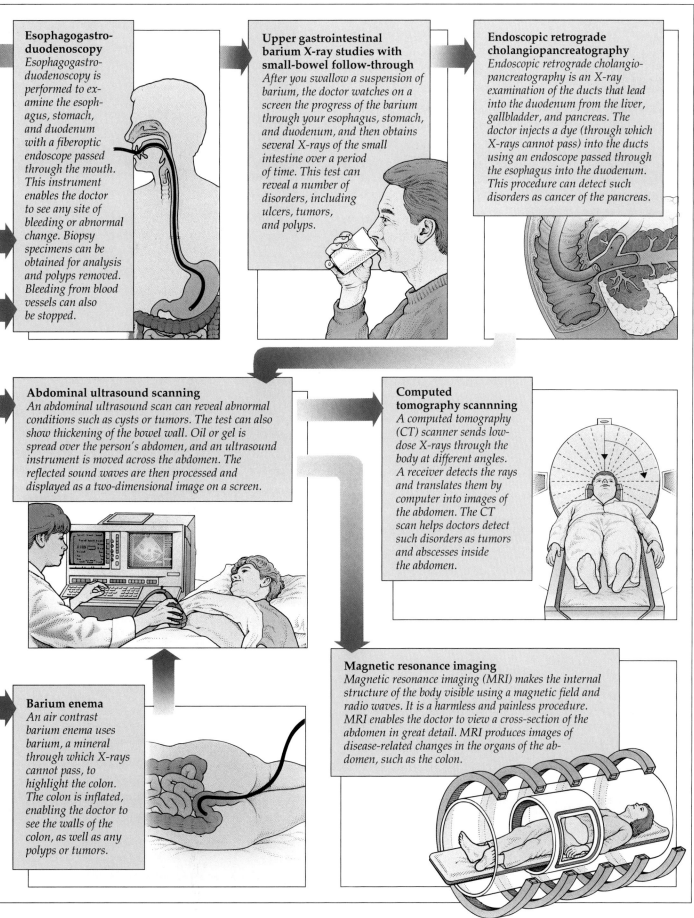

### Esophagogastro-duodenoscopy

*Esophagogastroduodenoscopy is performed to examine the esophagus, stomach, and duodenum with a fiberoptic endoscope passed through the mouth. This instrument enables the doctor to see any site of bleeding or abnormal change. Biopsy specimens can be obtained for analysis and polyps removed. Bleeding from blood vessels can also be stopped.*

### Upper gastrointestinal barium X-ray studies with small-bowel follow-through

*After you swallow a suspension of barium, the doctor watches on a screen the progress of the barium through your esophagus, stomach, and duodenum, and then obtains several X-rays of the small intestine over a period of time. This test can reveal a number of disorders, including ulcers, tumors, and polyps.*

### Endoscopic retrograde cholangiopancreatography

*Endoscopic retrograde cholangio-pancreatography is an X-ray examination of the ducts that lead into the duodenum from the liver, gallbladder, and pancreas. The doctor injects a dye (through which X-rays cannot pass) into the ducts using an endoscope passed through the esophagus into the duodenum. This procedure can detect such disorders as cancer of the pancreas.*

### Abdominal ultrasound scanning

*An abdominal ultrasound scan can reveal abnormal conditions such as cysts or tumors. The test can also show thickening of the bowel wall. Oil or gel is spread over the person's abdomen, and an ultrasound instrument is moved across the abdomen. The reflected sound waves are then processed and displayed as a two-dimensional image on a screen.*

### Computed tomography scannning

*A computed tomography (CT) scanner sends low-dose X-rays through the body at different angles. A receiver detects the rays and translates them by computer into images of the abdomen. The CT scan helps doctors detect such disorders as tumors and abscesses inside the abdomen.*

### Magnetic resonance imaging

*Magnetic resonance imaging (MRI) makes the internal structure of the body visible using a magnetic field and radio waves. It is a harmless and painless procedure. MRI enables the doctor to view a cross-section of the abdomen in great detail. MRI produces images of disease-related changes in the organs of the abdomen, such as the colon.*

### Barium enema

*An air contrast barium enema uses barium, a mineral through which X-rays cannot pass, to highlight the colon. The colon is inflated, enabling the doctor to see the walls of the colon, as well as any polyps or tumors.*

## CONSTIPATION

Like diarrhea, the term constipation is sometimes used imprecisely. Many people worry that they do not move their bowels completely or often enough. But regularity and ease of defecation are more important than frequency. Constipation refers to the difficult passage of hard, dry feces. In most cases, the condition is caused by eating a diet low in fiber or by not drinking enough fluids. A person may also repeatedly ignore the urge to defecate, which can lead to constipation. Other causes of constipation include taking narcotic analgesic drugs (such as codeine) and aluminum-containing antacids, depression, painful anal conditions, bodily immobility (as after surgery), and blockage and dehydration of stool from a cancer of the colon.

## OTHER TYPES OF ABNORMAL STOOLS

You should become familar with the way your stools usually look. If you look at your stools regularly, you will observe that they vary widely in consistency, size, color, and density. It is important to know which changes are normal and which changes indicate disease. If you notice a persistent change in your stools or in your bowel habits, inform your doctor. The importance of recognizing blood in the stools is discussed on page 80.

## Floating feces

You should not be concerned about stools that float in the toilet. Although pancreatic disease produces floating stools, these are usually pale, bulky, greasy, and offensive in odor. A much more common cause of floating stools is the presence of trapped gas, which makes the stools less dense than water. This gas is produced by the bacterial fermentation of fiber and starches in the colon. It is regarded as a sign of a healthy diet.

## HOW CONSTIPATION OCCURS

Constipation results in part from an increase in the time it takes for feces to pass through the colon. A prolonged time in the rectum allows more water to be absorbed from the feces than usual, making them hard and dry. Sometimes people ignore the urge to defecate, which causes soft stools entering the rectum to become hard and dry.

**Large, soft stools**
*The large, soft stools produced by a high-fiber diet stretch the muscles of the colon. These muscles propel the stool toward the rectum as the muscle fibers contract back to their normal length.*

**Small, hard stools**
*The small, hard stools produced by a low-fiber diet do not stimulate the muscles of the colon to contract and propel the stools forward. The colon continues to absorb water from the stools as long as they remain there.*

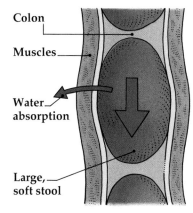

Colon
Muscles
Water absorption
Large, soft stool

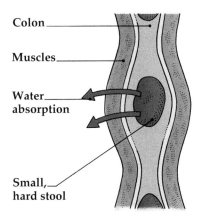

Colon
Muscles
Water absorption
Small, hard stool

## Mucous discharge

The digestive tract secretes mucus. This mucus serves to insulate the lining of the digestive tract from the chemical activity of its contents and also provides a protective lubricant for the passage of stools. Slimy feces that contain excessive mucus sometimes accompany irritable bowel syndrome (see page 123). Inflammatory bowel disease and some infections can also produce mucus in the feces, often accompanied by diarrhea and blood loss.

## ANAL PAIN

Pain that occurs in the anal region during defecation is usually caused by stretching of the anus from the passage of hard stools. The stools may also cause the lining of the anus to tear. Anal inflammation, hemorrhoids, or other diseases of

**IRRITABLE BOWEL SYNDROME**

Some people develop alternating bouts of constipation and diarrhea, along with other abdominal symptoms. If a doctor finds no abnormality, these people are diagnosed as having irritable bowel syndrome. New symptoms, such as abdominal pain, rectal bleeding, or poorly digested food in stools, should never be ignored. A doctor should investigate them to exclude cancer.

the anus can make passing a normal stool painful. Any pain that you experience for longer than a day should be reported to your doctor. Pain in the anal region that occurs at times other than during defecation is called proctalgia. Your doctor can usually identify the cause of the pain – which may be an infection, an abscess, or a more serious condition – by performing a rectal examination.

## FECAL INCONTINENCE

Fecal incontinence is the inability to retain feces in the rectum. Anyone can be temporarily incontinent during a severe attack of diarrhea. This type of incontinence usually stops as soon as the diarrhea goes away. In older people, the most common cause of fecal incontinence is an accumulation of impacted feces wedged in the rectum. This impaction irritates the rectal lining, causing fluid and newly formed feces to be passed around the impaction and out of the anus involuntarily. Less common causes include damage to the sphincter mechanism of the anus, as may occur during childbirth or surgery, and disorders of the nerves or muscles of the anus.

**EXCESSIVE GAS**

Passing gas almost never indicates the presence of a serious disease. Gas is almost always the result of the bacterial fermentation of food residue in the colon. The more fiber you eat, the greater the quantity of gas you will produce. In some societies, where the diet is naturally high in fiber, the passage of gas is regarded as an indication of healthy bowels. Some people experience excessive gas when they increase the amount of fiber they consume. This problem usually disappears within 3 or 4 weeks. Try to increase the amount of fiber you consume gradually to avoid excessive gas production.

## ASK YOUR DOCTOR
## BOWEL PROBLEMS

Q When I have a bowel movement, I notice blood in the toilet. My wife thinks I have hemorrhoids. What causes them?

A Hemorrhoids often occur when people strain to pass hard stools. They can cause bleeding. Occasionally, blood loss from the rectum can indicate a serious disease. Your doctor can exclude this possibility by performing a rectal examination. If you have hemorrhoids, sit in a tub of warm water to relieve the pain, swelling, and itching. Increase the amount of fiber in your diet to produce softer stools that will not be so difficult to pass.

Q I am constipated and take laxatives to keep myself regular. Is this harmful?

A It can be. Laxatives should almost never be used. Prolonged, regular use can cause the bowel to be overemptied, and you could become dependent on the drugs to have a bowel movement. To prevent constipation, eat a high-fiber diet, drink plenty of fluids, and defecate as soon as you feel the need.

Q To avoid constipation, I take an over-the-counter fiber supplement. Are such supplements safe?

A These bulk-forming preparations are safe, providing you drink plenty of water (4 to 6 glasses) every day. If you do not drink enough water, the fiber supplement can dry out and block up your intestine. The best way to achieve regular bowel activity is to consume fiber in your diet. Fresh fruits, vegetables, and whole-grain breads are good sources of fiber. They will add bulk to your stools, making them easier to pass.

**Anal protrusions**
*Lumps and bumps around the anus are relatively common. In most cases, the lumps are hemorrhoids, which are swollen veins that protrude from the surface of the anus, particularly when a person strains to pass stools (see right). Hemorrhoids can bleed and cause pain and itching. Other lumps that can occur in the anal region include tumors, warts, cysts, and abscesses. These conditions can be identified and treated by your doctor.*

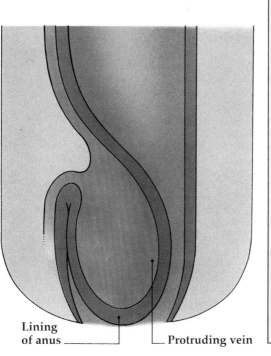

Lining of anus

Protruding vein

# CHAPTER FOUR

# DIGESTIVE SYSTEM DISORDERS

YOUR BODY IS A highly sophisticated organism. To function normally, it depends on nutrients obtained from the food you eat. Any disorder that prevents your digestive system from getting, processing, or absorbing nutrients will affect your general well-being. Disorders that can affect the digestive tract include obstruction, perforation, and twisting of the intestine. The stomach or intestines can also become inflamed. Any damage to the lining of the digestive tract can cause profuse bleeding because the tract has a rich blood supply to ensure that nutrients can enter the bloodstream quickly. When you eat food and drink liquids, a constant stream of nonsterile material enters your digestive tract, which can easily become infected or infested by microorganisms. The discomfort you experience from any of these digestive disorders can range from slight irritation to excruciating pain. Among the various diseases and conditions that can affect the digestive system are hiatal hernia, peptic esophagitis, peptic ulcer, irritable bowel syndrome, cholecystitis (inflammation of the gallbladder), pancreatitis (inflammation of the pancreas), gallstones, hepatitis (inflammation of the liver), appendicitis (inflammation of the appendix), inflammatory bowel disease, and hemor-

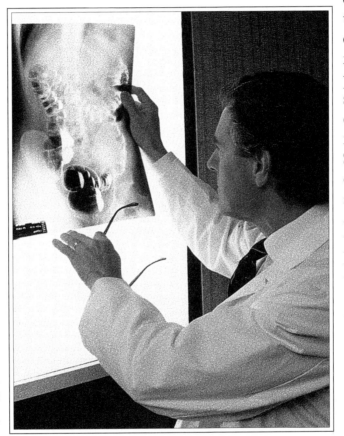

rhoids. Benign (noncancerous) or malignant (cancerous) tumors can also develop in the digestive system. The colon and rectum are especially common sites for cancer.

This chapter discusses the disorders that can affect the different parts of your digestive system: the esophagus, stomach, duodenum, colon, rectum, and anus. It also examines the causes and symptoms of these disorders and describes how your doctor evaluates and treats them. Because the digestive system fulfills so many important functions inside your body, its disorders can have far-reaching effects. Some disorders produce symptoms, such as vomiting, diarrhea, or constipation, that are clearly linked to the digestive system. Other disorders signal their presence indirectly. Examples of such disorders include pancreatitis, which produces symptoms of diabetes, and liver failure, which brings on drowsiness and confusion. Major advances in the diagnosis and treatment of gastrointestinal diseases have occurred during the last two decades. New techniques, such as endoscopy, imaging, and laser surgery, now enable doctors to examine and treat the digestive system with more precision and less discomfort and risk to the patient. These techniques are explained in several chapters throughout this volume.

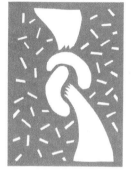

# ESOPHAGEAL DISORDERS

D AMAGE TO THE ESOPHAGUS usually produces difficult and painful swallowing and chest pain. Among the causes of such damage are reflux of stomach acid, disorders that affect the lining or muscle of the esophagus, outside pressure on the esophagus from a tumor or other swelling inside the chest, and corrosive substances, swallowed accidentally or intentionally.

Acid reflux (regurgitation of acidic fluid that also contains digestive enzymes from the stomach into the esophagus) is by far the most common irritant affecting the esophagus. The esophagus is also at risk for injury caused by swallowed corrosive substances, such as liquid drain cleaners, and items that lodge in the esophagus, such as small bones. Infection, inflammation, congenital defects, and cancer can also affect the esophagus.

## REFLUX ESOPHAGITIS

In some people, acid reflux produces inflammation and sometimes ulceration of the esophagus (reflux esophagitis). Chest discomfort is one of the first signs of reflux esophagitis. Doctors usually perform endoscopy (an internal examination with a fiberoptic instrument) to confirm the diagnosis of reflux esophagitis. Endoscopy allows a direct view of the lining of the esophagus.

To reduce the amount of reflux you experience, eat six small meals instead of three regular-sized meals, so you do not overfill your stomach. Do not bend over or lie down immediately after meals. Lose a few pounds if you are overweight. Avoid foods or drinks with a high concentration of sugar, such as syrups, honey, or liqueurs. Quit smoking, because smoking increases the acidity of the stomach's contents. Eliminate coffee and carbonated drinks. Sleep with your head elevated to prevent reflux at night. Your doctor may prescribe medication to neutralize acid or reduce acid secretion in your stomach, or to move the contents more quickly through your esophagus and stomach.

**Ulceration and bleeding in esophagitis**
*In severe cases of reflux esophagitis (below), ulceration occurs (arrow), sometimes causing bleeding from the damaged esophageal lining. Scarring of the lower esophagus may obstruct the passage of chewed food.*

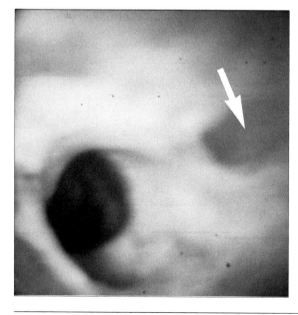

**Esophageal strictures**
*Esophageal strictures are narrowings of the esophagus that cause difficulty swallowing. Causes include scarring from chronic inflammation or a cancerous growth (right). With prolonged use, nonsteroidal anti-inflammatory drugs (including aspirin), the antibiotic tetracycline, and potassium supplements can produce ulcers that cause scarring and narrowing. Doctors treat benign (noncancerous) strictures by mechanical widening with specially designed tubes.*

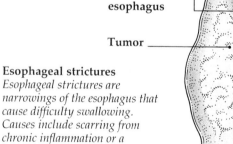

Walls of the esophagus

Tumor

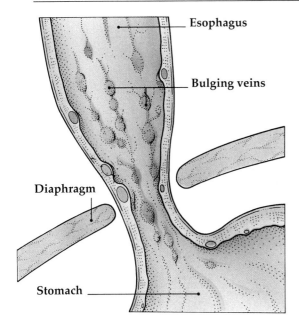

Esophagus

Bulging veins

Diaphragm

Stomach

**Esophageal varices**
*Varices result from portal hypertension – increased blood pressure in the portal vein (the blood vessel that carries blood from the stomach and intestine to the liver), most often due to liver disease. Blood traveling from the abdominal organs to the liver meets increased resistance. Some blood becomes diverted to the veins in the esophagus, causing them to bulge into the esophageal cavity (left).*

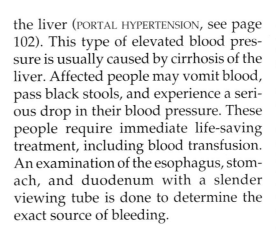

Trapped food

Contracted muscle

## ESOPHAGEAL SPASM

Esophageal spasm results from unco-ordinated contractions of the muscles in the esophagus. Disordered contractions can occur in several areas of the esophagus or in one area only. Spasm in several areas of the esophagus causes central chest pain similar to the kind of pain caused by a heart attack.

All types of esophageal spasm can be diagnosed by a barium X-ray, but more precise information can be obtained with a technique known as esophageal manometry. During this technique, doctors position a pressure-sensitive device in the person's esophagus that records changes in esophageal pressure at different points along its length. Esophageal spasm is difficult to control. The success of a variety of treatments, including drugs, has been inconsistent.

## ESOPHAGEAL VARICES

Varices are large, dilated veins in the lower part of the esophagus that sometimes burst and bleed into the esophagus and stomach. The cause is elevated blood pressure in the portal vein, which carries blood from the stomach and intestines to

the liver (PORTAL HYPERTENSION, see page 102). This type of elevated blood pressure is usually caused by cirrhosis of the liver. Affected people may vomit blood, pass black stools, and experience a serious drop in their blood pressure. These people require immediate life-saving treatment, including blood transfusion. An examination of the esophagus, stomach, and duodenum with a slender viewing tube is done to determine the exact source of bleeding.

### Treatment of varices

Treatment of esophageal varices may consist of compression of the veins with a balloon catheter that presses against the veins to stop the bleeding, followed by injection of a solution that shrinks and shuts off the veins. After several injections, the risk of bleeding decreases. The varices may form again.

**Achalasia**
*In a person with achalasia, both solids and liquids can become trapped in the esophagus because its lower segment fails to relax (above). This condition can cause regurgitation of food eaten the previous day or two. In some cases, the tight segment in the lower esophagus can be forced open by a balloon positioned in the lower esophagus or by an operation.*

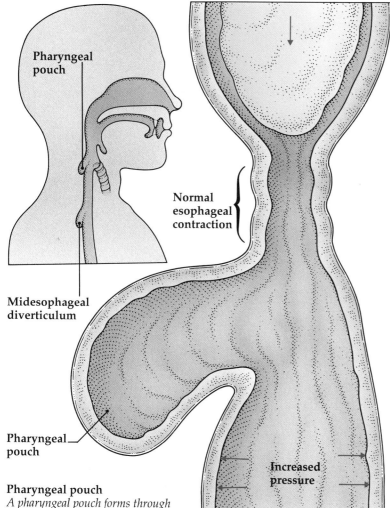

**Pharyngeal pouch**

**Normal esophageal contraction**

**Midesophageal diverticulum**

**Pharyngeal pouch**

**Increased pressure**

**Pharyngeal pouch**
*A pharyngeal pouch forms through the back wall of the lower part of the throat (pharynx). The pouch develops when the esophageal muscles fail to relax during swallowing, because of incoordination. This failure to relax creates pressure, causing the area above to bulge through the muscular layer of the esophagus.*

**Esophageal cancer**
*In a person with esophageal cancer, a malignant tumor of the esophagus (right) causes difficulty swallowing, which leads to reduced food intake and weight loss. Esophageal cancer is diagnosed by barium X-ray (see page 81), followed by analysis of samples obtained during endoscopy (see page 93). The cells are examined under a microscope to confirm malignancy.*

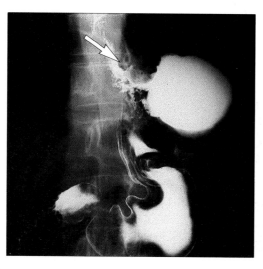

# ESOPHAGEAL DIVERTICULA

Outward bulges in parts of the esophageal wall are called esophageal diverticula. They can be caused by protrusion of the esophageal lining from a weakness in the muscle wall or by continuous pulling of a portion of the wall by scarring. Doctors can confirm the presence of a diverticulum by a barium X-ray. Two types of diverticula can occur – the pharyngeal pouch and the midesophageal diverticulum. Surgery is the only effective treatment for a pharyngeal pouch. The surgeon removes the pouch and partly cuts the esophageal sphincter to weaken it and prevent recurrence of the pouch. Midesophageal diverticula are pouches formed farther down in the esophagus. They rarely cause symptoms and usually require no treatment.

# ORAL AND ESOPHAGEAL CANCER

Oral cancer accounts for about 2 percent of all tumors in the US. Most oral tumors affect the lips and tongue and first appear as an ulcer or lump that gradually enlarges. These cancers occur more commonly in older people. High-risk factors include cigarette, pipe, and cigar smoking, use of chewing tobacco, and alcohol consumption.

About 10 new cases of esophageal cancer occur per 100,000 of the US population every year. People with reflux esophagitis and scarring of the esophagus are at slightly higher risk.

## Diagnosis and treatment
Diagnosis of both oral and esophageal cancer is reached after examination of a biopsy specimen from the affected area. Early detection, followed by surgery, provides the best chance for survival. Radiation therapy, anticancer drugs, or laser destruction of a tumor may temporarily alleviate symptoms.

# CASE HISTORY
## DIFFICULTY SWALLOWING

Edna's father was diagnosed with cancer of the esophagus 18 months ago and she cared for him until he died. She seemed to cope well with her father's death, and her husband was relieved at the speed of her recovery. But Edna recently noticed a lump in her throat and had some difficulty swallowing food. Worried that she too might have cancer, she decided to visit her doctor.

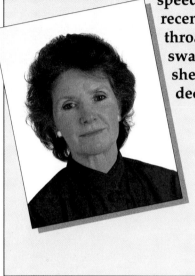

**PERSONAL DETAILS**
**Name** Edna Harris
**Age** 50
**Occupation** Manager, office supply company
**Family** Edna's mother died in an accident. Edna and her father ran the family business together after her mother's death.

## MEDICAL BACKGROUND
Edna had always been healthy. But her fears that her father was undermining his own health by drinking and smoking too much were confirmed by the development of his cancer of the esophagus.

## THE CONSULTATION
The family doctor notices that Edna has lost a lot of weight. Reviewing her medical history, he senses that her outer cheerfulness masks an anxious state of mind. He asks Edna if she has been depressed since her father's death. She confesses that she has been more upset than she has admitted to her husband and that she has been worried about the future of the family business. Edna tells her doctor that she feels as though she has a permanent lump in her throat and has had difficulty swallowing solid foods. She is afraid that she may have developed the same disease as her father.

## FURTHER INVESTIGATIONS
Although Edna is a nonsmoker and rarely drinks alcohol, her doctor does not rule out the possibility of physical disease. But he suspects that she

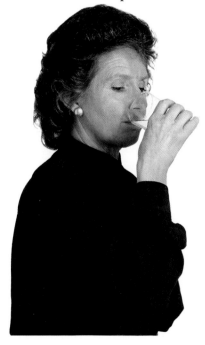

may have an anxiety disorder that developed after her father's death. To rule out the possibility of disease, he performs several blood tests and makes an appointment for Edna to undergo a barium X-ray (see page 81) at the local hospital.

## THE DIAGNOSIS
The results of the blood tests are normal and the barium X-ray reveals no abnormality in Edna's esophagus. Edna's doctor reaches a diagnosis of GLOBUS HYSTERICUS, an anxiety disorder in which increased tension in the muscles of the throat produces a sensation of a lump in the throat. The sensation is constant but becomes more noticeable when the person is swallowing. Globus hystericus occurs in some tense and anxious people. In Edna's case, the lump is probably a psychological expression of her fears about the business and the anxiety that she has about her father's death.

## THE TREATMENT
The doctor refers Edna to a psychotherapist who counsels her about her father's death and helps her overcome her fears of having esophageal cancer. After several visits, Edna begins to come to terms with her grief. The lump in her throat and her difficulty swallowing diminish.

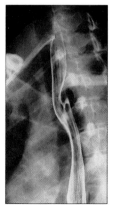

**The barium X-ray**
*Edna drinks a glass of barium, which is impervious to X-rays, mixed with flavored liquid. A number of X-rays are obtained. They provide clear images of her upper and lower digestive tracts. The barium X-ray at right shows no esophageal abnormality.*

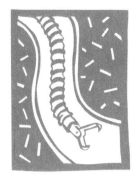

# STOMACH AND DUODENAL DISORDERS

A VARIETY OF AGENTS can damage the sensitive linings of the stomach and duodenum (the upper part of the small intestine), including infectious organisms, the acidic fluid produced by the stomach, and harmful substances in food and drugs. Disorders can affect the stomach's ability to store food and prepare it for digestion. The functions of both the stomach and the duodenum may also be affected by impaired blood supply.

The stomach secretes a powerful fluid composed of acid and the enzyme pepsin. Cells lining the inside of the stomach produce a layer of protective mucus that provides insulation from the damaging effects of this acidic mixture. An imbalance between the production of the acid/pepsin mixture and the production of the mucus can lead to inflammation of the lining of the stomach or duodenum (gastritis or duodenitis) and ulceration (gastric ulcers or duodenal ulcers). Other disorders of the stomach and duodenum include diverticula and cancer.

**Acute erosive gastritis**
*In people with acute gastritis, erosions (arrow) can cause internal bleeding. These erosions may be widespread in the stomach lining. A severe form of acute erosive gastritis can cause massive blood loss, sometimes resulting in death.*

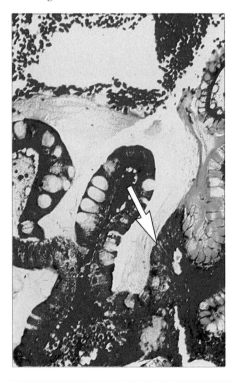

**Normal gastric glands**

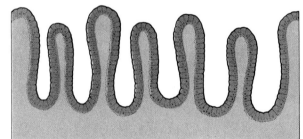

**Erosion of the stomach lining**
*Doctors confirm a diagnosis of gastritis by using gastroscopy (see page 93) to detect the abnormal appearance of the stomach lining. They also take samples of stomach tissue for examination under a microscope. Healthy stomach lining, called gastric mucosa (above left), shows a well-defined glandular structure. Acute erosive gastritis destroys areas of the mucosa and specialized glandular tissue (below left).*

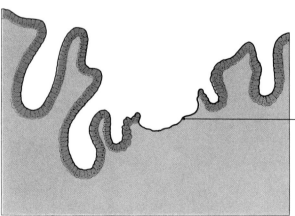

**Loss of glandular structure**

## GASTRITIS

Inflammation of the stomach lining is called gastritis. It may be acute (experienced as a sudden attack) or chronic (developing gradually over a long time). Drugs – such as nonsteroidal anti-inflammatory drugs (NSAIDs), including aspirin, and potassium or iron salts – can cause acute or chronic gastritis. So can drinking too much alcohol. In recent years, interest has focused on the bacterium *Helicobacter pylori* as a cause of gastritis, although the source of the bacterium is unknown. Many people with gastritis have no symptoms, but some develop indigestion, nausea, and vomiting. Erosive gastritis can cause acute bleeding that leads to vomiting of blood, a lowering of blood pressure, and the appearance of blood in the stools. Pernicious anemia, one form of vitamin $B_{12}$ deficiency anemia, occurs when chronic gastritis causes the stomach to lose the cells that release intrinsic factor, a substance essential for the absorption of vitamin $B_{12}$. For treatment, doctors administer vitamin $B_{12}$ injections.

## DUODENITIS

Duodenitis refers to inflammation of the uppermost part of the duodenum. Duodenitis is much less common than gastritis but frequently occurs in people with duodenal ulcers. Doctors don't know whether duodenitis predisposes people to ulcer formation. Some people with duodenitis also have gastritis, and infection with the bacterium *Helicobacter pylori* may play a role. In rare cases, other disorders – including Crohn's disease (see page 115), giardiasis (see page 127), liver disease, pancreatic disorders, chronic kidney failure, and tuberculosis – can cause inflammation of the duodenum. Microscopic evidence of duodenal inflammation also has been found in about 12 percent of healthy people who have no symptoms of duodenitis.

## HOW TO AVOID CHRONIC GASTRITIS

Prolonged irritation of the stomach lining by a number of factors can cause chronic gastritis. Avoid these factors and you will reduce your risk of developing chronic gastritis.

 Do not smoke. Tobacco smoking increases the acidity of the stomach's contents. This acidity increases the risk of inflammation and can lead to chronic gastritis over the long term.

 Do not take nonsteroidal anti-inflammatory drugs (NSAIDs), such as aspirin or ibuprofen, over long periods of time. NSAIDs have been shown to erode the stomach lining. Instead, take acetaminophen to reduce inflammation.

 Avoid alcohol. Although small amounts of alcohol stimulate the appetite and help you digest food, alcohol increases the production of gastric acid. Large amounts consumed over a long period cause gastritis by irritating the lining of the stomach.

### HELICOBACTER PYLORI

The bacterium *Helicobacter pylori* may be one of the causes of gastritis. Researchers think that the organism may be found in many people with gastritis. Rarely found in people under age 20, *Helicobacter pylori* may infect more than 60 percent of people over age 65 in the US. It is possible that infection with the organism precedes peptic ulcers, but this theory has not been confirmed. Doctors have attempted to treat ulcers with antibiotics, with or without drugs such as bismuth salts that are known to be toxic to *Helicobacter pylori*.

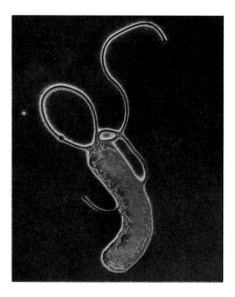

**The bacterium**
Helicobacter pylori *is an S-shaped bacterium with whiplike appendages that help the microorganism move through the inner surface of the stomach (right, magnified 7,080 times). Medical experts are unsure of the source of the bacterium. In infected persons, clusters of the bacteria adhere to cells that line the surface of the digestive tract. The way in which the bacterium damages the stomach lining remains unknown, but* Helicobacter pylori *produces a number of damaging enzymes that may cause erosion of the stomach lining.*

# HIATAL HERNIA

When the muscle of the diaphragm becomes weak, part of the stomach can protrude through the normal opening in the diaphragm. This condition is called hiatal hernia. The underlying cause remains unknown. Hiatal hernia occurs more frequently in women, overweight people, and smokers. Many people with hiatal hernia experience no symptoms, but some have acid reflux, which in turn causes esophagitis (see page 86) and heartburn. The pain caused by hiatal hernia becomes worse at night. The sliding hiatal hernia is the most common type and is accompanied by inflammation of the esophagus from stomach juices. Another type, paraesophageal hernia, causes no acid reflux.

## Diagnosis and treatment

A barium X-ray can confirm a diagnosis of hiatal hernia, but doctors usually perform endoscopy (see page 93) to determine the severity of esophageal inflammation and to look for ulcer formation. To alleviate symptoms, an affected person should avoid overfilling the stomach, sleep with the head elevated to reduce reflux at night, and quit smoking. Antacids can reduce stomach acidity and protect the esophagus against damage caused by acid reflux.

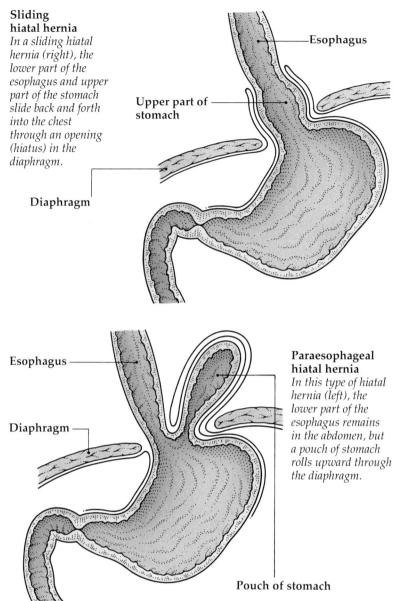

**Sliding hiatal hernia**
*In a sliding hiatal hernia (right), the lower part of the esophagus and upper part of the stomach slide back and forth into the chest through an opening (hiatus) in the diaphragm.*

Esophagus

Upper part of stomach

Diaphragm

Esophagus

Diaphragm

**Paraesophageal hiatal hernia**
*In this type of hiatal hernia (left), the lower part of the esophagus remains in the abdomen, but a pouch of stomach rolls upward through the diaphragm.*

Pouch of stomach

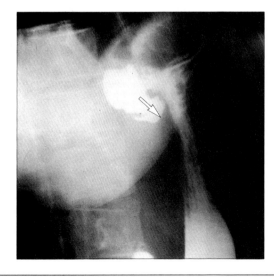

**Barium X-ray of a diverticulum**
*This barium X-ray shows a gastric diverticulum in the upper part of the stomach (arrow). Most gastric diverticula produce no symptoms.*

# GASTRIC DIVERTICULA

Gastric diverticula are small pouches located on the upper back wall of the stomach. Doctors don't know what causes diverticula, but most are present from birth. They rarely become inflamed. Some pouches occur in the pyloric region, near the entrance to the duodenum. False diverticula, or "pseudodiverticula," usually arise from scarring caused by peptic ulceration. Through an endoscope, a gastric diverticulum looks like a small, round opening with sharp edges.

# ENDOSCOPY

Endoscopy is the visual examination of inner body structures with an optical instrument. The procedure allows your doctor to see what is happening inside your body without surgery. Fiberoptic devices (which transmit images through thin, flexible glass or plastic threads) linked to monitors have replaced the rigid endoscopes used previously. Many specialized tools are available that can be passed through the endoscope to take tissue samples and to perform minor surgery. Esophagogastro-duodenoscopy (endoscopy of the upper digestive tract) has replaced barium X-rays in the investigation of reflux esophagitis, peptic ulcer disease, and stomach cancer.

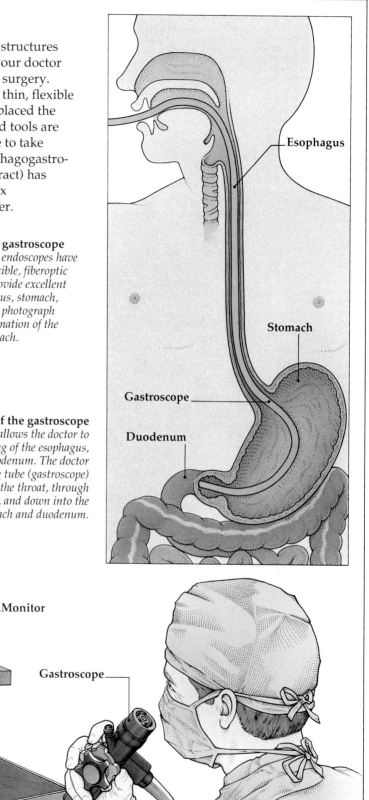

Esophagus

Stomach

Gastroscope

Duodenum

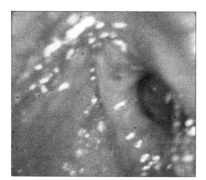

**View through the gastroscope**
*The older, semirigid endoscopes have been replaced by flexible, fiberoptic instruments that provide excellent views of the esophagus, stomach, and duodenum. The photograph at left shows inflammation of the outlet from the stomach.*

**Gastroscopy**
*Unlike surgery, gastroscopy does not require general anesthesia. Drugs, such as diazepam, are sometimes used to reduce anxiety and to allow the endoscope to pass into the gastroduodenal tract more easily. The doctor inserts the viewing tube through the mouth and follows its progress on a monitor.*

**Route of the gastroscope**
*Gastroscopy allows the doctor to examine the lining of the esophagus, stomach, and duodenum. The doctor passes a viewing tube (gastroscope) down the back of the throat, through the esophagus, and down into the stomach and duodenum.*

Monitor

Gastroscope

# WHAT IS A PEPTIC ULCER?

Each year, one in every 50 Americans develops a peptic ulcer. There are two main types of peptic ulcers – those found in the stomach (gastric ulcers) and those found in the duodenum (duodenal ulcers). Peptic ulcers can occur at any age. About 10 percent of men and 4 percent of women develop a duodenal ulcer at some time during their lives. Duodenal ulcers are four times more common than gastric ulcers, which occur with similar frequency in men and women.

## WHERE DO PEPTIC ULCERS OCCUR?

Gastric ulcers (a type of peptic ulcer) can occur anywhere in the stomach but they are usually found on the stomach's lesser curve and between the body of the stomach and its lower portion. Duodenal ulcers mainly affect the first part of the duodenum, known as the duodenal bulb. The diagram below shows the distribution of both types of peptic ulcers in the US population.

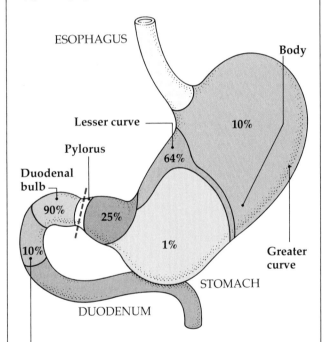

**Second part of duodenum**

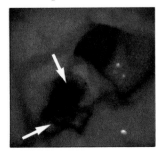

**"Kissing" ulcers**
*Duodenal ulcers occasionally occur on the front and back walls of the duodenum, opposite each other. These are known as kissing ulcers (see arrows at left).*

## HOW DOES A PEPTIC ULCER FORM?

1 A layer of mucus normally protects the lining of the stomach and duodenum from digestive secretions and other potentially harmful substances.

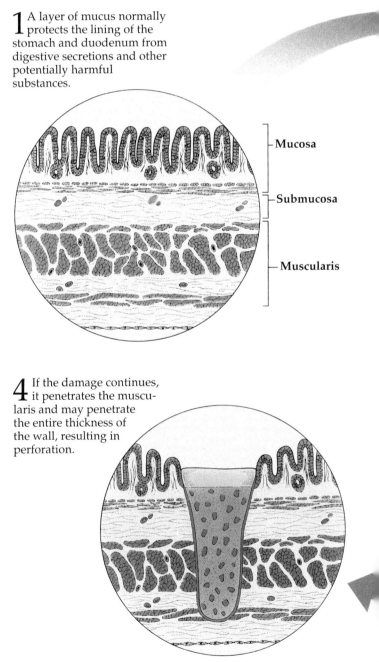

4 If the damage continues, it penetrates the muscularis and may penetrate the entire thickness of the wall, resulting in perforation.

**The role of acid and other digestive secretions**

*Normally, a layer of mucus protects the stomach lining from acid and other secretions, such as pepsin, an enzyme that digests protein. Gastric ulceration occurs when this protective barrier breaks down and stomach juice that contains acid and pepsin comes into contact with cells of the stomach lining. Ulceration of the duodenal lining occurs when excess acid secreted in the stomach passes into the duodenum and breaks through its protective mucous layer.*

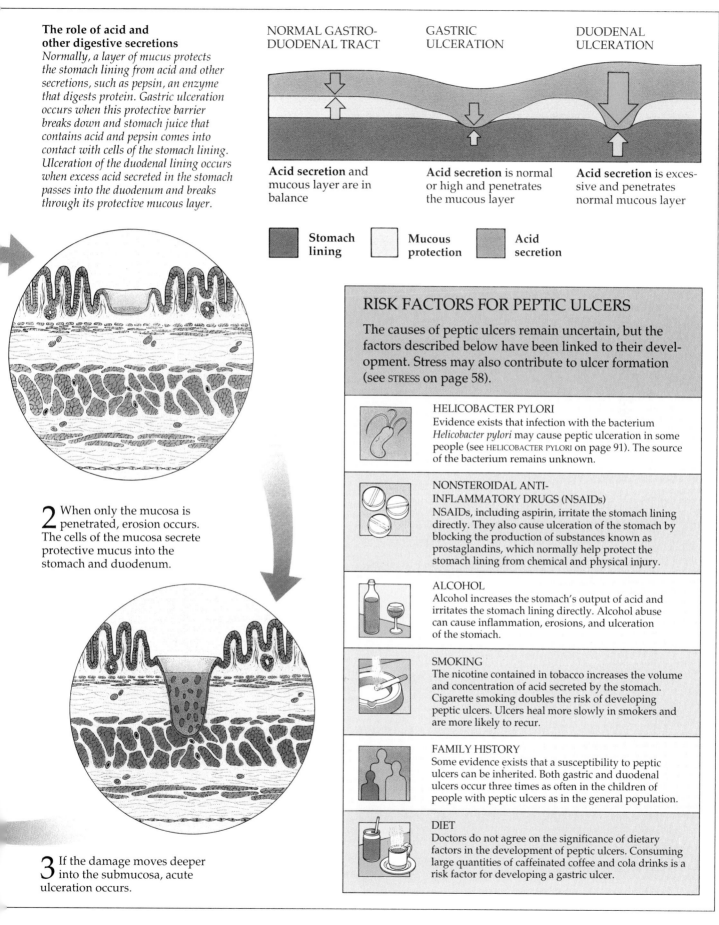

NORMAL GASTRO-DUODENAL TRACT

GASTRIC ULCERATION

DUODENAL ULCERATION

**Acid secretion** and mucous layer are in balance

**Acid secretion** is normal or high and penetrates the mucous layer

**Acid secretion** is excessive and penetrates normal mucous layer

- Stomach lining
- Mucous protection
- Acid secretion

**2** When only the mucosa is penetrated, erosion occurs. The cells of the mucosa secrete protective mucus into the stomach and duodenum.

**3** If the damage moves deeper into the submucosa, acute ulceration occurs.

## RISK FACTORS FOR PEPTIC ULCERS

The causes of peptic ulcers remain uncertain, but the factors described below have been linked to their development. Stress may also contribute to ulcer formation (see STRESS on page 58).

**HELICOBACTER PYLORI**
Evidence exists that infection with the bacterium *Helicobacter pylori* may cause peptic ulceration in some people (see HELICOBACTER PYLORI on page 91). The source of the bacterium remains unknown.

**NONSTEROIDAL ANTI-INFLAMMATORY DRUGS (NSAIDs)**
NSAIDs, including aspirin, irritate the stomach lining directly. They also cause ulceration of the stomach by blocking the production of substances known as prostaglandins, which normally help protect the stomach lining from chemical and physical injury.

**ALCOHOL**
Alcohol increases the stomach's output of acid and irritates the stomach lining directly. Alcohol abuse can cause inflammation, erosions, and ulceration of the stomach.

**SMOKING**
The nicotine contained in tobacco increases the volume and concentration of acid secreted by the stomach. Cigarette smoking doubles the risk of developing peptic ulcers. Ulcers heal more slowly in smokers and are more likely to recur.

**FAMILY HISTORY**
Some evidence exists that a susceptibility to peptic ulcers can be inherited. Both gastric and duodenal ulcers occur three times as often in the children of people with peptic ulcers as in the general population.

**DIET**
Doctors do not agree on the significance of dietary factors in the development of peptic ulcers. Consuming large quantities of caffeinated coffee and cola drinks is a risk factor for developing a gastric ulcer.

# MANAGEMENT OF PEPTIC ULCERS

Life-style changes, antacid and other drug treatment, and surgery are all part of managing peptic ulcers. If you have been diagnosed with an ulcer and you are a smoker, the first thing you should do is to quit smoking. If your ulcer is chronic (constant), try to eat small meals regularly and avoid spicy or greasy foods, alcohol, coffee, and aspirin. They all can irritate the stomach lining.

A number of effective drugs have been developed to treat peptic ulcers. These drugs can be broadly divided into four groups. Some drugs reduce the secretion of acid by parietal cells in the stomach lining (see below). Mucosal protectors prevent acid from reaching the ulcer by coating the lining of the stomach and duodenum with a protective layer. Another older group, antacids, neutralizes acid. There is also a group of drugs that at least temporarily eradicates the bacterium *Helicobacter pylori* (see HELICOBACTER PYLORI on page 91).

## DRUGS THAT REDUCE ACID SECRETION

Three types of drugs work by reducing acid secretion from the parietal cells that line the stomach – histamine ($H_2$) blockers, proton pump inhibitors, and anticholinergic agents. Each type of drug acts on a different part of the parietal cell to reduce acid secretion.

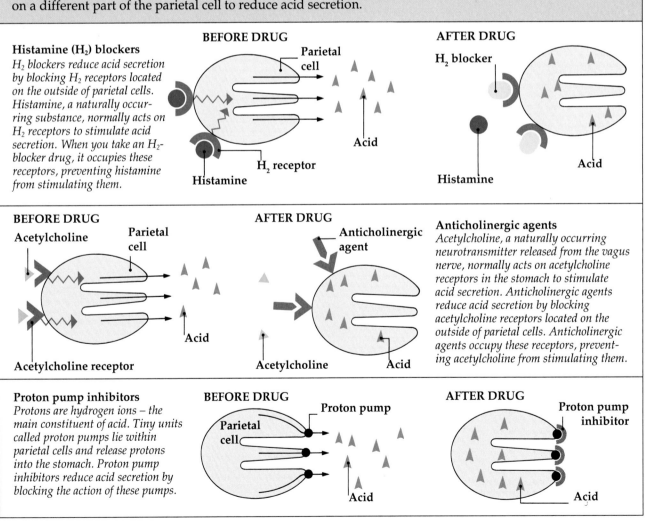

**Histamine ($H_2$) blockers**
*$H_2$ blockers reduce acid secretion by blocking $H_2$ receptors located on the outside of parietal cells. Histamine, a naturally occurring substance, normally acts on $H_2$ receptors to stimulate acid secretion. When you take an $H_2$-blocker drug, it occupies these receptors, preventing histamine from stimulating them.*

BEFORE DRUG — Parietal cell, Histamine, $H_2$ receptor, Acid

AFTER DRUG — $H_2$ blocker, Histamine, Acid

BEFORE DRUG — Acetylcholine, Parietal cell, Acetylcholine receptor, Acid

AFTER DRUG — Anticholinergic agent, Acetylcholine, Acid

**Anticholinergic agents**
*Acetylcholine, a naturally occurring neurotransmitter released from the vagus nerve, normally acts on acetylcholine receptors in the stomach to stimulate acid secretion. Anticholinergic agents reduce acid secretion by blocking acetylcholine receptors located on the outside of parietal cells. Anticholinergic agents occupy these receptors, preventing acetylcholine from stimulating them.*

**Proton pump inhibitors**
*Protons are hydrogen ions – the main constituent of acid. Tiny units called proton pumps lie within parietal cells and release protons into the stomach. Proton pump inhibitors reduce acid secretion by blocking the action of these pumps.*

BEFORE DRUG — Parietal cell, Proton pump, Acid

AFTER DRUG — Proton pump inhibitor, Acid

## ANTACIDS

Many people with symptoms of peptic ulcer or indigestion seek relief with over-the-counter antacids. They may see their doctor only when such treatment fails. Antacids taken under medical supervision are safe and effective in treating peptic ulcers or indigestion. But the drugs that reduce acid secretion have largely replaced antacids (see page 96). Prolonged, unsupervised use of antacids may result in a serious disruption of the body's chemical balance.

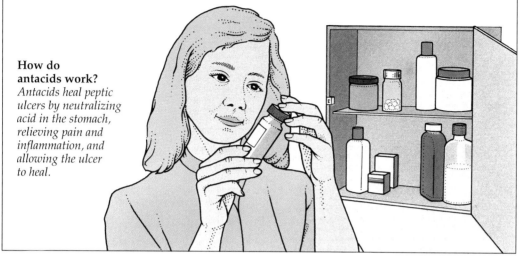

**How do antacids work?**
*Antacids heal peptic ulcers by neutralizing acid in the stomach, relieving pain and inflammation, and allowing the ulcer to heal.*

**PROSTA-GLANDIN ANALOGUES**

Prostaglandins are substances made by the body that have many functions. For example, they cause pain and inflammation in damaged tissue. They also protect the stomach and duodenal linings from ulceration. Prostaglandin analogues are drugs that act like naturally occurring prostaglandins. Most are still classified as investigational drugs and the way in which they help ulcers heal remains unknown.

## Surgery

New drug treatment has reduced the number of operations performed for the complications of peptic ulcers. But roughly 20 percent of people with an ulcer ultimately require surgery because of scarring and obstruction, uncontrolled bleeding, or perforation of the ulcer. The most commonly performed procedures are called the Billroth I and II partial gastrectomies for gastric and duodenal ulceration and the highly selective vagotomy combined with pyloroplasty for duodenal ulceration (see right). In Billroth I partial gastrectomy, surgeons remove the lower part of the stomach, including the ulcer. They then stitch the remaining part of the stomach onto the upper end of the duodenum. In Billroth II partial gastrectomy, 80 percent of the lower part of the stomach may be removed. Surgeons close the duodenum and join the cut end of the stomach to the jejunum about 20 inches from the closed end of the duodenum. The procedure can produce side effects, such as diarrhea, vomiting, and weight loss.

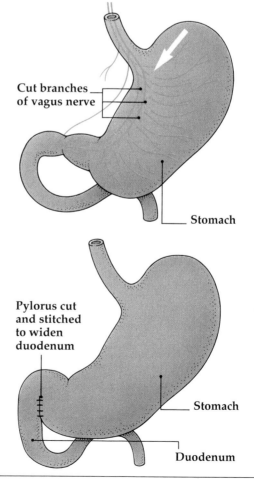

Cut branches of vagus nerve

Stomach

Pylorus cut and stitched to widen duodenum

Stomach

Duodenum

**Highly selective vagotomy and pyloroplasty**
*In the operation called highly selective vagotomy, surgeons cut some branches of the vagus nerve (arrow, above left). This action prevents nerve signals from stimulating acid secretion by the stomach lining, reducing acid secretion. The operation is usually combined with pyloroplasty, which involves cutting the pylorus and the duodenum and sewing them up so that the upper end is wider (lower left). This procedure allows the contents of the stomach to flow through the duodenum more quickly and minimizes the impaired emptying of the stomach contents that can be brought on by vagotomy.*

## STOMACH CANCER

**Dietary factors**
*Various additives in pickled, smoked, or salted foods, such as bacon, may cause stomach cancer, but doctors have no proof of the link as yet. High concentrations of the contaminant nitrate – used as a preservative in foods such as hot dogs or sausage, or found in drinking water – may also be a factor. The incidence of stomach cancer is high in countries where the consumption of smoked and nitrate-cured foods is high.*

Until the 1940s, stomach cancer was common in the US. Since then, there has been a dramatic and unexplained reduction in the annual death rate from the disease, from around 22 to less than seven per 100,000 of the population. The highest incidence of stomach cancer occurs in people aged 55 to 65, and the male-to-female ratio is 3 to 2.

No conclusive evidence about the cause of stomach cancer exists, but research suggests that dietary factors may be involved. Some factors, such as pernicious anemia, previous gastric surgery, and polyps of the stomach, have been identified as potentially precancerous conditions. Doctors do not know whether genetic factors play a role in the development of stomach cancer. But the disorder is slightly more common in people with blood group A, and clusters of the condition have been detected in families. Stomach cancer may arise from an interaction between diet and a genetic predisposition to the condition.

## Symptoms of stomach cancer

In its early stages, stomach cancer usually causes no symptoms. If the cancer is ulcerated, it may produce symptoms that are indistinguishable from those of a stomach ulcer. This fact has prompted doctors to perform early investigation of symptoms that suggest an ulcer in people over age 45. People with advanced stomach cancer may develop abdominal pain, loss of appetite, weight loss, and abdominal swelling. Advanced stomach cancer may spread to other parts of the body, such as the liver or bones. When the cancer is located in the lower part of the stomach, it may obstruct the outflow of stomach contents, causing severe and uncontrollable vomiting. Cancer near the gastroesophageal junction may block this opening, making it increasingly difficult to swallow solid foods.

**Diagnosing stomach cancer**
*Doctors can confirm the diagnosis of stomach cancer by barium X-ray (arrow near right) or esophagogastroduodenoscopy (arrow far right). The second procedure allows tissue samples to be removed without surgery for examination under a microscope, increasing diagnostic accuracy. After diagnosis, more investigations may be needed to determine the extent of any spread of the cancer.*

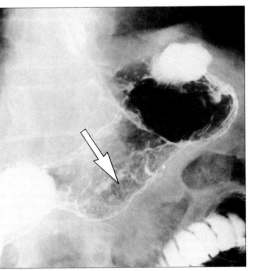
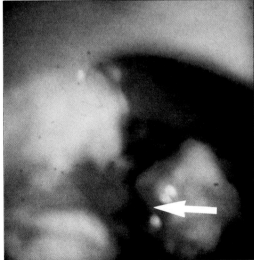

## TREATING STOMACH CANCER

In its early stages, before stomach cancer spreads, surgery can cure the condition. Once the cancer has spread, it cannot be cured, but symptoms produced by obstruction from a tumor can be relieved surgically. Chemotherapy (treatment with anticancer drugs) may prolong life and reduce symptoms. The overall survival rate for people with stomach cancer is poor – only about 7 percent of people survive 5 years after diagnosis. Early diagnosis and surgery are essential to reduce the death rate from this disease.

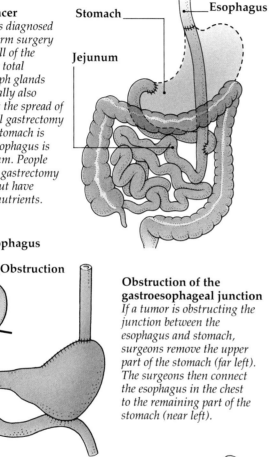

**Surgery can cure stomach cancer**
*If stomach cancer is diagnosed early, doctors perform surgery to remove part or all of the stomach (partial or total gastrectomy). Lymph glands in the area are usually also removed to prevent the spread of cancer. With a total gastrectomy (right), the entire stomach is removed and the esophagus is joined to the jejunum. People who have had total gastrectomy can swallow food but have trouble absorbing nutrients.*

Stomach
Esophagus
Jejunum

Esophagus
Obstruction
Stomach

**Obstruction of the gastroesophageal junction**
*If a tumor is obstructing the junction between the esophagus and stomach, surgeons remove the upper part of the stomach (far left). The surgeons then connect the esophagus in the chest to the remaining part of the stomach (near left).*

Obstruction
Stomach
Duodenum

**Obstruction at the lower end of the stomach**
*Obstruction at the lower end of the stomach can be relieved by removal of the lower portion of the stomach (near right). The remaining part of the stomach is then attached to the duodenum (far right) or the jejunum.*

## ASK YOUR DOCTOR
## STOMACH PROBLEMS

**Q** My husband has been experiencing abdominal pain. His doctor ordered a test called a GI series. What is this test?

**A** A GI series is an X-ray examination of the gastrointestinal (GI) tract that uses barium, an element through which X-rays cannot pass. There are two types of GI series: upper and lower. To conduct an upper GI series, the doctor gives the person a mixture of barium and water to drink. A series of X-rays are then taken of the esophagus, stomach, and duodenum as the barium moves through these organs. In a lower GI series, the person is given a barium enema. Doctors then take X-rays of the large intestine.

**Q** My mother has a stomach ulcer. Her doctor told her that she must have it monitored even though her symptoms are gone. She is taking an ulcer-healing drug. Why must she see the doctor again?

**A** In a small number of cases, an ulcer can develop on a stomach cancer. Your mother's doctor is simply making sure that if her ulcer does not heal completely, or if there is any evidence it is cancerous, it can be treated as early as possible.

**Q** I have been having indigestion and I see that many antacids are available. Which is the best?

**A** Take the antacid that works best for you. Like most drugs, antacids can produce side effects. Products containing too much magnesium can cause diarrhea. Those with aluminum only can produce constipation. Sodium bicarbonate may be dangerous if you have liver, heart, or kidney disease.

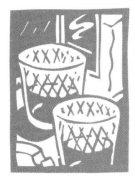

# LIVER AND GALLBLADDER DISORDERS

EXCESSIVE ALCOHOL CONSUMPTION is the most common cause of liver disease in developed countries. But serious liver disease can also be caused by viral infection of the liver (viral hepatitis); poisoning by toxic chemicals, drug sensitivities, or drug overdoses; or an immune system disorder. Most disorders of the gallbladder and bile ducts occur after gallstones develop.

Alcohol can damage the liver in several ways. Alcoholic liver disease progresses through stages of increasing severity, from accumulation of fat inside liver cells (fatty liver), to acute (sudden, short-term) alcoholic hepatitis, to cirrhosis of the liver. People with fatty liver or alcoholic hepatitis can develop cirrhosis of the liver if they continue to drink. But cirrhosis can also occur on its own.

## ALCOHOLIC LIVER DISEASE

People with fatty liver may not have symptoms, but the liver becomes tender and enlarged and blood test results for liver function are abnormal.

Mild alcoholic hepatitis may not produce symptoms either, but people with

## HOW DOES ALCOHOL DAMAGE THE LIVER?

Your body has no storage capacity for alcohol. The chemical is either excreted unchanged in the urine or breath or becomes converted into a substance called acetaldehyde in the liver cells. Acetaldehyde is toxic and can damage the outer membranes of liver cells, eventually killing them.

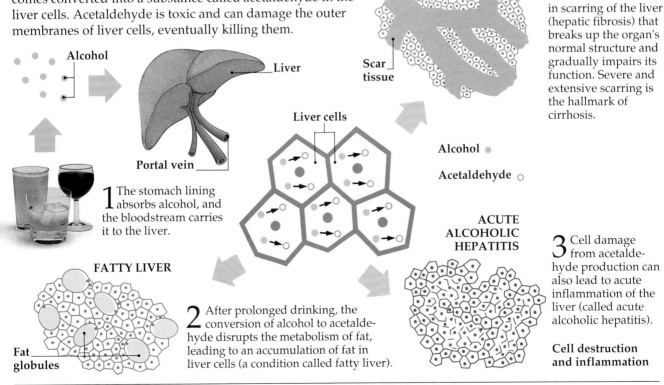

**FIBROSIS/CIRRHOSIS**

4 Chronic damage to the cells results in scarring of the liver (hepatic fibrosis) that breaks up the organ's normal structure and gradually impairs its function. Severe and extensive scarring is the hallmark of cirrhosis.

Scar tissue

Alcohol ●

Acetaldehyde ○

Liver

Portal vein

Liver cells

**ACUTE ALCOHOLIC HEPATITIS**

3 Cell damage from acetaldehyde production can also lead to acute inflammation of the liver (called acute alcoholic hepatitis).

**Cell destruction and inflammation**

1 The stomach lining absorbs alcohol, and the bloodstream carries it to the liver.

**FATTY LIVER**

2 After prolonged drinking, the conversion of alcohol to acetaldehyde disrupts the metabolism of fat, leading to an accumulation of fat in liver cells (a condition called fatty liver).

Fat globules

## WHO IS AT RISK FOR ALCOHOLIC LIVER DISEASE?

The death rate from cirrhosis of the liver is closely correlated with the amount of alcohol consumed. Cirrhosis is a common cause of death in the US – in 1984, about 27,000 people died of cirrhosis and chronic liver disease. Shown here are important risk factors for alcoholic liver disease, including cirrhosis:

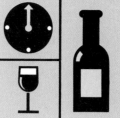

**Pattern of alcohol consumption**
Continued daily drinking is dangerous, but intermittent use can also be damaging.

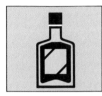

**Average daily alcohol consumption**
People who develop cirrhosis usually consume large amounts of hard liquor, wine, or beer every day. Although the risk increases the longer and the more you drink, virtually any level of alcohol consumption is potentially damaging to the liver.

**Gender**
Women are more susceptible to liver damage from alcohol than are men, partly because of their smaller size and partly because they lack special stomach enzymes that break down alcohol.

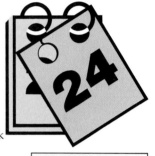

**Duration of consumption**
Significant liver damage is uncommon in people who drink to excess for less than 5 consecutive years.

the disorder may develop loss of appetite, weight loss, fatigue, and an enlarged liver. More severe alcoholic hepatitis can cause symptoms such as fever; an enlarged, tender liver; bleeding inside the gastrointestinal tract; accumulation of fluid in the abdominal cavity (called ascites); and liver failure.

## Cirrhosis of the liver

In people who have cirrhosis of the liver, bands of scar tissue break up the normal structure of the liver. The organ can no longer remove toxic substances from the blood. These toxic substances build up in the bloodstream and can affect brain function. High blood pressure develops in the portal vein, which carries blood from the abdominal organs to the liver (see PORTAL HYPERTENSION on page 102). Cirrhosis also increases the risk of liver cancer (see page 106).

## Treatment and outlook

Total and permanent abstinence from alcohol is essential for a complete recovery from fatty liver and acute alcoholic hepatitis. People with severe alcoholic hepatitis need intensive hospital treatment and may need several months to fully recover. This illness can be fatal.

Cirrhosis of the liver is irreversible. Only about half of all people diagnosed with alcoholic cirrhosis will be alive 5 years after diagnosis. This average increases to 60 percent with abstinence from alcohol and declines to 40 percent with continued heavy drinking.

Some complications of alcoholic liver disease respond to treatment. Varicose veins in the esophagus, a complication of portal hypertension, can be improved by injection of a solution that shrinks and blocks off the affected veins. But new varicose veins often form.

### IS CIRRHOSIS ALWAYS CAUSED BY ALCOHOL?

Alcohol consumption is the most common cause of cirrhosis. But some people develop cirrhosis following long-term hepatitis (inflammation of the liver) caused by a viral infection or by an immune system disturbance. Other causes of cirrhosis include disorders of the bile ducts (the channels through which bile travels from the liver to the gallbladder and duodenum) and metabolic disorders (disturbances of body chemistry). Most metabolic disorders affecting liver cells are inherited.

## PORTAL HYPERTENSION

The portal vein carries blood from the digestive tract, spleen, and pancreas to the liver. Blood flow to the liver can become obstructed, most often from cirrhosis but sometimes from a blood clot in the portal vein or one of its tributaries, or from narrowing of the vein at birth. This obstruction leads to portal hypertension, an increase in blood pressure in the portal vein. Reverse pressure throughout the system of veins that feeds the portal vein can lead to the conditions shown at right.

**Blood flow** ⟹

**Reverse pressure** →

**Fluid** →

**Fluid collection in the abdomen**
*In some people with portal hypertension, pressure forces fluid into the abdomen, where it collects. This condition is called ascites.*

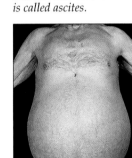

### CHRONIC ACTIVE VIRAL HEPATITIS

Several different viruses can infect the liver and cause viral hepatitis (inflammation of the liver from a viral infection). People contract type A hepatitis from contaminated food or water. They contract types B and C hepatitis through sexual intercourse, contaminated blood, or needle sharing related to drug abuse. Types B and C can lead to a type of liver inflammation called chronic active hepatitis and eventually to cirrhosis and/or liver cancer. Chronic active hepatitis may be treated with interferon-alpha, a genetically engineered protein that fights infection.

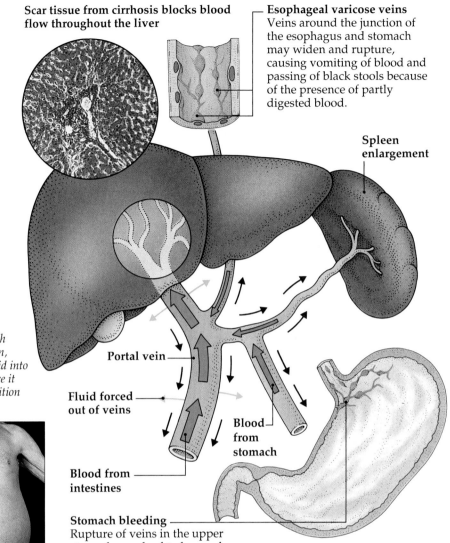

**Scar tissue from cirrhosis blocks blood flow throughout the liver**

**Esophageal varicose veins**
Veins around the junction of the esophagus and stomach may widen and rupture, causing vomiting of blood and passing of black stools because of the presence of partly digested blood.

**Spleen enlargement**

**Portal vein**

**Fluid forced out of veins**

**Blood from stomach**

**Blood from intestines**

**Stomach bleeding**
Rupture of veins in the upper stomach may lead to hemorrhage.

Ascites (fluid in the abdomen), also a complication of portal hypertension, can be treated with diuretic drugs, restricted sodium intake, and drainage if breathing becomes impaired. Affected brain function responds to treatments that decrease the absorption of toxic substances from the colon. These treatments include laxatives, such as lactulose, and oral antibiotics, such as neomycin, to kill bacteria in the colon that form toxins.

## JAUNDICE

Bilirubin is a normal breakdown product of hemoglobin, the oxygen-carrying pigment in red blood cells. Liver cells collect bilirubin and excrete it into bile. Jaundice develops when bilirubin levels increase in the blood. The pigment is deposited throughout the body, causing yellowish discoloration.

### Causes

In hepatitis, inflammation impairs excretion of bilirubin, causing jaundice. Obstruction of bile flow from the liver to the gallbladder can also produce jaundice. Gallstones, cancer, and scarring from surgery can obstruct the ducts outside the liver. Some drugs and a disease called primary biliary cirrhosis can interrupt bile flow inside the liver. Increased bilirubin production from greater red blood cell breakdown (hemolytic anemia) can also produce jaundice.

# CASE HISTORY
# ITCHING AND JAUNDICE

J ANE HAD BEEN TROUBLED for some time by itching all over her body. For many months, she had coped with the situation by applying a soothing lotion. But the itching got worse, and Jane became alarmed when a friend told her that the color of her complexion had been yellow-green lately. She decided to see her doctor.

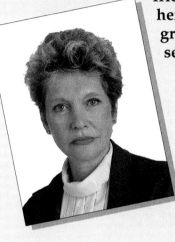

**PERSONAL DETAILS**
**Name** Jane Martin
**Age** 52
**Occupation** Chemist
**Family** Jane's father died of a heart attack 3 years ago. Her mother has rheumatoid arthritis.

## MEDICAL BACKGROUND
Jane has had no serious illnesses and has never had itchy skin. She doesn't smoke or drink much alcohol.

## THE CONSULTATION
The doctor examines Jane's skin and the whites of her eyes. She notices a distinct yellowish discoloration and many scratch marks on Jane's arms and chest. When she examines Jane's abdomen, she notices that her liver is enlarged and tender.

The doctor takes a blood sample so that some blood tests can be performed. The results show that Jane has a high level of the pigment bilirubin in her blood as well as high levels of some enzymes produced by the liver. These results confirm that Jane has cholestasis – an interference with the flow of bile out of her liver. Bilirubin has accumulated in her blood, causing the jaundice, or yellowing of her skin. The deposit of bile salts in her skin has caused the itching. Jane's doctor is uncertain of the underlying cause, so she refers Jane to a hepatologist, a doctor who specializes in liver disorders.

## THE DIAGNOSIS
The hepatologist orders more blood tests, which show that Jane's blood contains antibodies (substances produced by the immune system) that are attacking her liver tissue. An ultrasound scan shows no obvious obstruction of bile flow. But results of a liver biopsy confirm the specialist's suspicions.

**The physical examination**
*During the initial visit, Jane's doctor examines her upper abdomen and notices that her liver is enlarged.*

The specialist tells Jane that she has PRIMARY BILIARY CIRRHOSIS. This condition is an autoimmune disorder in which the body's immune system attacks and destroys the small bile ducts in the liver. Unlike the more common forms of liver cirrhosis, it is not caused by alcohol.

## THE TREATMENT
The specialist tells Jane that there is no medical treatment that can stop the progression of her disease. She may become a candidate for liver transplantation in the future. He prescribes a drug (cholestyramine) to help reduce her itching.

During the next 2 years, Jane's jaundice gets worse, and she has intermittent abdominal pain and ascites (fluid collection in the abdomen from liver disease). The doctor refers her to a transplant center. Two months later, she undergoes a successful liver transplant operation.

## THE OUTCOME
Fully recovered from her illness, Jane can now look forward to years of active life.

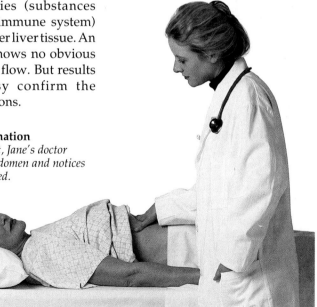

# SURGICAL PROCEDURES
# LIVER TRANSPLANT

SURGEONS PERFORMED **the first successful liver transplant in 1967. The survival period for recipients of transplanted livers was disappointingly short until 1981, when a new drug called cyclosporine debuted that prevented rejection of the transplanted liver. Today, there are more than 70 transplant centers in the US. Reports show that more than 80 percent of people who undergo a liver transplant operation can resume their usual level of activity.**

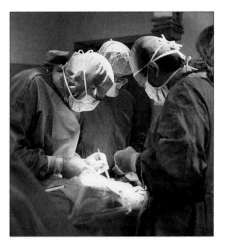

People with certain terminal liver diseases are the most likely candidates for a liver transplant. Such diseases can include chronic active hepatitis (see page 102), primary biliary cirrhosis (see page 103), and a number of other liver diseases. Doctors do not usually do transplants for people with alcoholic cirrhosis unless they have totally abstained from alcohol. For children whose biliary systems have failed to develop, a liver transplant may be the only chance for survival. The recipient should be free of infection and of significant heart and lung diseases.

## The donor
The donor may be a person between 1 and 55 years of age who is free of infection or cancer. The liver must be removed immediately after the donor's death, although it can be stored in an ice-cold preserving solution for up to 24 hours.

## Compatibility
The liver is remarkably resistant to rejection by the recipient's immune system. Although doctors try to match the blood groups of the donor and recipient, successful transplants have been made between people of different blood groups. The size of the donor liver is very important in the selection of a recipient. An oversized or small donor liver can cause technical difficulties in transplantation, especially in a child.

**1** The donor liver is obtained from a person who has been pronounced brain dead, usually as the result of an accident. The liver is removed carefully, with its blood vessels and biliary drainage system intact. The vessels and the organ itself can be trimmed to fit the recipient at the time of surgery.

**2** The liver is stored in a solution that helps preserve liver cells. The solution may contain drugs to prevent clotting, infection, and tissue damage while the liver is being transported.

**3** The recipient is anesthetized and fully monitored throughout the procedure. Blood loss may be severe, so the surgical team uses suction machines to return the patient's blood into circulation.

**4** The surgeons make an incision in the upper part of the abdomen to expose the operation site. They extend the incision into the chest if needed.

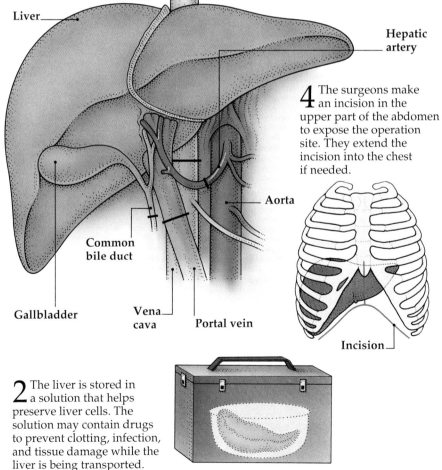

Liver

Hepatic artery

Aorta

Common bile duct

Gallbladder

Vena cava

Portal vein

Incision

**5** The surgeons then clamp the vena cava, the main vessel returning blood to the heart, above and below the recipient's diseased liver. The clamps interfere with the patient's blood flow, so the surgeons construct a bypass. They remove the liver after cutting the hepatic artery, portal vein, and bile duct.

**6** The surgeons then begin to connect the new liver to the vena cava. Next, the hepatic artery and portal vein are rejoined. Finally, the patient's and the donor bile ducts can be joined directly with a tube shaped like a T. The tube's short arms are attached to the bile ducts, and its long arm runs out through the abdomen to remove bile. The tube can be removed later. The bile ducts can also be joined indirectly by way of the gallbladder to the jejunum, the middle part of the small intestine.

**8** Rejection of the new liver can occur as early as the fifth day after the operation, so doctors start immuno-suppressive therapy immediately. A drug called cyclosporine is the most effective immunosuppressive agent now available. Use of the drug must be monitored carefully, because it can be toxic to the kidneys and can cause other problems.

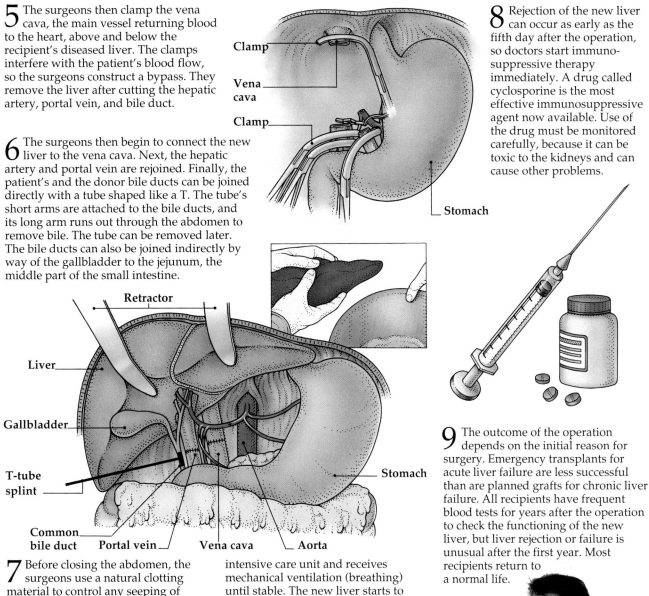

Clamp
Vena cava
Clamp
Stomach

Retractor
Liver
Gallbladder
T-tube splint
Common bile duct
Portal vein
Vena cava
Aorta
Stomach

**9** The outcome of the operation depends on the initial reason for surgery. Emergency transplants for acute liver failure are less successful than are planned grafts for chronic liver failure. All recipients have frequent blood tests for years after the operation to check the functioning of the new liver, but liver rejection or failure is unusual after the first year. Most recipients return to a normal life.

**7** Before closing the abdomen, the surgeons use a natural clotting material to control any seeping of blood and insert large drainage tubes. The incision is then sewn shut, and drainage tubes are put in place. After surgery, the patient is placed in an intensive care unit and receives mechanical ventilation (breathing) until stable. The new liver starts to function soon. Drainage tubes are removed as soon as the flow of fluid stops. The patient begins consuming a light diet as soon as possible.

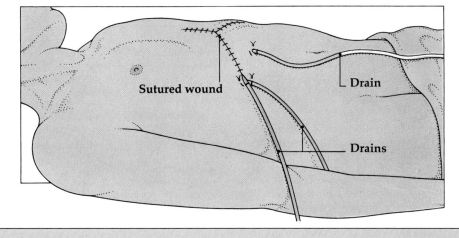

Sutured wound
Drain
Drains

## Diagnosis and treatment of jaundice

Jaundice may be accompanied by dark urine. Instead of being excreted by the liver, bilirubin builds up in the bloodstream and is excreted by the kidneys. Jaundice can also occur with pale stools if less bilirubin reaches the person's digestive tract. Blood tests, ultrasound or computed tomography (CT) scanning, a liver biopsy, and a procedure called endoscopic retrograde cholangiopancreatography (ERCP, see page 81) help doctors establish the cause of jaundice.

Treatment depends on the cause. Most forms of hemolytic anemia can be treated. Some types of hepatitis heal on their own. Some forms of chronic hepatitis and primary biliary cirrhosis are curable only by liver transplantation. Children whose biliary systems fail to develop also require a liver transplant.

## LIVER CANCER

The liver is a common site of secondary cancer (cancer that spreads from other parts of the body); it is less common for cancer to originate in the liver itself (primary liver cancer). Primary liver cancer, including bile duct cancer, causes about 11,500 deaths per year in this country. In some parts of the world, primary liver cancer is much more common. Known risk factors include infection with the hepatitis B and C viruses, the consumption of peanuts contaminated by certain molds, and the presence of parasites in the liver (such as liver flukes). In the US, a high percentage of people with primary liver cancer have cirrhosis.

Loss of the sense of well-being, weight loss, abdominal pain, an enlarged liver, and ascites (fluid in the abdomen) are common manifestations of liver cancer. Doctors confirm the diagnosis by ultrasound scanning and a liver biopsy. The outlook is poor. Occasionally, tumors confined to a certain area can be removed to improve the chances of survival.

## EXTERNAL SIGNS OF LIVER DISEASE

Examination of the skin, eyes, and hands can often reveal signs of liver disease to a doctor.

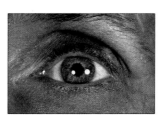

**Jaundice in the eyes**
*This person has obstructive jaundice – yellowing of the skin and whites of the eyes from the obstruction of bile flow from the liver. He also has fatty deposits in his eyelids from obstructive jaundice.*

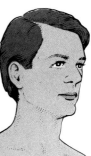

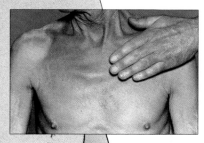

**Jaundice in the skin**
*The yellow discoloration of this person's trunk is clearly apparent when compared with the color of the doctor's hand.*

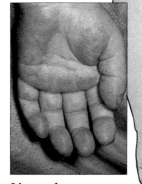

**Liver palm**
*Reddening of the palms of the hands is a common feature of alcoholic liver disease.*

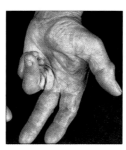

**Dupuytren's contracture**
*One or more fingers bent in a fixed position is a characteristic that is common in (although is not restricted to) people with liver cirrhosis.*

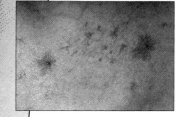

**Spider nevi**
*Large numbers of these raised, pinhead-sized, bluish points, from which small blood vessels radiate, may be a sign of liver disease.*

## GALLSTONES

Gallstones are solid lumps of various sizes that can develop in the gallbladder when an imbalance arises in the chemical composition of bile. The most common type consists mainly of cholesterol. Women are at greater risk of developing cholesterol gallstones than are men, especially women who are overweight.

Gallstones are very common. But only a small proportion of people with gallstones ever experience symptoms from the stones. Gallstones that produce no symptoms do not require treatment.

### Gallstone-related disorders

Adverse effects caused by stones in the gallbladder or common bile duct include inflammation of the gallbladder (acute cholecystitis), severe, cramping pain (biliary colic), infection of the biliary tract (cholangitis), and jaundice.

Doctors can detect acute cholecystitis (sudden inflammation of the gallbladder) with ultrasound scanning. Surgeons usually remove the gallbladder (cholecystectomy) within 48 hours. If the person is not a good candidate for surgery, doctors treat the condition with intravenous fluids, painkillers, and antibiotics until the inflammation subsides. Then the gallbladder is removed. Sound wave disintegration of some stones (lithotripsy, see page 108) has been attempted with some success.

A stone that is obstructing the common bile duct may pass on its own into the duodenum. But usually the stone must be removed by surgery or via an endoscope (see page 108). The gallbladder is sometimes also removed because the person often has more stones.

Infection of the common bile duct is a medical emergency. Doctors treat it with antibiotics. Sometimes they drain infected material from the bile ducts, or perform surgery or endoscopic retrograde cholangiopancreatography (ERCP, see page 81).

## COMPLICATIONS OF GALLSTONES

**Acute cholecystitis**
When a gallstone becomes lodged in the cystic duct, it can cause infection of bile and the development of acute cholecystitis (sudden inflammation of the gallbladder). This condition causes a severe, sharp pain over the gallbladder in the upper right area of the abdomen that can spread into the back and right shoulder blade. The pain is often accompanied by fever and vomiting and usually subsides with treatment or when the stone passes into the duodenum or falls back into the gallbladder.

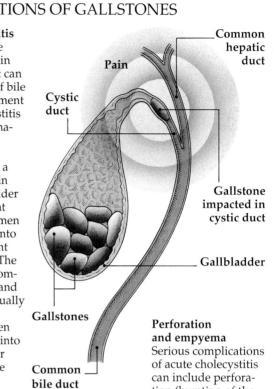

Pain

Common hepatic duct

Cystic duct

Gallstone impacted in cystic duct

Gallbladder

Gallstones

Common bile duct

**Chronic cholecystitis**
Repeated attacks of acute cholecystitis of varying severity may lead to chronic cholecystitis, in which the gallbladder becomes shrunken and thick-walled and ceases to function, producing recurrent attacks of abdominal pain.

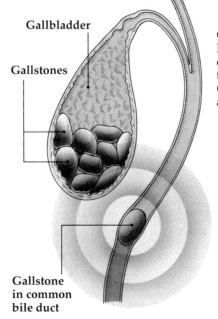

Gallbladder

Gallstones

Gallstone in common bile duct

**Perforation and empyema**
Serious complications of acute cholecystitis can include perforation (bursting of the gallbladder, causing inflammation of the membrane lining the abdominal cavity) or empyema, in which the gallbladder fills with pus. In either case, the person becomes extremely sick and needs immediate surgery.

**Cholangitis**
In some people with bile duct obstruction, the biliary tract becomes infected (cholangitis) and causes a high fever and chills.

**Bile duct obstruction**
Passage of gallstones in the common bile duct can cause jaundice and biliary colic. Biliary colic is a severe, cramping pain in the upper right part of the abdomen that may radiate to the back. It is accompanied by nausea and vomiting. Tests, such as ultrasound scanning, can establish the cause of the pain.

## Treating gallstones

Doctors use various methods to treat gallstones. The most common are removal of the gallbladder and surgical or endoscopic removal of stones obstructing the common bile duct. When small cholesterol stones are present in a functioning gallbladder, they can sometimes be dissolved with the drugs chenodeoxycholic acid or ursodeoxycholic acid. In another technique, doctors introduce a strong solvent directly into the gallbladder to dissolve cholesterol.

Gallstones can also be crushed during a procedure called lithotripsy. This procedure can be performed with a mechanical crushing instrument passed through an endoscope. More recently, a technique called extracorporeal shockwave lithotripsy has emerged that pulverizes stones in the gallbladder and common bile duct by means of externally applied multiple shock waves. The crushed gallstones are then excreted in the bile. Today, when doctors use this technique, they supplement it with drug treatment and endoscopic removal of duct stones. Gallstones recur in about half of all people who have any form of nonsurgical treatment.

### REMOVING A GALLSTONE WITH AN ENDOSCOPE

A gallstone in the lower part of the common bile duct can usually be removed with an endoscope (a tubelike viewing instrument) passed down the esophagus, through the stomach, and into the duodenum. The entrances of the pancreatic and bile ducts are investigated with probes.

**Gallstones**
*The photograph at upper right shows the intricate surface detail of a gallstone removed from the gallbladder (magnified 23,000 times), revealing its crystalline structure. The X-ray at lower right shows a gallbladder containing gallstones. Stones can also be seen in the bile ducts.*

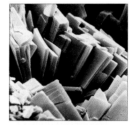

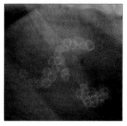

**Gallbladder**

**Endoscope**

**Stomach**

**Duodenum**

**1** Doctors detect the presence and location of the gallstone with X-ray imaging after introducing a dye into the bile duct and pancreatic duct through a channel in the endoscope. This technique is called endoscopic retrograde cholangiopancreatography (ERCP).

**2** The surgeon passes a snaring device down another channel of the endoscope to remove the stone, after mechanically crushing it if it is too big.

**Common bile duct**

**Gallstone**

**Snare**

**Contrast medium**

**Pancreatic duct**

# SURGICAL PROCEDURES
## LAPAROSCOPIC CHOLECYSTECTOMY

**L**APAROSCOPIC CHOLECYSTECTOMY
**is a commonly used surgical
technique for removing the gallbladder, using a fiberoptic
viewing instrument called a
laparoscope. The procedure does
not require a large abdominal
incision, so recovery after the
operation is relatively rapid.
In some cases, the surgeon must
open the abdominal cavity with a
scalpel to remove the gallbladder.**

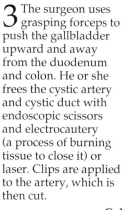

**3** The surgeon uses
grasping forceps to
push the gallbladder
upward and away
from the duodenum
and colon. He or she
frees the cystic artery
and cystic duct with
endoscopic scissors
and electrocautery
(a process of burning
tissue to close it) or
laser. Clips are applied
to the artery, which is
then cut.

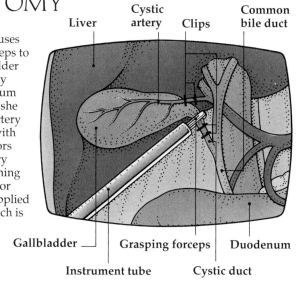

Liver   Cystic artery   Clips   Common bile duct

Gallbladder   Grasping forceps   Duodenum

Instrument tube   Cystic duct

**4** The surgeon clips the cystic duct close to the gallbladder so that no stones can escape. An operative
cholangiogram (an X-ray image that shows the bile ducts
after they have been filled with a dye through which X-
rays cannot pass) is obtained by passing a slender tube
through the cystic duct into the main bile duct to ensure
that the bile duct does not contain any hidden stones.
The cystic duct is cut and tied.

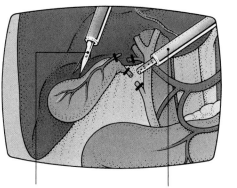

**5** The surgeon uses
microscissors to release
the gallbladder from the
liver. Any blood vessels are
coagulated. Special tubes
enable the surgeon to
introduce fluid into and
suction fluid out of the
operative area so
that the image on the
monitor remains clear.

Microscissors   Irrigation/suction tube

Incisions

**1** The patient receives general anesthesia.
The surgeon inserts a spring-loaded needle
through an incision near the patient's navel (1)
and pumps carbon dioxide through this needle
until the abdomen is distended by the gas. The
doctor inserts the laparoscope into the same
incision. The abdominal cavity appears on a
monitor as the operation proceeds.

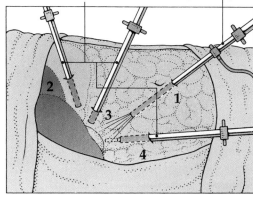

Instrument tubes   Laparoscope

**2** Three additional tubes are inserted into the
right side of the abdomen (2, 3, 4) to help the
surgeon gain access to different parts of the
abdomen with instruments and the laparoscope.

Removed gallbladder

**6** The surgeon with-
draws the freed gall-
bladder from the abdomi-
nal cavity through the
navel after crushing the
stones or extracting them.
He or she may place a
drain in the former
gallbladder site, if needed.
The carbon dioxide is
released from the abdomi-
nal cavity, and the four
incisions are sewn up.

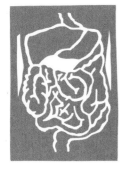

# PANCREATIC DISORDERS

THE PANCREAS is a complex organ that plays several important roles in the body. Disorders of the pancreas usually have far-reaching effects. The most common pancreatic disorders include inflammation, pseudocysts, and cancer. Symptoms arising from these conditions can include pain and discomfort, digestive problems, and disruption of the hormone balance in the bloodstream.

Exocrine tissue accounts for the bulk of the pancreas. This tissue produces enzymes that are secreted into a duct that empties into the duodenum. These enzymes are essential for the digestion of food. Scattered throughout the exocrine tissue are endocrine glands called the islets of Langerhans, which secrete hormones such as insulin directly into the bloodstream. If the pancreas becomes inflamed, or if the main pancreatic duct is blocked by a tumor, the digestive enzymes may leak out of the duct into the pancreas and cause inflammation.

**Healthy pancreatic tissue**
*Tissue in a healthy pancreas (right) shows endocrine glands (the pale area in the center). These glands release the hormones insulin and glucagon. The darker tissue surrounding the endocrine glands consists mainly of exocrine glands that produce digestive enzymes.*

**Acute pancreatitis**
*In acute pancreatitis, the normal structure of the endocrine and exocrine glands is disrupted. Pus cells (see arrow) have invaded the pancreatic tissue and indicate that the pancreas is acutely inflamed.*

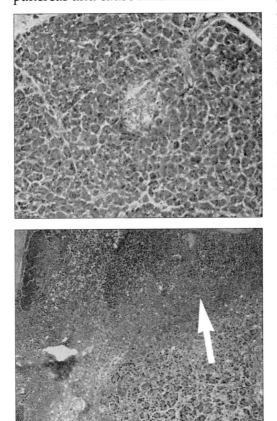

## PANCREATITIS

Inflammation of the pancreas is called pancreatitis. The condition may be acute, if the symptoms appear suddenly and severely, or chronic, if the symptoms are less severe but continue for a long period of time. Pancreatitis can also flare up in recurrent acute episodes.

### What causes pancreatitis?
Many cases of pancreatitis follow progressive damage to the pancreas from alcohol abuse. Another form of acute pancreatitis often accompanies gallstones, but inflammation can occur with no obvious explanation. The incidence of acute pancreatitis is about 10 per 100,000 of the population in the US and is equally divided between men and women. Chronic pancreatitis occurs in about four per 100,000 of the population, with a male-to-female ratio of 3 to 1. Most cases of pancreatitis occur in people between ages 40 and 60. Chronic pancreatitis also occurs in children with cystic fibrosis, an inherited disease.

### What are the symptoms?
In an acute attack of pancreatitis, the person suddenly develops a strong, steady pain in the upper part of the abdomen, which then penetrates to the back. Nausea, vomiting, and abdominal distention also occur. A fever is often present. In severe, hemorrhaging attacks, the patient may have a rapid pulse and low blood pressure and can go into shock.

# CASE HISTORY
## ABDOMINAL PAIN AND VOMITING

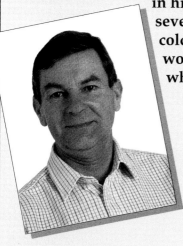

A FTER AN EXCEPTIONALLY STRESSFUL **board meeting, at which David presented his firm's financial statements, he came home, ate a large, rich meal, and drank heavily. The next day at work, David felt severe pain in his upper abdomen, vomited several times, and began to feel cold, clammy, and faint. His co-workers called an ambulance, which rushed him to the hospital.**

**PERSONAL DETAILS**
**Name** David Lomax
**Age** 50
**Occupation** Accountant for a real estate development firm
**Family** David's father died when David was a teenager. His mother is alive and healthy.

**MEDICAL BACKGROUND**
David has had periods of depression since his 20s. This depression, compounded by the stresses of his job, has led David to steadily increase his alcohol consumption. He now drinks up to two bottles of vodka and a case of beer a week. His drinking is beginning to affect his work and family.

**THE EXAMINATION**
When he arrives at the emergency room, David is in severe pain and has a rapid pulse and low blood pressure, which are symptoms of shock. The medical staff admit him to the intensive care unit, give him an injection to relieve the pain, and set up an intravenous infusion to restore his blood volume and correct his low blood pressure. Later, the doctors perform an abdominal X-ray and take blood samples.

**THE DIAGNOSIS**
The X-ray shows some dilation of the bowel, which means the intestines are swelling and are unable to propel their contents. The analysis of David's blood confirms that his pancreas is acutely inflamed. An ultrasound scan shows that his pancreas is swollen. Based on these results and David's history and symptoms, the doctor diagnoses ACUTE PANCREATITIS brought on by David's high alcohol intake.

**THE TREATMENT**
Eating aggravates the inflamed pancreas, so David is given no food for several days. After some time, the pain begins to diminish, and David is able to start eating a light diet. After a week, the pain has disappeared completely, and he is allowed to go home. Subsequent ultrasound scans show that he has developed a fluid-filled sac called a pseudocyst (see page 112) because his pancreatic ducts have become blocked and swollen. During the next 3 months, repeated ultrasound scans indicate that the pseudocyst is subsiding. But David has a hard time giving up alcohol, and his doctor urges him to seek help from an alcohol support group. David finds that attending group meetings and talking about his alcohol addiction gives him the support he needs to live a day at a time without alcohol.

**Ultrasound scan**
*By pressing the ultrasound transducer on David's abdomen and moving it slowly in a circular motion, the doctor can see on the ultrasound monitor that David's pancreas is inflamed and contains a pseudocyst.*

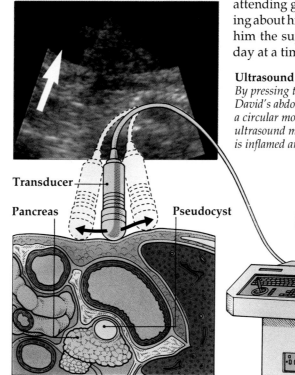
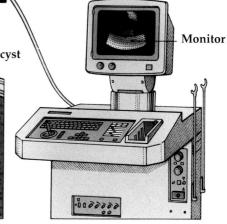

Transducer
Pancreas
Pseudocyst
Monitor

A bluish discoloration of the skin can appear on the sides or around the navel.

Recurrent attacks of chronic pancreatitis cause a deficiency of enzymes and hormones, producing malabsorption (see page 114) and diabetes mellitus. Doctors diagnose the condition with blood tests, ultrasound scanning, computed tomography (CT) scanning, and endoscopic retrograde cholangiopancreatography (ERCP, see page 81).

## How is pancreatitis treated?

During an acute attack of pancreatitis, doctors give the affected person painkillers and other drugs that suppress the production of stomach acid. Doctors sometimes remove the stomach contents through a tube inserted into the nose or mouth. Severe complications are treated if they arise. Surgery may be necessary to drain an abscess. People with chronic pancreatitis may receive digestive enzyme replacements or insulin.

## CYSTS AND PSEUDOCYSTS

True cysts are rare. They have a lining of protective cells and occur in the pancreas, the liver, and the kidneys. True cysts are sometimes congenital (present from birth) but do not occur in the pancreatic duct system. True cysts rarely cause problems. Pseudocysts, fluid-filled sacs in the pancreas, are much more common. Pseudocysts usually appear as a complication of pancreatitis and may cause pain, nausea, and vomiting. Computed tomography (CT) scanning (a diagnostic technique that uses X-rays and a computer to produce body images) can often detect the presence of pseudocysts. Some pseudocysts shrink as acute pancreatitis subsides. Others require surgical drainage. Another group of pancreatic cysts are called cystic tumors. These cysts can be benign (cystadenoma) or cancerous (cystadenocarcinoma).

# CANCER OF THE PANCREAS

Pancreatic cancer accounts for just over 5 percent of all deaths from cancer. Its incidence is increasing, but the reason for the increase remains unknown. More than 75 percent of cases occur in people over 60. Symptoms can include pain in the upper abdomen (often penetrating to the back), weight loss, and jaundice. The outlook for most kinds of pancreatic cancer is poor, but if the tumor is confined to the area around the pouch called the ampulla of Vater, the chances of being cured are much higher.

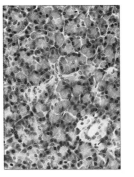
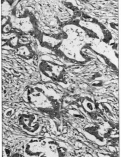

**Cancer of the pancreas**
*Healthy pancreatic tissue (above left) has been replaced by groups of malignant cells (above right).*

**Cystadenoma**
*The cystadenoma (benign cyst) in the head of the pancreas at right has obstructed the pancreatic duct and caused it to widen.*

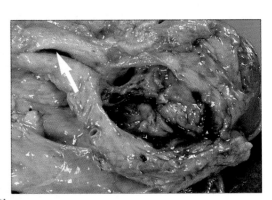

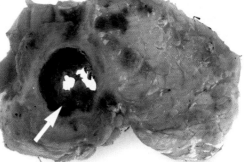

**Pseudocyst**
*A pseudocyst (see arrow) can be clearly seen in this severed tail of the pancreas at left. The cyst is filled with fluid.*

**DUODENAL DIVERTICULA**
Duodenal diverticula, small pouches that occur in the duodenum, generally cause no symptoms. But if they are close to the ampulla of Vater, the passageway at the junction of the common bile duct and the pancreatic duct, the diverticula may increase a person's risk of developing inflammation of the biliary and pancreatic ducts.

**Ampulla of Vater**
**Diverticulum**

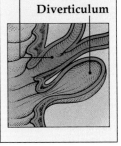

# SURGICAL PROCEDURES
# DRAINAGE OF A PSEUDOCYST

Accumulations of **fluid that occur in the pancreas when it becomes inflamed are called pseudocysts. Many pseudocysts disappear when the inflammation subsides. But very large pseudocysts can cause severe symptoms and are usually drained. The most successful method is internal drainage. Surgeons create an opening between the cyst and the stomach or between the cyst and the intestine to allow drainage. Some pseudocysts can be drained through a tube inserted in the abdominal wall.**

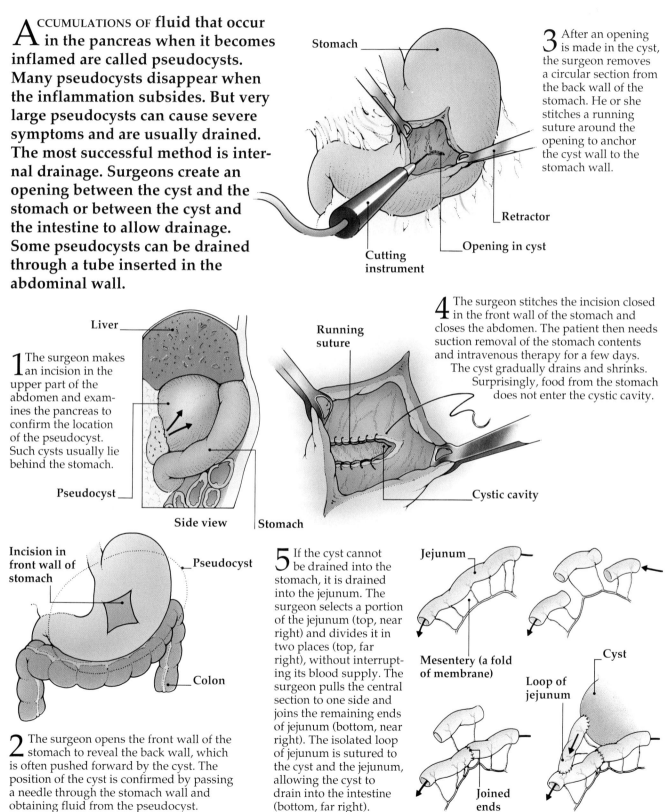

**3** After an opening is made in the cyst, the surgeon removes a circular section from the back wall of the stomach. He or she stitches a running suture around the opening to anchor the cyst wall to the stomach wall.

Stomach

Cutting instrument

Opening in cyst

Retractor

**1** The surgeon makes an incision in the upper part of the abdomen and examines the pancreas to confirm the location of the pseudocyst. Such cysts usually lie behind the stomach.

Liver

Pseudocyst

Side view

Stomach

Running suture

**4** The surgeon stitches the incision closed in the front wall of the stomach and closes the abdomen. The patient then needs suction removal of the stomach contents and intravenous therapy for a few days. The cyst gradually drains and shrinks. Surprisingly, food from the stomach does not enter the cystic cavity.

Cystic cavity

Incision in front wall of stomach

Pseudocyst

Colon

**2** The surgeon opens the front wall of the stomach to reveal the back wall, which is often pushed forward by the cyst. The position of the cyst is confirmed by passing a needle through the stomach wall and obtaining fluid from the pseudocyst.

**5** If the cyst cannot be drained into the stomach, it is drained into the jejunum. The surgeon selects a portion of the jejunum (top, near right) and divides it in two places (top, far right), without interrupting its blood supply. The surgeon pulls the central section to one side and joins the remaining ends of jejunum (bottom, near right). The isolated loop of jejunum is sutured to the cyst and the jejunum, allowing the cyst to drain into the intestine (bottom, far right).

Jejunum

Mesentery (a fold of membrane)

Cyst

Loop of jejunum

Joined ends

# INTESTINAL DISORDERS

T HE INTESTINES ARE SUSCEPTIBLE to a range of diseases, including infection, inflammation, tumor formation, and immune system disturbance. Diseases of the intestines can affect the speed at which the contents pass, impair absorption of nutrients in the small intestine, or change the amount of water and mineral salts absorbed or secreted by the colon. These processes produce symptoms such as diarrhea, constipation, or pain.

**Malabsorption caused by lactose intolerance**
*If a lactose-intolerant person consumes dairy products, undigested lactose accumulates in the small intestine, increasing the concentration of the intestinal contents and reducing water absorption. Fermentation of lactose by bacteria in the colon causes gas, bloating, and diarrhea. Water secretion by the colon adds to diarrhea. Some people become lactose intolerant as children. Others develop intolerance after inflammation of the intestines.*

Diarrhea can be caused by food poisoning from toxins and infections, celiac sprue (see page 115), and diverticular disease of the small intestine (see page 120). Intolerance to foods that contain lactose (see below and page 11), increased muscular activity from inflammatory bowel diseases (Crohn's disease and ulcerative colitis), and irritable bowel syndrome can also bring on diarrhea.

⬡⬡ Undigested lactose

Bacteria

⬅ Secretion of water

◯◯◯ Gas

💧💧 Diarrhea

➡ Reduced absorption of water

## MALABSORPTION

Malabsorption refers to the impaired absorption of nutrients, including vitamins and minerals, through the lining of the small intestine. The unabsorbed food residue passes out in the feces. Conditions causing malabsorption include celiac sprue, extensive Crohn's disease, pancreatitis, and surgery that removes part of the stomach or small intestine. Common effects of malabsorption are diarrhea, weight loss, and, in severe cases, malnutrition. The diagnosis is confirmed by blood tests, barium X-ray of the small intestines, and biopsy of the jejunum. Treatment of malabsorption depends on the underlying disorder, but often includes vitamin and mineral supplements and sometimes replacement of enzymes from the pancreas.

### Lactose intolerance
Inability to digest lactose, the sugar found in milk, is a common malabsorption disorder. Some people cannot eat or drink most dairy products without experiencing abdominal symptoms. Temporary lactose intolerance following gastroenteritis occurs because cells in the stomach lining that produce the enzyme that digests lactose may have been damaged. Intestinal production of this digestive enzyme takes some time to return to normal. People with temporary lactose intolerance may have to eliminate milk from their diets for a while.

# INFLAMMATORY BOWEL DISEASE

Inflammatory bowel disease is the general term for Crohn's disease and ulcerative colitis, two recurring inflammatory disorders. Ulcerative colitis is more common in the US, with an annual incidence of 5.7 per 100,000 of the population. The incidence of Crohn's disease is 4.8 per 100,000, but the rate appears to be increasing. The peak age of onset for both disorders is late adolescence.

The cause of both diseases remains unknown, but several theories have been proposed. The cause does not appear to be exposure to an infectious agent. Inflammatory bowel disease may arise after diarrhea caused by a bacterium or an ameba or after a reaction to antibiotic treatment. Doctors theorize that the disease may represent an abnormal immune reaction to the body's own tissues. Both diseases are more common in developed countries, which has led some researchers to suspect a dietary or stress factor. There also seems to be a genetic predisposition to both diseases.

## Symptoms of inflammatory bowel disease

Both types of inflammatory bowel disease usually cause diarrhea, fever, and abdominal pain. In ulcerative colitis, the diarrhea contains blood and mucus, and sometimes pus. In some cases of Crohn's disease, the symptoms are the same as in ulcerative colitis. In Crohn's disease, fistulas (abnormal channels) can develop between the intestines and other abdominal organs or between the intestines and the outer surface of the body.

**Sites of inflammatory bowel disease**
*Crohn's disease (near right) can affect any part of the digestive tract, from the mouth to the anus, but is usually found at the junction of the small and large intestines (terminal ileum). Inflammation is patchy, with areas of normal tissue lying between inflamed areas. Chronic inflammation may cause stricture. Ulcerative colitis (far right) can affect the entire colon or only parts of it.*

## CELIAC SPRUE

Celiac sprue is a disorder in which the lining of the small intestine becomes damaged by an allergic reaction to gluten, a protein found in wheat, rye, and some other grains. The damage causes malabsorption, a failure to absorb important nutrients from the intestine. The most common symptoms include weight loss, weakness, and diarrhea from the malabsorption of fat. The stools look pale and bulky and are offensive in odor because fat passes through the intestine unabsorbed and can be seen in the feces. Celiac sprue can occur at any age, depending on when cereals are first eaten, and can be successfully treated with a gluten-free diet. Celiac sprue tends to run in families, although some family members experience no symptoms.

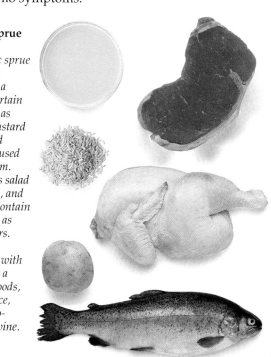

**Treating celiac sprue**
*The only effective treatment for celiac sprue is to avoid all foods containing gluten, a protein found in certain grains. Foods such as beer, pasta, and mustard are also not allowed because grains are used to manufacture them. Some foods, such as salad dressings, vinegars, and some margarines, contain hidden gluten used as binders or thickeners. Apart from these restrictions, people with celiac sprue can eat a varied diet of safe foods, such as potatoes, rice, fish, poultry, unprocessed meats, and wine.*

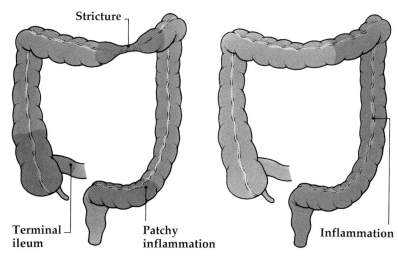

Stricture

Terminal ileum

Patchy inflammation

Inflammation

# EFFECTS OF INFLAMMATORY BOWEL DISEASE

Crohn's disease and ulcerative colitis have many features in common. But they differ from one another in several respects, including the segments of gastrointestinal tract they affect and the type of inflammation they cause. The diseases can sometimes be distinguished by barium X-ray, endoscopy, and microscopic analysis of samples of inflamed tissue. Both Crohn's disease and ulcerative colitis damage the digestive tract, but they can also cause a number of complications that affect other parts of the body.

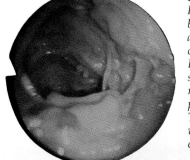

**Endoscopy of Crohn's disease**
*In Crohn's disease, the intestine becomes inflamed in some segments and not others, so endoscopy of the colon may reveal only normal tissue. But affected areas often contain scattered ulcers with patches of normal mucosa in between. The ulcers often penetrate the wall of the intestine. The inflammation can lead to scarring, which can cause narrowing and obstruction of the intestine.*

**Investigating Crohn's disease with a microscope**
*In Crohn's disease, inflammation produces ulcers on the surface of the intestine that enlarge and penetrate the deep muscle layers (below). Groups of inflammatory cells called granulomas (see arrow) occur in many cases of Crohn's disease. Cancerous changes sometimes appear.*

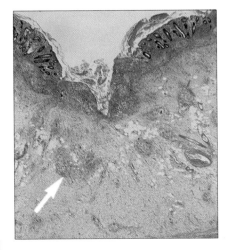

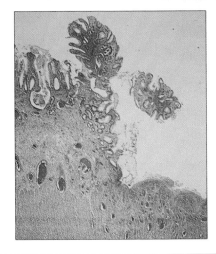

**Investigating ulcerative colitis with a microscope**
*In contrast to Crohn's disease, the inflammation caused by ulcerative colitis is confined to the mucosa (inner surface of the colon). Granulomas are not present. In many cases, the mucosa is severely damaged and loses mucus-producing cells (goblet cells). Healing and scarring cause the formation of pseudopolyps. Cancerous cell changes sometimes occur with ulcerative colitis.*

**Endoscopy of ulcerative colitis**
*Inflammation of the lining of the intestine (mucosa) is always visible during endoscopic examinations of active ulcerative colitis. The affected mucosa usually looks granular, and inflammatory pseudopolyps are often seen.*

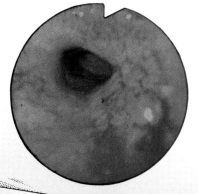

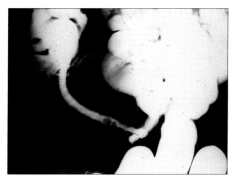

**Barium X-ray of Crohn's disease**
*When Crohn's disease affects only the colon, it looks similar to ulcerative colitis. The barium X-ray of Crohn's disease (above) shows superficial ulceration along the transverse colon and deep fissuring ulceration in the descending colon. Fissures often become deep cracks in the intestinal wall.*

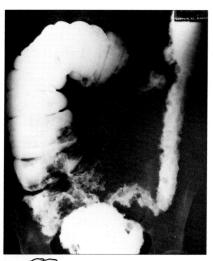

**Barium X-ray of ulcerative colitis**
*Bleeding ulcers occur in ulcerative colitis. The ulcers are usually shallow and widespread, with no areas of healthy colon. The X-ray above clearly shows the transition from damaged lining to healthy lining in the descending colon.*

# COMPLICATIONS OF INFLAMMATORY BOWEL DISEASE

The inflammatory conditions described below, which strike areas of the body far from the affected bowel, can accompany both Crohn's disease and ulcerative colitis. Doctors do not fully understand why. One theory suggests that an autoimmune disorder, in which the body's immune system attacks itself, is active in inflammatory bowel disease. An agent that provokes these complications may be produced in the affected bowel. Most of these conditions subside when the bowel disorder improves.

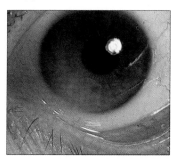

**Iritis**
*Iritis (inflammation of the iris, above) is one of the most common disorders complicating inflammatory bowel disease.*

**Erythema nodosum**
*Erythema nodosum is a skin condition characterized by red areas of swelling on the legs (below). It is often accompanied by fever and muscle and joint pain.*

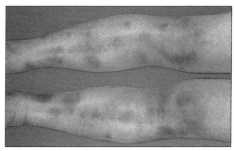

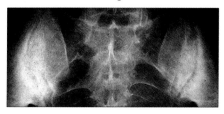

**Sacroiliitis**
*Common joint disorders linked to inflammatory bowel disease include arthritis, ankylosing spondylitis (inflammation of the vertebrae of the spine), and sacroiliitis. This condition (inflammation of the sacroiliac joint, above) causes pain in the lower back, buttocks, and thighs.*

# CASE HISTORY
# RECURRENT DIARRHEA

FOR ALMOST 2 YEARS, **Peter has been having periods of abdominal cramping and diarrhea that come and go. In recent weeks, he has lost his appetite, has begun losing weight, and has felt increasingly tired and irritable. His girlfriend finally persuades him to see his doctor.**

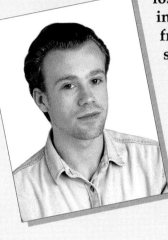

**PERSONAL DETAILS**
**Name** Peter Miller
**Age** 21
**Occupation** Medical student
**Family** Peter's parents are both healthy, but some other relatives have a history of gastrointestinal problems.

## THE CONSULTATION
Peter tells the doctor about his fatigue and abdominal symptoms. The doctor notices that he looks thin and pale. Peter has a temperature of 99.8°F. The doctor feels Peter's abdomen and notices an area of tenderness in the lower right quadrant.

## FURTHER INVESTIGATION
Blood test results reveal that Peter is anemic. A barium enema X-ray shows irregularities in the lining of Peter's cecum (the beginning of his colon) and in two areas in his small intestine. During an endoscopic examination of his colon (colonoscopy), a sample of tissue is obtained for microscopic examination.

## THE DIAGNOSIS
The results of these tests show that Peter has CROHN'S DISEASE, a chronic inflammatory digestive tract disease of unknown cause. Crohn's disease can cause the diarrhea, fever, and other symptoms that Peter has experienced. The inflammation has caused minor blood loss. This loss, combined with Peter's poor nutrition and a suppression of blood cell production also caused by the inflammation, has led to anemia.

## THE TREATMENT
The doctor admits Peter to the hospital and puts him on a bland, low-fiber diet. He prescribes a mild sedative, an antispasmodic drug for the cramping, and corticosteroid drugs for the inflammation. As Peter's condition improves, the doctor stops the sedative and antispasmodic drugs and reduces the dosage of the corticosteroids. After Peter's discharge from the hospital, the lowered corticosteroid dosage is replaced by an anti-inflammatory drug with fewer side effects.

## THE OUTCOME
After 18 months, Peter suddenly develops severe, cramping abdominal pain and vomiting. His doctor gives him corticosteroid drugs, and a barium X-ray reveals a narrowing in his small intestine from the continued activity of his Crohn's disease. Peter's doctor recommends surgery, telling him that medication will not improve his scarred, thickened bowel enough to relieve the obstruction. Peter agrees to the operation. Surgeons cut out the narrowed area of his small intestine, and Peter's condition improves dramatically.

**Colonoscopy**
*Colonoscopy reveals that most of the lining of Peter's colon appears to be normal. But the region near its junction with the small intestine is red and inflamed and has a cobblestone appearance.*

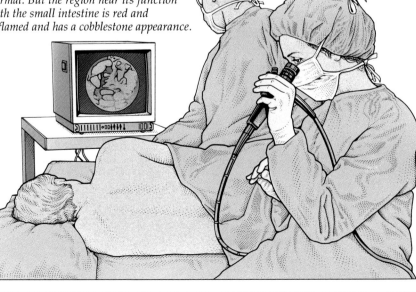

## TREATING INFLAMMATORY BOWEL DISEASES WITH DRUGS

Treatment of both Crohn's disease and ulcerative colitis attempts to suppress the inflammatory process so the body can repair itself. Anti-inflammatory drugs often succeed, and aspirin-derived agents, such as sulfasalazine, or newly available medications called osalazine and mesalamine, which have fewer unwanted side effects, are the drugs of choice for people with mild to moderate disease. These drugs also reduce the frequency of relapses of both diseases. For people who do not respond to aspirin, powerful anti-inflammatory drugs called corticosteroids are used alone or with other drugs. The side effects of corticosteroid drugs can be more serious than those of the salicylates, so they are usually stopped or reduced as soon as symptoms improve. Certain antibiotics are often given as well. In both Crohn's disease and ulcerative colitis, surgery is performed only in cases of severe internal hemorrhage, perforation, fistula (abnormal channel) formation, or obstruction.

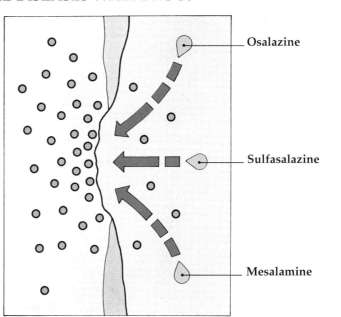

Osalazine

Sulfasalazine

Mesalamine

**How the drugs work**
*Several naturally occurring chemicals trigger inflammation, including some called prostaglandins, which are derivatives of fatty acids that act like hormones in your body. Sulfasalazine, osalazine, and mesalamine prevent the formation of prostaglandins in the intestinal wall. This process halts further inflammation, allowing the area to heal. Sulfasalazine can cause kidney problems or a rash. The other two drugs can treat inflammation with fewer side effects.*

## COLON CANCER

Cancer of the large intestine, or colon, accounts for about 53,000 deaths each year in the US. It is the second most common cancer in women (after breast cancer) and the third most prevalent cancer in men (after lung and prostate cancers). Cancer of the small intestine is rare, accounting for less than 2 percent of all digestive tract tumors.

The underlying cause of colon cancer is not yet known, but a number of risk factors have been identified. Risk factors include adenomatous polyps (see page 122) and certain forms of inflammatory bowel disease, a high-fat and/or low-fiber diet, a family history of polyposis (multiple polyps) or cancer of the colon, and age (most cases occur in people who are in their 60s or 70s). Researchers have

recently found a gene that identifies people who are predisposed to colon cancer. The most common sign of cancer of the colon is a change in the normal pattern of bowel function. Any persistent change should be investigated promptly by your doctor.

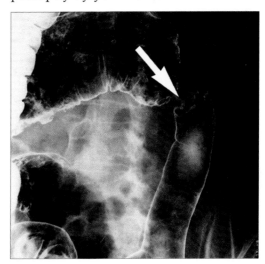

**Diagnosing colon cancer**
*An air contrast barium X-ray investigation, in which air is introduced into the colon along with barium to produce an image of surface abnormalities, can reveal a tumor (see arrow at left). Colonoscopy enables biopsy specimens of the tumor to be obtained which can confirm the diagnosis. To find out whether the cancer has spread to other areas of the body, such as the lungs, liver, or bones, doctors may also perform X-rays, computed tomographic (CT) scanning, and ultrasound scanning.*

## Treatment of colon cancer

Surgery is the principal treatment for cancer of the colon. After the surgeons have removed the tumor and the surrounding segment of colon, they rejoin the ends of the colon. An abdominal opening (colostomy) must be constructed if the cancer is low in the rectum. But the use of surgical staples instead of sutures has reduced the need for colostomy, because the remaining part of the colon can usually be joined to the rectum to form an outlet for stools.

The survival rate of people with colon cancer depends on how far it has progressed. If it is confined to the inner lining of the colon, the 5-year survival rate is close to 90 percent. But if the cancer has spread to other nearby organs, this rate falls to 40 percent. Chemotherapy (treatment with anticancer drugs) is sometimes used with surgery.

**The cause of diverticular disease**
*Diverticula appear when the muscles of the intestinal wall exert too much pressure. This can occur, for example, when pushing against small, hard stools to force them toward the rectum. This increased pressure pushes small areas of the intestinal lining through points of weakness in the muscular wall, usually where blood vessels penetrate the wall (right).*

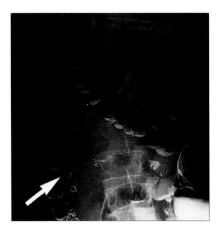

**Diagnosing diverticular disease**
*Doctors can diagnose diverticula easily by barium X-ray examination of the colon or by colonoscopy. In a barium X-ray, diverticula (arrow above) appear as knobs along the outer surface of the intestinal wall. In colonoscopy, pouches that may contain fecal residue can be seen in the intestinal lining.*

# DIVERTICULAR DISEASE

Diverticular disease includes both diverticulosis and diverticulitis. Diverticulosis refers to the presence of diverticula – small sacs created by protrusion of the intestinal wall's inner lining through the muscular layers of the wall. Thickening of the muscle layer may cause pain in some people with the disease. Diverticulitis occurs when these sacs or protrusions become infected and inflamed. Diverticula can occur anywhere along the digestive tract but usually affect the lower end of the colon. Diverticula in the colon occur mainly in older people, while diverticula in the stomach and small intestine (which are uncommon) are not age-related. The disease is common in the US, where low-fiber diets and constipation are important contributing factors.

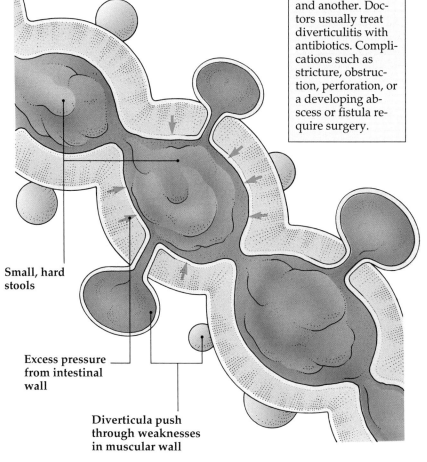

Small, hard stools

Excess pressure from intestinal wall

**Diverticula push through weaknesses in muscular wall**

## DIVERTICULITIS

Diverticulitis refers to the inflammation and infection of diverticula. The inflammation causes swelling and muscle spasm, which bring on acute pain, tenderness, and fever. Occasionally, an abscess can develop around the diverticulum and can burst, causing inflammation of the membrane that lines the abdominal cavity (peritonitis). Other complications include the formation of strictures (narrowings of the intestine) and the development of an abnormal channel (fistula) between one part of the intestine and another. Doctors usually treat diverticulitis with antibiotics. Complications such as stricture, obstruction, perforation, or a developing abscess or fistula require surgery.

# SURGICAL PROCEDURES
## COLOSTOMY

COLOSTOMY IS AN OPERATION **that joins part of the colon to a hole cut in the surface of the abdomen, creating a stoma, an opening through which feces can pass into a collecting bag. A colostomy may be temporary or permanent. A temporary colostomy allows waste to be discharged while sections of colon beyond the exit point recover from inflammation or surgery. When the colon has healed, the stoma can be closed. A permanent colostomy is performed when the rectum and anus are entirely removed.**

### CREATING A PERMANENT COLOSTOMY

**1** Before the operation, the doctor asks the patient to stand so the doctor can see any scars or bony protuberances on the patient's abdomen. The doctor chooses a site for the stoma that is free from such areas to ensure that the colostomy bag will fit securely. The usual location is in the lower left part of the abdomen, between the navel and the hip bone. The site must be placed where the patient can easily see it.

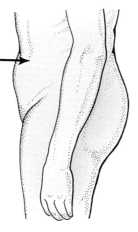

**Incision**

**2** The surgeon makes a long vertical incision to begin the surgery. After the rectum and anus have been removed, the colon is held with a clamp.

**Site of stoma**

**3** The surgeon removes a circular area of skin and underlying fat from the site and splits the abdominal muscles to create a vertical tunnel.

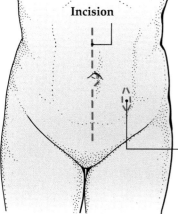

**Site of stoma**

**4** The end of the colon is pulled through this tunnel onto the skin. Then the main incision is closed.

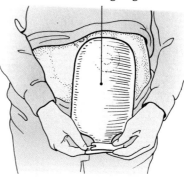

**Colon**

**Sutures**

**5** The surgeon joins the end of the colon to the skin with a series of absorbable sutures.

**Collecting bag**

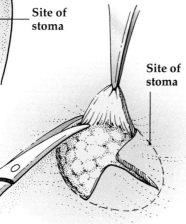

**6** The stoma appliance has a flat square of gum that is pressed onto the skin around the stoma. The collecting bag clips onto this square. The patient changes the disposable bag when needed, but the gum square can be left on for a few days to minimize skin damage.

---

### LIVING WITH A COLOSTOMY

Bowel function recovers quickly. At first, the stoma discharges continuously. Then the patient begins to have regular bowel movements that discharge into the collecting bag.

---

### CREATING A TEMPORARY COLOSTOMY

A temporary colostomy can be formed like a permanent one, or it can be formed from a loop of colon that is not completely cut in two. This type of temporary colostomy is usually located in the upper right part of the abdomen. Its closure is a simpler procedure. The surgeon frees the colon from the skin and closes the opening in the loop. The repaired bowel is pushed back inside the abdomen. The muscles and skin are sewn shut.

## Symptoms and treatment

Most people with diverticulosis have no symptoms, but 20 percent of them experience abdominal pain, constipation, and/or diarrhea, bloating, and gas. This pattern of symptoms is similar to that of irritable bowel syndrome. In rare cases, diverticular bleeding may occur. Uncomplicated diverticulosis responds well to a high-fiber diet. Doctors may prescribe antispasmodic drugs to relieve abdominal pain. Bleeding usually subsides without treatment, but surgery is occasionally needed to remove the diseased part of the intestine.

## POLYPS

Growths that project from the lining of the intestine into the digestive tract are called polyps. Three types of polyps can occur in the colon – adenomatous, inflammatory, and hamartomatous polyps. Adenomatous polyps are the most important type because they can develop into cancers. People with inherited multiple polyps (see FAMILIAL POLYPOSIS on page 47) also have an increased risk of cancer. Inflammatory polyps are not precancerous. These growths are not true polyps. They usually appear after inflammation of the colon heals. Hamartomatous polyps accompany both the form of polyposis that arises in children and Peutz-Jeghers syndrome (see GLOSSARY OF DISORDERS on page 141). These forms do not become cancerous.

## Diagnosis and treatment

Polyps usually cause no symptoms, although bleeding can occur. Doctors often detect polyps during an unrelated examination. They are sometimes found during an air contrast barium X-ray examination (see page 81). To remove polyps during colonoscopy, surgeons snare them with a wire loop that burns them as it cuts them away (electrocauterization). If the polyp is too broadly attached, or if there are too many polyps, the doctor examines tissue specimens taken from the colon. If any suspicious areas are found, the surgeon removes the section of colon containing the polyp.

**Adenomatous polyps**

*Adenomatous polyps are the result of excessive growth of epithelial cells in the mucosa. The polyps are not cancerous as long as these cells grow in an orderly pattern. But if the growth of these cells becomes disorganized, and the cells break through the mucosa, the polyps are considered cancerous.*

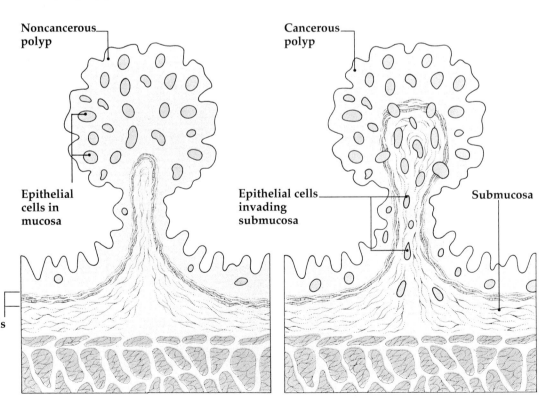

Noncancerous polyp

Epithelial cells in mucosa

Intact muscularis mucosa

Cancerous polyp

Epithelial cells invading submucosa

Submucosa

## WHAT IS VOLVULUS?

Volvulus is the term doctors use to describe a loop of intestine that becomes twisted, obstructing the passage of the intestinal contents. This twisting also blocks off the intestine's blood supply, which can cause gangrene of the bowel. The obstruction causes severe pain and vomiting. Volvulus can occur at many sites in the intestine, but the most common site is the sigmoid colon, the S-shaped portion of the colon. Doctors can often untwist the loop of a volvulus in the sigmoid colon without major surgery. After a sigmoidoscope (a form of endoscope, or fiberoptic instrument, see page 93) is passed into the colon, a tube is eased through the twisted section of intestine, unraveling it and releasing obstructed gas and feces.

**Diagnosing volvulus**
*Volvulus of the colon causes massive distention of the abdomen. A huge dilated length of intestine can be seen on this X-ray (see arrow, left). Doctors sometimes suspect volvulus of the small intestine from an X-ray but can diagnose the condition at this site with certainty only by surgery.*

**Surgical treatment**
*Volvulus of the sigmoid colon often recurs, and surgery eventually may be necessary. During the operation, the surgeon opens the abdomen and manually untwists the loop (left). If there is any damage, the affected tissue is removed.*

## IRRITABLE BOWEL SYNDROME

A combination of abdominal discomfort that comes and goes, irregular bowel habits (constipation or alternating constipation and diarrhea), or indigestion that occurs without the presence of any disease is known as irritable bowel syndrome, especially if the person is under considerable stress. It is the most common disorder of the digestive tract. Other symptoms of irritable bowel syndrome include bloating, excessive gas, temporary relief of pain after passing gas or feces, a feeling of incomplete bowel emptying, and mucus in the feces.

### Managing irritable bowel syndrome
Irritable bowel syndrome is a chronic disorder linked to anxiety and stress. People affected by it may benefit from relaxation techniques. Doctors recom-

mend a high-fiber diet for those who experience constipation. People with diarrhea must follow a low-fiber diet. Antispasmodic drugs or antacids can relieve abdominal discomfort. But laxatives and antidiarrheal drugs should be avoided because these drugs may perpetuate symptoms.

**What causes irritable bowel syndrome?**
*The cause of irritable bowel syndrome is not fully understood, but many doctors see a link between emotional stress and the disorder (see STRESS on page 58). The underlying abnormality is a disturbance of muscle movement in the large intestine.*

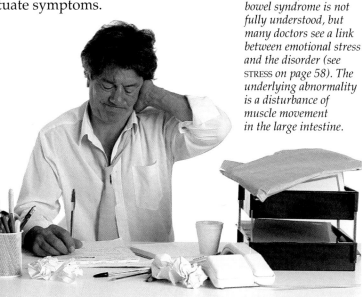

# SURGICAL PROCEDURES
## APPENDECTOMY

T HE APPENDIX **is a small tube connected to the large intestine in the lower right part of the abdomen, near the cecum. Its function is unknown. Doctors remove the appendix when they suspect appendicitis, an inflammation of the appendix. The appendix can easily become inflamed and infected because bacteria from the large intestine can enter it and become trapped inside. Appendectomy prevents the inflamed appendix from causing further complications, such as rupture and infection of the abdominal cavity.**

1 The surgeon makes an incision in the lower right section of the abdomen and exposes the large intestine.

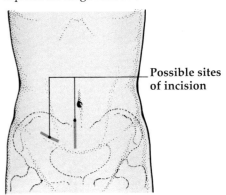

Possible sites of incision

2 The surgeon gently draws the appendix to the surface of the abdomen and clamps it at the base, where it joins the cecum. The appendix is then tied off.

Tie

Clamp

Appendix

Cecum

3 Next, the surgeon draws a purse-string suture tightly around the base of the appendix to seal it and cuts the appendix away.

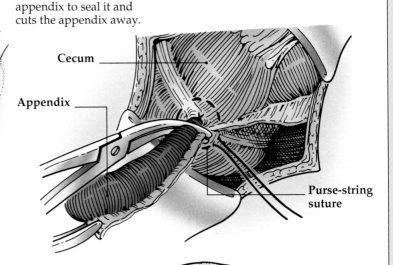

Cecum

Appendix

Purse-string suture

4 After tucking the stump into the cecum, the surgeon sutures it in place. This procedure prevents the incision from leaking into the abdominal cavity.

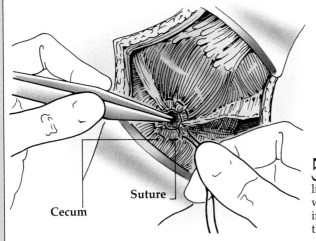

Suture

Cecum

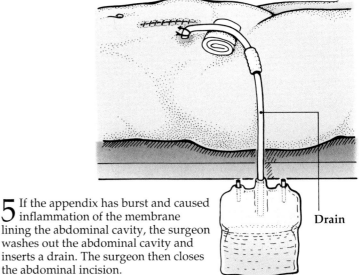

5 If the appendix has burst and caused inflammation of the membrane lining the abdominal cavity, the surgeon washes out the abdominal cavity and inserts a drain. The surgeon then closes the abdominal incision.

Drain

## INTESTINAL INFECTIONS

When certain bacteria or viruses invade and colonize your intestines, they can cause abdominal discomfort, vomiting, diarrhea, and tissue damage. The term doctors use to describe this condition is gastroenteritis. Gastroenteritis is very common, especially in children. The condition usually clears up within a few days without any treatment other than replacement of lost body fluids. But if diarrhea and/or vomiting persists, or blood appears in the stools, you should seek medical advice.

Most organisms that cause gastroenteritis reach your body by the fecal-oral route. This means that you have swallowed food or water contaminated with organisms from the feces of an infected person or animal. High standards of sanitation usually prevent outbreaks of infection. In countries where water supplies can be contaminated and sanitation may be difficult to maintain, travelers from other countries are especially at risk of contracting gastroenteritis.

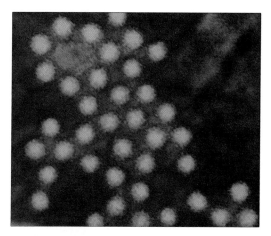

**The Norwalk virus**
*This color-enhanced photograph (right, magnified 62,650 times) shows the Norwalk virus. This virus causes about 30 percent of all outbreaks of viral gastroenteritis in the US, affecting people of all ages. The Norwalk virus was first discovered in 1968, following an outbreak of "winter vomiting disease" in Norwalk, Ohio.*

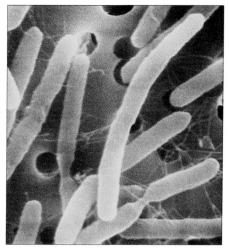

**Invasive bacteria**
*Several types of bacteria can invade the wall of the digestive tract to cause infective diarrhea. The bacterium* Helicobacter jejuni *is the most common type of invasive bacterium. Its usual source is farm animals or contaminated farm products, such as milk and eggs. Several species of* Salmonella *bacteria also cause severe infective diarrhea, including* Salmonella typhi, *the cause of typhoid fever (see color-enhanced microscopic photograph at left, magnified 2,860 times).*

**Toxigenic bacteria**
*One toxin-secreting bacterium is* Vibrio cholera *(right, magnified 2,850 times), the cause of cholera. Severe diarrhea caused by choleralike bacteria contained in shellfish is still common in the US. Food poisoning from toxins produced by* Staphylococcus aureus *(below, magnified 3,000 times) and* Bacillus cereus *(below right, magnified 960 times) is also very common in the US. Both organisms easily grow and produce toxins on unrefrigerated foods.*

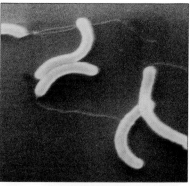

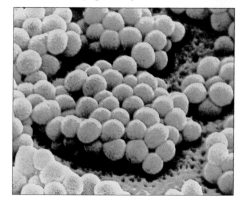

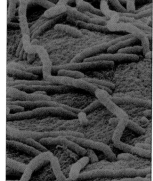

## Viral infections

Several groups of viruses can cause gastroenteritis, including adenoviruses, coxsackieviruses, and polioviruses. Rotaviruses and the Norwalk virus are common causes of gastroenteritis in infants. These viruses multiply inside the cells that line the digestive tract, causing inflammation, malabsorption of nutrients, and an outpouring of water and minerals, such as sodium and potassium, from the intestine.

## Bacterial infections

Bacteria that cause gastroenteritis fall into two categories – the toxigenic type and the invasive type. Toxigenic bacteria produce toxins that inflame the lining of the intestine. Invasive bacteria invade and infect the intestinal wall, causing fever and watery diarrhea that sometimes contains pus and blood.

# CASE HISTORY
# TRAVELERS' DIARRHEA

FOUR WEEKS AGO, Stephen went on a short business trip to Mexico. To avoid the risk of infection during the trip, he had been careful not to drink any tap water. But 2 weeks after his return, Stephen began to feel sick. He developed a fever, severe diarrhea containing blood and mucus, and cramping abdominal pain. Alarmed by his symptoms, he decided to see his doctor.

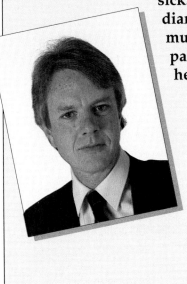

**PERSONAL DETAILS**
**Name** Stephen Krause
**Age** 43
**Occupation** Management consultant
**Family** Married with two children. His father and mother are both healthy.

## MEDICAL BACKGROUND
Stephen had appendicitis at age 14 and had an operation to remove his appendix. Apart from this illness, he has been healthy.

## THE CONSULTATION
Stephen tells his doctor that his symptoms started 2 weeks after his return from Mexico. He also describes how careful he was to drink only bottled water while he was away. The doctor sees that Stephen is dehydrated and finds tenderness along his colon and over his liver. She asks Stephen whether he drank any beverages containing ice cubes while he was away. Stephen remembers that he did.

## FURTHER INVESTIGATION
The doctor admits Stephen to the hospital for further investigation and orders intravenous fluids to treat his dehydration. An endoscopic examination of his colon reveals ulcers on the colon lining. Microscopic examination of a sample of feces reveals large numbers of amebae (a type of single-celled parasite). An ultrasound scan of his liver does not show an abscess (a pus-filled sac).

### A parasitic infection
*Stephen describes his symptoms to the doctor. A sample of feces, sent to the hospital laboratory for examination under a microscope, reveals the parasite* Entamoeba histolytica *(see photograph above right). Sometimes this organism travels to the liver to form abscesses.*

## THE DIAGNOSIS
Stephen's symptoms, and the presence of amebae in his stools after his trip to Mexico, lead the doctor to a diagnosis of AMEBIC DYSENTERY. This disease is caused by the parasite *Entamoeba histolytica*, which can invade the colon walls and cause ulceration of the lining, bleeding, excess mucus secretion, and diarrhea. The parasite reaches the body when particles of feces containing the organism are ingested in contaminated drinking water or food. Stephen was probably infected by the ice cubes in his drinks, which were made from the local water.

## THE TREATMENT
The doctor gives Stephen the antiparasitic drug metronidazole for 2 weeks. He recovers quickly, and samples of his feces examined during the next 2 months show no evidence of the parasite.

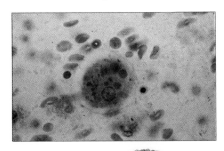

## PARASITIC WORMS

Several species of parasitic worms live in the human intestines. Conditions caused by worms commonly seen in the US include pinworm and whipworm infestations, ascariasis, and toxocariasis. In many cases (except fish tapeworms), worm infestations cause few or no symptoms and a person may be unknowingly infected for many years. But if infection is heavy, worms can cause chronic and debilitating symptoms, such as abdominal pain and diarrhea. Most types of worms can be eliminated with drugs called anthelmintics.

# INTESTINAL PARASITES

A parasite is an organism that lives in or on another living creature. Human intestinal parasites include certain protozoa and worms. Many parasites spread between individuals by the fecal-oral route, which means that something you have eaten or drunk has been contaminated by traces of the feces of an infected person or animal, probably through poor hygiene affecting food or water. Good personal hygiene and scrupulous sanitation in food preparation are essential to prevent infection from parasites.

## Protozoal infection

Protozoa are the simplest type of animal, consisting of a single cell. Two types of protozoa can cause intestinal infections – *Giardia lamblia* and *Entamoeba histolytica* (see TRAVELERS' DIARRHEA on page 126). The organism *Giardia lamblia* infects the small intestine. Spread by contaminated food or water or by direct personal contact, it attaches to the surface of the intestine but does not invade the tissues. *Giardia lamblia* may produce no symptoms. When symptoms occur, they start 2 or 3 days after infection and include violent diarrhea, excess gas, abdominal cramps, and nausea. Giardiasis sometimes goes away without treatment, but infection can become chronic, causing violent attacks of diarrhea and gas and abdominal pain that require medical treatment.

**Giardia lamblia**
*The photograph at right shows the protozoan* Giardia lamblia *(see arrow).* Common in the tropics, Giardia lamblia *has also been found in the mountain streams of some Western states. It is common among groups of children who may pass on the infection in places such as day-care centers. The disease is spread by contaminated food or water, or by direct personal contact.*

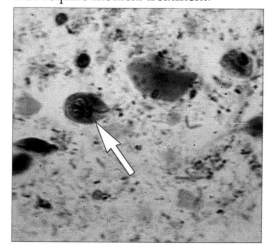

# ASK YOUR DOCTOR
## GASTROENTERITIS

**Q** **I plan to travel to South America this fall. Should I be vaccinated against gastroenteritis?**

**A** There is no vaccination available against gastroenteritis. Certain preventive drugs can be taken before your trip, but they all have unwanted side effects. The best precaution against gastroenteritis is to avoid consuming local tap water and uncooked vegetables and fruits. They may be contaminated with infective organisms. Also, make sure you have had a recent typhoid booster shot.

**Q** **My 8-month-old son has vomited his last two feedings. He was weaned 2 months ago and had no problems adjusting to formula. What could be the problem?**

**A** Your son probably has viral gastroenteritis (inflammation of the stomach and intestines caused by a virus), which is common in infants. Replace his feedings with rehydration fluids (see REPLACING LOST BODY FLUIDS on page 78). If he continues to vomit and his condition does not improve, call your doctor.

**Q** **I am 26 years old and have had diarrhea and abdominal pain for 2 months. I have also lost about 10 pounds. Someone told me antibiotics might help. Is this true?**

**A** Antibiotics are drugs used only to treat infection caused by bacteria. Your symptoms may signal inflammatory bowel disease or some other serious disorder that is not caused by a bacterial infection. You should see your doctor immediately. He or she will take your medical history and perform a thorough examination and will then decide the best course of treatment.

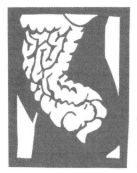

# RECTAL AND ANAL DISORDERS

MANY DISORDERS of the rectum and anus are minor. They can be corrected by maintaining regular bowel habits, increasing your intake of fluids, and including high-fiber foods, such as whole-grain cereals, fruits, and vegetables, in your diet. Some more serious disorders require medical treatment. Most problems that affect the rectum and anus have characteristic symptoms that should prompt you to see your doctor for diagnosis and treatment.

**Types of hemorrhoids**
*Hemorrhoids are divided into two categories – internal and external. Internal hemorrhoids occur inside the anal canal and may move out of place during defecation. External hemorrhoids develop on the rim of the anus. Either kind of hemorrhoid can become blocked by a blood clot, reducing its blood supply and causing severe pain.*

One of the most common symptoms of a rectal or anal disorder is bleeding during defecation. A sudden but lasting change in your usual bowel habits, such as reduced frequency of defecation or the passing of abnormal-looking stools, can also indicate a serious rectal or anal disorder. These symptoms should always be investigated by your doctor. Itching and pain during defecation can also signal a treatable rectal or anal disorder.

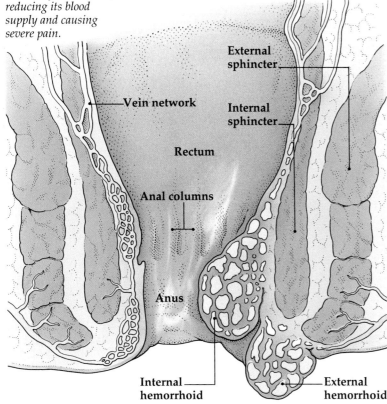

External sphincter

Vein network

Internal sphincter

Rectum

Anal columns

Anus

Internal hemorrhoid

External hemorrhoid

## HEMORRHOIDS

Protrusions from the lining of the anus caused by distended (varicose) veins are called hemorrhoids. The reason hemorrhoids occur remains unclear. Some people have a weakness of the anal veins from birth that predisposes them to hemorrhoids later in life. A diet that does not include enough fiber-containing foods can lead to constipation, and then to hemorrhoids, in part because a constipated person must strain harder during defecation. One of the most common symptoms of hemorrhoids is bleeding from the distended veins, which are damaged by the passage of hard, dry stools. The bleeding comes and goes, occurring mainly during defecation, and can be seen on toilet paper or on the surface of the stool in the toilet bowl. Some people with hemorrhoids develop a mucous discharge from the anus that can stain underclothes and cause itching of the skin around the anus.

### Diagnosis and treatment
Doctors diagnose hemorrhoids by examining the rectum with a finger. Proctoscopy (direct visual examination of the inside of the rectum and anal canal with a fiberoptic instrument called an endoscope) usually confirms the diagnosis and excludes the possibility of

cancer. Hemorrhoids may shrink in people who switch to a high-fiber diet. The application of a preparation containing an anesthetic or corticosteroid can reduce discomfort and irritation. Such preparations also help lubricate the anal canal, reducing damage during defecation. If protruding, internal hemorrhoids are especially painful – or if they bleed – they may be removed by elastic band ligation. In this process, elastic bands are applied to the neck of a hemorrhoid, constricting it tightly so that it withers and drops off painlessly. Alternatively, cryosurgery (which destroys tissue by freezing) or electric currents may be used to shrink the veins. In severe cases of protruding external hemorrhoids, doctors may remove them surgically or destroy them with a laser.

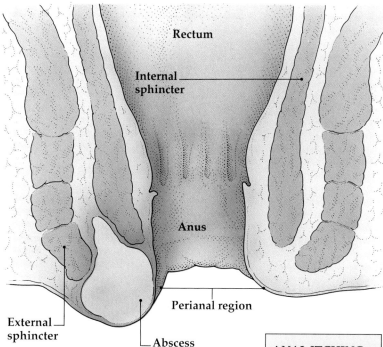

**Formation of an abscess**
*A perianal (near the anus) abscess usually follows an infection of the skin or glands of the anus. Pus may spread to form deeper pockets of pus between the internal and external sphincters, the muscular rings surrounding the anus.*

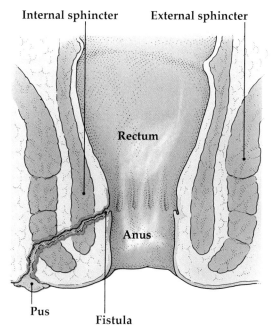

**Anal fistula**
*An anal fistula is an abnormal channel that connects the inside of the anal canal to the skin surrounding the anus. Most anal fistulas are caused by abscesses that have spread to the skin surface, producing pain and the discharge of pus and feces onto the skin. When the abscess does not heal, a channel develops between the internal infected anal gland and the skin. Doctors treat a chronic anal fistula by cutting out the channel and its lining so the area can heal.*

## PERIANAL ABSCESS

A perianal (near the anus) abscess is a collection of pus beneath the skin around the anus that develops after an infection, usually by bacteria in the colon. The condition usually affects people in their 30s and 40s and is more common in men than in women. Perianal abscesses are usually very painful. Doctors may not be able to diagnose them for a few days after the pain starts, because it takes time for the pus to move out of the sweat- and oil-producing glands in the anus and to produce swelling under the skin around the anus. A painful lump develops around the anal canal, producing redness, heat, and swelling. Treatment includes taking analgesic drugs (painkillers) and warm baths and draining the abscess. Antibiotics are prescribed to kill the bacteria responsible for the abscess and to reduce the spread of infection to other tissues.

### ANAL ITCHING
Itching and irritation around the anus (called pruritus ani) is a symptom of many rectal and anal disorders, including hemorrhoids, anal fistulas (see caption at lower left), and anal fissures (tears in the lining of the anal canal). Itching can also be caused by pinworm infestation or a skin disorder such as eczema. In more than 50 percent of cases, no underlying cause can be found. In such cases, doctors advise affected people to avoid overly aggressive wiping of the anus after defecation and to keep the area clean. A corticosteroid cream applied directly to the anal region can also be helpful if used sparingly.

Anal intercourse and other sexual acts involving the anus or rectum increase the risk of sexually transmitted diseases – especially human immunodeficiency virus (HIV) and genital warts caused by the human papillomavirus – leading to an increased risk of anal cancer. Anal intercourse also increases the risk of diseases not usually transmitted through sexual activity, such as amebic dysentery. Many of the diseases contracted through anal intercourse damage the lining of the anal canal and rectum, producing symptoms such as rectal pain, discharge, and a sensation that the rectum is full. Some signs of an anal or rectal disease, such as the sores caused by syphilis or gonorrhea, can be mistaken for signs of inflammatory bowel disease. The risk of infection is greater for the anally receptive partner but both partners are at risk. Blood and stool tests help to reach a diagnosis. Such sexually transmitted anal or rectal diseases can be avoided by refraining from anal intercourse or by using condoms.

# ANAL FISSURE

An anal fissure is a tear in the lining of the anal canal that extends inward from the anal opening. It is fairly common, and often first produces a swollen area of skin near the anus. The cause of anal fissures remains unclear, but the strain and pressure of passing hard, dry stools may contribute to their development. Anal fissures also occur in people with chronic diarrhea, in part from overly vigorous wiping. Fissures most commonly affect people in their 20s and 30s. Both sexes are equally affected. A fissure can cause a sharp or burning pain during or just after defecation that can persist for several hours. The pain often causes affected people to suppress the urge to defecate, and they may become constipated. Other symptoms include spasm of the anal muscles, bloody discharge that stains the toilet paper after defecation, and sometimes a chronic discharge. Most anal fissures can be detected by examination of the anus, but spasm of the anal sphincter and pain often prevent adequate rectal examination. Some anal fissures go away by themselves after a few days. Doctors treat persistent or recurrent anal fissures with a high-fiber diet and sometimes minor surgery to cut the internal anal sphincter muscle.

## RECTAL PROLAPSE

Rectal prolapse refers to the protrusion of the rectal lining and muscle wall through the anal canal, usually from straining to defecate. Prolapse usually occurs in older people in whom the tissues that support the perineum (the area between the anus and the genital organs) have weakened. In early rectal prolapse, a doctor's examination of the perineum may not reveal any abnormality, but the anus may have poor sphincter tone. Sigmoidoscopy (see page 80) may show only mild inflammation of the rectal lining. Later, the rectum may protrude farther with straining, but the person can easily reposition it with a finger. Rectal prolapse can also become permanent.

Surgery may be recommended for people with permanent rectal prolapse. During the procedure, the surgeon may insert wire or nylon to tighten the anal sphincter or raise and reposition the rectum. This complicated surgery is not always successful, and recurrence of the rectal prolapse is common. Rectal prolapse is usually temporary in children and corrects itself once a high-fiber diet has relieved the child's constipation.

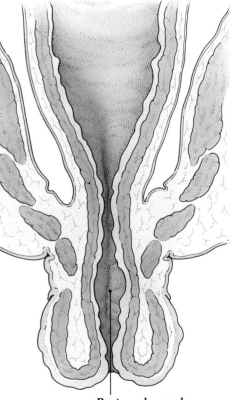

Rectum descends
through anal canal and
protrudes through anus

**Symptoms of rectal prolapse**
*A rectum that has protruded through the anus rarely causes pain. Major symptoms include fecal incontinence, a discharge of mucus, rectal bleeding, and discomfort.*

# CASE HISTORY
## INTERMITTENT RECTAL BLEEDING

JOHN HAS ALWAYS BEEN **healthy. During his 50 years in business and since retirement, he has rarely needed to see a doctor. In the past few months, he has become constipated and has noticed some blood on the surface of his stools. When the bleeding became more apparent, John decided to have it checked by his doctor.**

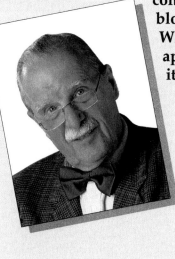

**PERSONAL DETAILS**
**Name** John Sulenski
**Age** 81
**Occupation** Retired
store owner
**Family** Both of John's
parents died in their 70s.
John's wife is healthy.

### MEDICAL BACKGROUND
John has been healthy all his life. He has seen his doctor only once in the last 20 years, when he had two unusual-looking moles removed from his back. Fortunately, results of tissue sample tests showed these moles to be benign (noncancerous).

### THE CONSULTATION
The doctor listens to John's description of his symptoms and asks him about his bowel habits. John replies that, although his stools appear to be normal aside from the blood, over the past 4 months they have become hard and difficult to pass. He also tells his doctor that he often feels as if he has not completely emptied his bowels after defecation. John says he has become worried about the blood that sometimes appears on the surface of his stools and on the toilet paper after defecation. The doctor performs a rectal examination and notices that John has hemorrhoids. The doctor initially thinks they may be responsible for the bleeding, al-though the hemorrhoids do not explain his change in bowel habits. When the doctor feels a hard lump farther inside John's rectum, he refers John to a gastroenterologist (a doctor who specializes in digestive tract disorders) for an examination.

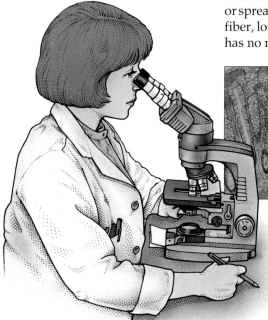

### THE GASTROENTERO-LOGIST'S CONSULTATION
The gastroenterologist examines John's colon and rectum with a colonoscope (a flexible viewing instrument inserted into the anus). He confirms that there is an irregular mass, which is bleeding slightly, high in John's rectum. The gastroenterologist obtains a small biopsy specimen of the mass for microscopic examination in the laboratory.

### THE DIAGNOSIS
The results of John's colonoscopy and biopsy confirm that he has RECTAL CANCER, a malignant tumor of the upper part of the rectum.

### THE TREATMENT
John has surgery, during which the tumor and surrounding part of his rectum are removed. The surgeon then brings the colon down and joins it to the remaining part of John's rectum (see SURGICAL PROCEDURES on page 132). After John recovers from surgery, he sees the gastroenterologist for regular examinations to ensure that the tumor has not recurred or spread. He also switches to a high-fiber, low-fat diet. A year later, John has no more symptoms.

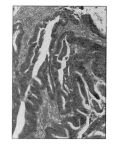

**Confirming the diagnosis**
*A stained section of the specimen (above right) taken from John's rectum is examined under a microscope. It shows the highly disrupted organization of the cancerous tissue, compared with normal tissue (above left).*

# SURGICAL PROCEDURES
## ANTERIOR RESECTION OF THE RECTUM

ANTERIOR RESECTION of the rectum is the surgical removal of a part of the rectum, usually done to treat rectal cancer. The surgeon cuts out the diseased section of the rectum and rejoins the healthy ends of the large intestine. Anterior resection is possible only when the tumor is located in the upper portion of the rectum. If the tumor is close to the anus, the anus and the rectum are removed, and the surgeon creates an artificial exit for feces (a colostomy).

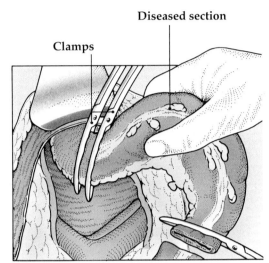

Clamps

Diseased section

**3** The diseased part of the rectum is clamped at each end and cut away from its supporting structures.

Incision

**1** Doctors prepare the patient for surgery by giving him or her oral antibiotics and laxative solutions and inserting a catheter into the bladder. After the patient is anesthetized, the surgeon makes a long vertical incision in the abdomen. The surgeon examines the abdominal cavity for signs of any other tumors.

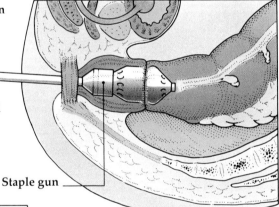

Staple gun

**4** The surgeon rejoins the two healthy ends of the large intestine with a staple gun. The staple gun is inserted into the bowel by way of the anus and delivers a ring of tiny metal staples that hold the two cut edges together.

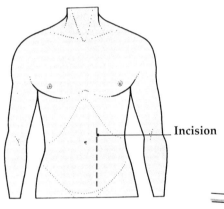

Rectum

Catheter in bladder

Tumor

Drainage tubes

**2** The surgeon locates the tumor with his or her hand and decides which portion of the rectum should be removed. If the tumor has spread into adjoining organs or tissues, surgery may not cure the condition.

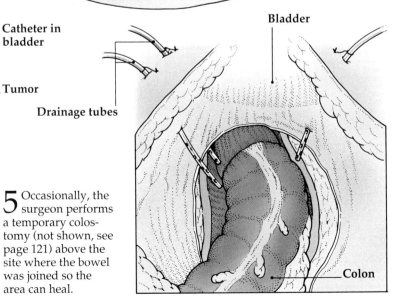

Bladder

Colon

**5** Occasionally, the surgeon performs a temporary colostomy (not shown, see page 121) above the site where the bowel was joined so the area can heal.

## RECTAL CANCER

Cancer of the rectum accounts for about one fourth of the tumors that affect the large intestine. About 3,000 new cases are diagnosed each year in the US. The high incidence of rectal cancer in developed countries has been linked to a diet that is low in fiber and high in fat. Genetic factors also contribute to rectal cancer. The disease affects men and women in equal numbers and its incidence peaks in people over 60. Evidence shows that some disorders of the colon (large intestine) increase the risk of rectal cancer. These disorders include adenomatous polyps of the rectum (see page 122) and longstanding ulcerative colitis (see page 115). Symptoms of rectal cancer include a sudden, sustained change in bowel habits along with rectal discomfort or a feeling of fullness, and bleeding through the anus. The pattern of rectal bleeding may be identical to that of hemorrhoids.

### Treatment of rectal cancer

Surgery is the treatment of choice for rectal cancer. If the tumor lies in the upper part of the rectum, the surgeon removes this part and the adjacent colon and rejoins the two ends of healthy intestine. If the tumor lies in the lower part of the rectum, the surgeon cuts the colon above the rectum and removes both the rectum and anus. After the operation, an exit for feces no longer exists. The surgeon must create an exit, called a permanent colostomy (see page 121).

After surgery, doctors use endoscopy to detect signs of recurrence. To reduce the chances of recurrence, doctors often use radiation therapy and chemotherapy (treatment with anticancer drugs). In people for whom surgery is unsuitable, the tumor may be destroyed by electrocautery (burning) or laser. Survival depends on whether cancerous cells have spread. Radiation therapy and chemotherapy may improve chances of survival in advanced cases of rectal cancer.

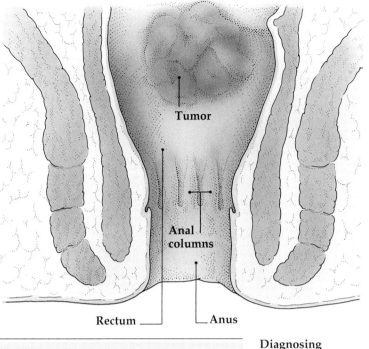

Tumor

Anal columns

Rectum

Anus

## ANAL CANCER

Cancer of the anus is uncommon. But a number of different malignant tumors can affect the anus, including squamous cell carcinoma, malignant melanoma, and basal cell carcinoma (the three most common types of skin cancer). These tumors may arise following genital warts, a sexually transmitted disease caused by the human papillomavirus. The most common symptoms include bleeding, pain, itching, and a detectable lump in the anus. A diagnosis of anal cancer can be reached by rectal examination and endoscopy. Surgery is the primary treatment, with or without radiation therapy or chemotherapy.

**Diagnosing rectal cancer**
*If you have a lump in your rectum, your doctor can feel it with a finger during a rectal examination. He or she may refer you for an examination with a sigmoidoscope (see page 80) to confirm the presence of a tumor, measure its size, and determine whether it can cause an obstruction.*

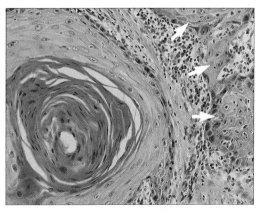

**Appearance of anal cancer**
*The most common type of tumor affecting the anus is squamous cell carcinoma. Microscopic examination confirms the diagnosis. The slide at left shows the characteristic collections of malignant cells in the skin lining (see arrows) in a biopsy specimen from a tumor of this type.*

# ABDOMINAL EMERGENCIES

Abdominal emergencies, such as peritonitis (inflammation of the membrane lining the abdominal wall), perforation of the intestine, or intestinal obstruction, are life-threatening disorders. They usually come on quickly. The symptoms produced by different abdominal emergencies are often similar, so it can be difficult for doctors to diagnose the exact cause of the problem without a thorough evaluation of the patient.

If you experience severe abdominal symptoms (see box at right), you must seek immediate medical treatment. Your doctor will first control any life-threatening complications and then try to determine the cause of the underlying disorder.

**Bleeding from
the digestive tract**
*Bleeding can occur from
many sites in the digestive
tract. The diagram below
shows the disorders that can
cause bleeding and the areas
most commonly affected.*

**Key**

**Cancers**

**Peptic ulcers**

**Esophageal
varicose veins**

**Diverticular
disease**

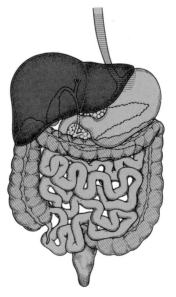

## BLEEDING

Vomiting blood and passing dark, bloody stools signal life-threatening emergencies. The digestive tract bleeds when the blood vessels in its wall become damaged. If a person vomits blood or passes black stools, the disorder may lie in the upper part of the digestive tract. If a person passes bright or dark red bloody stools, the problem probably lies in the lower part of the digestive tract.

## Causes of bleeding

The digestive tract can bleed at many sites. The duodenum (the first part of the small intestine) can bleed severely if a peptic ulcer erodes through a blood vessel in the duodenal wall. The stomach can also bleed heavily if a peptic ulcer or an ulcerating cancer invades the vessels in the stomach or duodenal lining. Erosive gastritis (severe inflammation of the stomach lining) also causes severe bleeding. Esophageal varicose veins are distended veins in the esophagus caused by portal hypertension (see page 102). These veins can rupture, causing massive blood loss. Esophageal varicose veins can develop following cirrhosis of the liver.

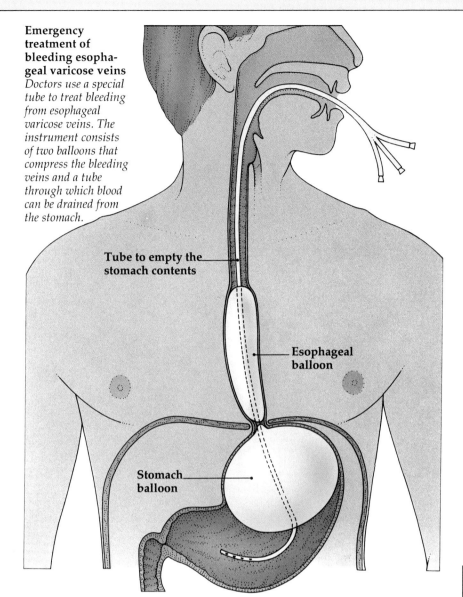

**Emergency treatment of bleeding esophageal varicose veins**
*Doctors use a special tube to treat bleeding from esophageal varicose veins. The instrument consists of two balloons that compress the bleeding veins and a tube through which blood can be drained from the stomach.*

**Tube to empty the stomach contents**

**Esophageal balloon**

**Stomach balloon**

## PERFORATION

A perforation is a hole that develops in a hollow organ, such as the stomach, intestine, or gallbladder, that allows fluid, air, or both to enter the abdominal cavity. This condition usually produces sudden, severe pain, peritonitis (inflammation of the lining of the abdominal cavity), and shock. Any part of a person's digestive tract can perforate, but the most common sites are the stomach, duodenum, and sigmoid colon (the S-shaped part of the colon just above the rectum). The stomach and duodenum can perforate if a peptic ulcer penetrates the organ's wall. Perforation in the sigmoid colon most often results from a ruptured diverticulum (see page 120).

In intestinal perforation, doctors first treat the life-threatening shock, begin antibiotic treatment, and relieve distention by passing a tube into the intestine from the nose or mouth to remove gas and fluid. They then treat the underlying cause. If the perforation lies in the large intestine, a colostomy (see page 121) is created. The affected area is usually removed. The colostomy may be closed after recovery.

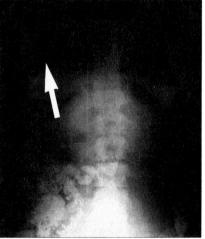

**Perforation of the digestive tract**
*In the chest X-ray above, an abnormal gas bubble can be seen under the diaphragm on the person's right side. This gas has escaped into the abdominal cavity through a perforation in the intestine.*

Bleeding in the digestive tract can also be caused by erosion of a polyp, ulceration in a diverticulum (see page 120), or ulceration of a cancerous tumor. Loss of a large quantity of blood may cause shock (circulatory collapse) from the reduced volume of blood in the circulation.

Doctors treat shock primarily with intravenous fluids or blood transfusions. They then try to identify the location of the bleeding. Doctors use endoscopy of the upper part of the gastrointestinal tract (see page 93) to identify bleeding sites in the upper part of the intestine, and colonoscopy (see page 80) and angiography (X-rays that display blood vessels filled

with a dye that is opaque to X-rays) to explore sites in the colon. Most ulcers stop bleeding when medical treatment begins, but surgery is sometimes needed to stop the bleeding. Varicose veins in the esophagus may initially be treated by compression. An inflatable, two-part balloon and tube is inserted into the esophagus to compress the veins. Then injections of corrosive chemicals that coagulate and seal the affected veins may be given. Bleeding farther down in the intestinal tract may stop on its own, but the affected section of bowel may need to be surgically removed if life-threatening bleeding continues.

135

## PERITONITIS

Peritonitis refers to inflammation of the peritoneum, the membrane that lines the abdominal cavity and protects the stomach and intestines. Peritonitis can be caused by infection or perforation of the digestive tract. Perforation of the intestine can cause the contents to leak into the peritoneal cavity. People with peritonitis vomit and have severe abdominal pain, which becomes worse if they move. They often have a high fever. Without treatment, peritonitis is almost always fatal. Doctors treat the underlying cause of the peritonitis. For example, if the peritonitis is caused by a ruptured appendix, surgeons perform an appendectomy to remove the source of infection. Antibiotics are also given.

## APPENDICITIS

Appendicitis – acute inflammation of the appendix – is a common abdominal emergency. The disorder begins as a vague pain in the region above or around the navel that soon worsens and moves to the lower right part of the abdomen. The pain is accompanied by loss of appetite, nausea, vomiting, and mild fever. Untreated appendicitis can cause gangrene and the appendix can rupture, causing peritonitis. Appendicitis can also cause a large abscess, which may surround the appendix. The infection can move to another part of the abdominal cavity and develop into an abscess there. Appendicitis can be difficult to diagnose. No tests exist that definitely confirm the condition. The symptoms of other diseases, such as infection of the lymph glands around the intestine and diseases of the female reproductive organs, can often mimic those of appendicitis. But if your doctor strongly suspects appendicitis, he or she will probably surgically remove the appendix to avoid complications such as peritonitis or an abscess.

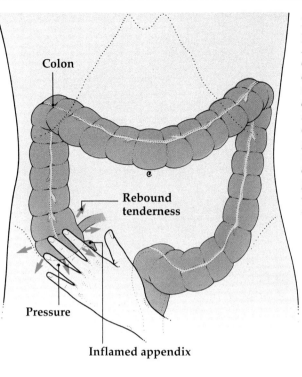

Colon

Rebound tenderness

Pressure

Inflamed appendix

**Investigating suspected appendicitis**
*In making a diagnosis of appendicitis, your doctor may press on the right side of your abdomen and ask if it hurts more when he or she lets go. This phenomenon is called rebound tenderness and occurs because the peritoneum (see page 31) is inflamed and hurts when it is moved.*

**Signs and symptoms of appendicitis**
*Appendicitis begins with a vague pain in the center of the abdomen that later moves to the lower right part of the abdomen. The person may also experience nausea, vomiting, and fever.*

**Inflamed appendix**
*The magnified photograph below of tissue from an inflamed and gangrenous appendix shows pus inside the appendix. The pus is about to create a hole through the dead tissue in the muscle wall of the appendix.*

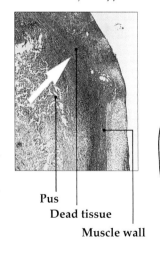

Pus
Dead tissue
Muscle wall

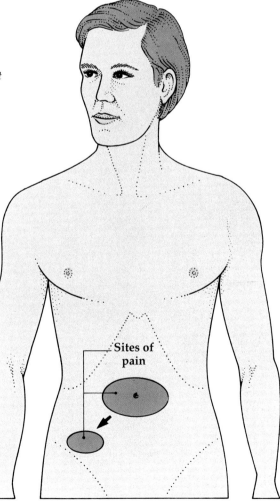

Sites of pain

# INTESTINAL OBSTRUCTIONS

Intestinal obstructions cover a group of abdominal emergencies with a variety of causes. Symptoms include pain, distention of the abdomen, vomiting, and complete cessation of the passage of gas or feces. The position of the obstruction can be indicated by the person's symptoms. Blockage of the upper part of the digestive tract causes profuse vomiting without distention of the abdomen. Obstruction of the large intestine produces severe distention without passage of gas or feces. Vomiting may occur somewhat later in the course of the illness. All cases of obstruction bring on severe, cramping pain and dehydration from vomiting or leakage of fluid into the channel of a nonfunctioning bowel. Treatment first relieves the pain and replaces lost fluids. Some people with obstructions respond to treatment with a long tube passed from the nose or mouth into the intestine to empty the bowel and reduce distention. Many times the obstruction does not go away without surgery to remove the blockage.

## Distention of the digestive tract

Obstruction of the digestive tract can occur at various sites. The degree of abdominal swelling depends on where the blockage occurs. The swelling arises from a buildup of gas inside the obstructed digestive tract that is unable to escape past the blocked area. The degree of the distention can vary from a small area of swelling to a massive bloating of the entire abdomen. Distention of the abdomen from obstruction is considered an abdominal emergency.

## Malignant obstruction

Cancers of the colon often do not produce obvious symptoms until a sudden blockage of the bowel occurs. Diagnosis can be confirmed by

## TYPES OF INTESTINAL OBSTRUCTIONS

**Obstruction high in the small intestine**
*If an obstruction occurs in the region of the upper end of the small intestine, distention is often absent, except in the stomach and sometimes the duodenum.*

Site of obstruction

Small intestine is not distended

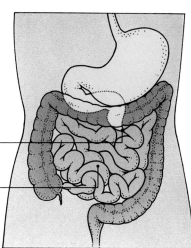

**Obstruction low in the small intestine**
*An obstruction at the lower end of the small intestine causes distention of the small intestine. Trapped fluid is often visible on an X-ray.*

Fluid in the small intestine

Site of obstruction

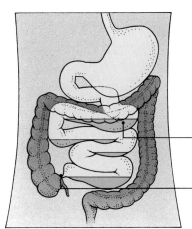

**Obstruction in the large intestine**
*Obstruction in the large intestine produces massive distention of the large intestine.*

Distended large intestine

Site of obstruction

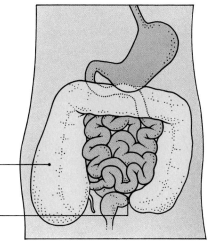

a barium X-ray (see page 81). If the obstruction is caused by a tumor, surgeons first perform a colostomy (see page 121) to release the obstruction. During a second operation, the tumor is removed. The colostomy may or may not be closed during this second operation. If the extent of the cancer makes removal

of the tumor impossible, the colostomy may be left open permanently. Sometimes the bowel is cut and rejoined so that the cancerous section is bypassed. This bypass procedure is called a palliative operation because it is performed only to relieve symptoms (the obstruction) and not to attempt to cure the cancer.

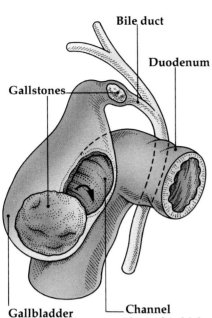

**Bile duct**

**Duodenum**

Gallstones

Gallbladder

**Channel through which gallstone passes**

**Gallstone ileus**
*In older people, mostly women, a large gallstone can enter the duodenum directly through an abnormal channel (fistula) created by repeated inflammation of the gallbladder. The channel penetrates the duodenum. The gallstone moves through the intestine until it reaches a narrow portion where it blocks the intestine.*

## Adhesions

After any type of abdominal surgery or inflammation of the membrane that lines the abdominal wall, bands of scar tissue called adhesions can form between the loops of the intestine or between the intestine and the abdominal wall. These adhesions rarely cause problems, but if a loop of the small intestine slips under an adhesion, it can become trapped and kinked, causing an obstruction in the intestine. If the blood supply to that part of the intestine is cut off, gangrene can develop. Doctors treat an obstruction caused by adhesions with an operation during which they open the abdomen and cut away the adhesions, releasing the trapped bowel. If the obstruction has caused the intestine to become gangrenous, the surgeon must remove that portion and rejoin the intestine. More

bands of scar tissue always form after the operation to correct adhesions, but most cause no problems.

## Volvulus

A volvulus is a loop of bowel that becomes twisted around itself. It usually develops in the loops of the small intestine, in the sigmoid colon (see page 46), or in the cecum. The twisted loop of bowel swells rapidly, and the chances of cutting off the blood supply of the bowel are much higher than in a simple obstruction. A volvulus is an abdominal emergency and usually requires an operation to untwist the bowel. If the condition is diagnosed early, the surgeon may be able to save the piece of bowel. But if the blood supply has been cut off for a long time, this section of the bowel must be removed and the healthy ends rejoined.

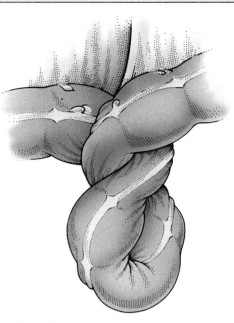

**Sigmoid volvulus**
*A volvulus twists both ends of the intestine closed so that its contents cannot move in either direction. It occurs most frequently in the sigmoid colon.*

## GALLBLADDER EMERGENCIES

The gallbladder is susceptible to medical emergencies. Gallstones are common and often block the bile duct, which can lead to biliary colic (intense cramping pain that comes and goes), cholecystitis (inflammation of the gallbladder), gangrene, perforation, empyema (in which the gallbladder's bile is replaced by pus), or a mucocele, a swollen sac filled with mucus. All these conditions, except mucocele, require immediate treatment (see page 108).

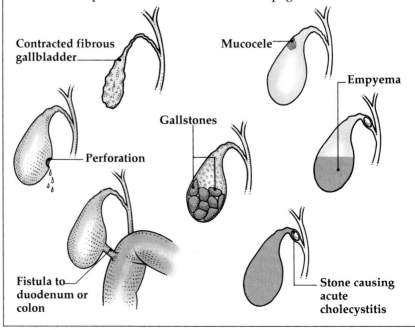

Contracted fibrous gallbladder

Mucocele

Empyema

Gallstones

Perforation

Fistula to duodenum or colon

Stone causing acute cholecystitis

# HERNIA

A hernia is the protrusion of the omentum (the fatty apron that covers the intestines) or of a loop of intestine through a defect in the abdominal wall. Hernias occur most frequently in the groin, where they are called inguinal or femoral, depending on their position. Many hernias cause little or no discomfort. But sometimes the protrusion becomes stuck (incarcerated), causing pain. An intestinal obstruction can follow. An incarcerated loop of intestine can become so twisted that its blood supply is cut off (strangulation), causing gangrene and perforation. Surgery must be performed immediately to release the intestine and repair the hernia. If gangrene is present, the surgeon removes the affected section and rejoins the healthy ends of the bowel. Because of these possible complications, doctors generally recommend surgery to repair a hernia.

Hernias can occur at weak points other than in the groin. Umbilical hernias, most common in infants, can develop around the navel. These hernias rarely cut off the blood supply and usually disappear around the age of 5 years. An incisional hernia can develop at the site of a previous abdominal operation. Such hernias range from a small defect to a large area of weakness through which almost the entire small intestine can pass. Incisional hernias are repaired surgically and a strong mesh gauze is placed over the hernia for strength. An epigastric hernia arises from weakness in the muscles of the central, upper part of the abdomen. This type of hernia occurs three times more commonly in men than in women. The blood supply of the intestine inside a hernia in any area may be cut off, but strangulation is most common in the groin.

> ### WARNING
>
> Hernias affect almost 2 percent of men in the US. Most hernias cause few problems. But hernias can strangulate, blocking off the blood supply to the intestine inside the hernia, so be aware of the danger signs. See your doctor or go to a hospital emergency room if:
>
> ◆ You cannot push the hernia back into place
>
> ◆ The area over the hernia becomes red, hot, and swollen
>
> ◆ The hernia becomes very tender and painful

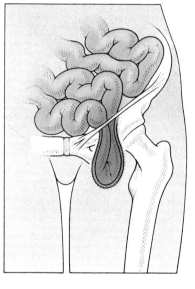

**Femoral hernia**
*Femoral hernias pass through a weakness close to the femoral vein in the groin. Because the femoral canal is a narrow structure, these hernias can strangulate more easily than inguinal hernias can.*

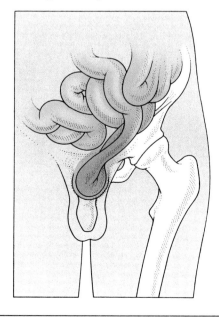

**Inguinal hernia**
*Inguinal hernias are more common than femoral hernias, especially in men. Men have a weakness in the inguinal canal through which their testicles descend. A loop of bowel can easily pass through this weak area and may become trapped.*

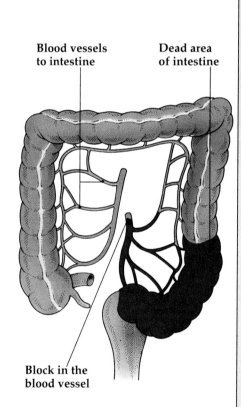

Blood vessels to intestine

Dead area of intestine

Block in the blood vessel

**Mesenteric infarction**
*A rare type of intestinal emergency occurs when the blood supply to part of the bowel is blocked – for example, by a blood clot – killing the bowel. This condition is called mesenteric infarction. The death rate from this condition is very high.*

# GLOSSARY OF DISORDERS

This glossary describes a number of disorders that affect the digestive tract. These disorders are not discussed elsewhere in this volume. Terms in italics refer to other entries in the glossary. For disorders discussed in other parts of the book, see the INDEX on pages 142 to 144.

## A

**Anal stenosis**
Tightness of the anus, also called anal stricture, in which the anus is too small to allow the normal passage of feces. This disorder often causes constipation and pain during defecation. Anal stenosis may be present from birth or can be caused by conditions that scar the anus, such as Crohn's disease or colitis.

## B

**Barrett's esophagus**
A condition in which the cells of the mucous membrane lining the lower part of the esophagus become similar to those found in the stomach lining. It usually follows prolonged acid reflux in the lower part of the esophagus. The condition may be precancerous.

**Bezoar**
A ball of food, mucus, vegetable fiber, hair, or other indigestible material in the stomach. Bezoars are rare in adults, except after partial gastrectomy (removal of part of the stomach). Trichobezoars (composed of hair only) occur in children who chew on or pull out and swallow their hair or in adults with severe emotional disturbances who eat hair. Bezoars can cause loss of appetite, nausea, vomiting, and abdominal pain. They can sometimes be removed with enzymes that digest protein or by surgery.

**Biliary atresia**
A rare disorder, present from birth, in which the bile ducts outside or inside the liver either fail to develop or develop abnormally. As a result, bile cannot flow through the ducts to the duodenum and becomes trapped in the liver. Unless surgery is performed, the condition is often fatal.

**Budd-Chiari syndrome**
A rare disorder in which the veins that drain blood from the liver are blocked or narrowed. This condition causes swelling of the liver, portal hypertension (elevated pressure in the portal vein, which carries blood from the intestines to the liver), and liver failure. The veins may be blocked by a blood clot, pressure from a tumor, or a congenital abnormality. If not treated, the condition is often fatal.

## C

**Carcinoid syndrome**
A rare condition characterized by bouts of facial flushing, diarrhea, and wheezing. It is caused by a tumor, called a carcinoid, in the intestine or the lung. This tumor secretes excess quantities of the substance serotonin, which performs a variety of functions in the body.

**Cystic fibrosis**
An inherited disease caused by a defective gene. People with the disease have repeated lung infections. They cannot absorb fats and other nutrients from food because the pancreas does not produce the required enzymes.

## D

**Duplication of the intestinal tract**
Any part of the digestive tract can be duplicated when it develops in the embryo. These duplications are most frequently found in the ileum, the final section of the small intestine. The condition is treated only if problems arise.

**Dumping syndrome**
A condition that brings on symptoms including sweating, faintness, and heart palpitations, caused by the rapid passage of food from the stomach to the upper intestine. The syndrome mainly affects people who have had stomach operations.

## F

**Familial polyposis**
An inherited disease causing multiple polyps in the colon and sometimes tumors in the bone and soft tissues. Affected people frequently develop bowel cancer by their late 20s.

## H

**Hemochromatosis**
An inherited disease, in which too much iron is absorbed and accumulates in the liver, pancreas, heart, testicles, and other organs. The iron that accumulates in the liver often causes cirrhosis.

**Hemosiderosis**
A general increase in the body's iron stores, usually as a result of multiple blood transfusions or of taking too many iron supplements.

**Hirschsprung's disease**
A rare disorder, present from birth, in which the nerve cells that control the rhythmic contractions in a section of the intestine fail to develop. The affected segment of intestine cannot propel feces, so the bowel above it becomes distended with feces. To treat the disease, the affected segment of intestine is usually removed.

## I

**Imperforate anus**
A disorder, present at birth, in which the anal canal fails to develop correctly. An affected infant may have a mild defect, with a membrane over the anus, or a more severe disorder, in which the rectum has no opening and the lower end of the bowel opens into the vagina or urethra. The condition is treated with surgery.

**Inborn errors of metabolism**
A group of genetic disorders in which the body cannot process certain amino acids obtained from food. In severe forms, such as Tay-Sachs disease, toxic chemicals accumulate in the brain, causing profound mental retardation, blindness, and often death at an early age.

**Intussusception**
A condition in which one part of the intestine telescopes inside another part. Occurring most commonly in infants, it usually has an obvious cause, such as a *Meckel's diverticulum* or a polyp. The condition may be corrected surgically.

**Intestinal lipodystrophy**
A rare digestive disorder of unknown cause. Common symptoms include malabsorption of nutrients, diarrhea, abdominal pain, and progressive weight loss. Intestinal lipodystrophy usually affects middle-aged men. Taking antibiotics for many months is the treatment.

# L

**Lymphomas**
A group of cancers that can be found in the lymphatic tissue of the digestive tract. Treatment of bowel lymphomas consists of radiation therapy and anticancer drugs (chemotherapy) rather than surgery.

# M

**Mallory-Weiss syndrome**
A condition in which violent vomiting tears the lower end of the esophagus, causing vomiting of blood. It is particularly common in alcoholics but may also occur with violent coughing, a severe asthma attack, or epileptic seizures.

**Meckel's diverticulum**
A common malformation of the digestive tract, present at birth, in which a small, wide-mouthed sac opens from the ileum, the final part of the small intestine. The diverticulum causes no problems unless it becomes infected, obstructed, or ulcerated.

**Megacolon**
A grossly distended colon, usually accompanied by severe, chronic constipation. In children, megacolon may be caused by *Hirschsprung's disease*, tears in the anus, or psychological factors that may have developed at the time of toilet training. In the elderly, it may be caused by constipation and long-term use of powerful laxatives. In severe cases, a segment of colon must be removed surgically. Often, however, the colon can be emptied by saline enemas.

**Mesenteric lymphadenitis**
An acute abdominal disorder, thought to be caused by a viral infection, in which lymph glands in the mesentery (a membrane that attaches various organs to the abdominal wall) of the digestive system become inflamed. It usually affects young children and often mimics acute appendicitis.

**Mucocele**
A swollen sac or cavity that is filled with mucus secreted from cells in its inner lining. A mucocele of the appendix is caused by constriction of the opening of the appendix into the intestine. A mucocele of the gallbladder may be caused by a gallstone obstructing its outlet.

# P

**Paralytic ileus**
A condition in which the waves that move food through the intestines slow down or stop. Fluid and gas collect in the intestine, with no passage of gas or stool. The condition can occur after intestinal or prostate surgery or can be caused by infection.

**Peutz-Jeghers syndrome**
An inherited condition in which many small polyps occur in the intestine, accompanied by small, flat spots on the lips. The polyps may bleed, cause abdominal pain, or result in an *intussusception*, but cancerous changes are rare.

**Pilonidal sinus**
A pit in the skin, usually containing hair, in the upper part of the cleft between the buttocks, caused by hair follicles burrowing inward. A pilonidal sinus may become infected, producing pain and discharge of pus. Treatment involves surgical removal of the sinus with a wide incision.

**Plummer-Vinson syndrome**
Difficulty swallowing caused by the formation of webs of tissue across the upper part of the esophagus. This condition accompanies iron deficiency anemia and usually affects women in their 40s.

**Pseudomembranous enterocolitis**
A severe inflammatory condition of the colon, caused by infection with the bacterium *Clostridium difficile*, that arises as a complication of the use of oral antibiotics (which kill the bacteria that normally live in the colon). The condition leads to necrosis (death of the lining of the colon), profuse watery diarrhea, toxemia (the presence of bacterial toxins in the bloodstream), shock, and collapse. Treatment consists of intravenous fluid replacement and the use of the antibiotic vancomycin, which combats the causative bacteria.

# R

**Rectocele**
A protrusion of the rectum through the back wall of the vagina. Rectocele, caused by a weakness in the muscles of the vaginal wall, is most common in postmenopausal women.

# S

**Scleroderma**
An autoimmune disorder (one in which the body's immune system attacks its own tissues) occurring more often in women than in men that can affect the digestive tract and some other organs. A common problem is difficulty swallowing because of replacement of the muscle of the esophagus by fibrous tissue.

**Situs inversus**
A very rare condition in which the internal organs, including the intestines, lie in a mirror image of their usual position. In this condition, inflammation of the appendix or gallbladder occurs on the left side.

# T

**Tropical sprue**
Chronic fatty diarrhea caused by malabsorption of nutrients occurring in a person who has visited a tropical area but who does not have parasites or other infection. The cause is unknown, but the disease improves with antibiotic treatment.

# W

**Wilson's disease**
A rare, inherited disorder in which copper accumulates in the liver and is slowly released into other parts of the body. It causes severe liver and brain damage. Lifelong treatment with an agent that binds to the copper can prevent such damage from occurring.

# INDEX

Page numbers in *italics* refer to illustrations and captions.

**Photograph sources:**
Audio Visual Services, St. Marys Hospital **106** (top left); **106** (center); **106** (bottom right)
Biophoto Associates **33** (top); **42**; **112**; **135**; **116** (bottom right)
Camera M.D. Studios **32**
Mr Richard Cummins **58**; **71** (top left); **77**; **94**; **98**; **116** (top center); **117** (top left)
Dr Stephen Gwyther **33** (bottom left); **63** (bottom left); **69**; **88**; **98**; **117**; **118**; **123**
The Hutchison Library **10** (top right)
The Image Bank **9**; **77** (top left); **85**
Institute of Orthopaedics **117** (bottom right)
KeyMed (Medical & Industrial Equipment) Ltd **61**
Dr G. de Lacey **63** (bottom right); **73**
Dr R. W. Lees **111**
Living Technology **55**
The Mansell Collection **10** (bottom left)
National Medical Slide Bank, UK

**58** (center); **75**; **102**; **120**; **126**; **127**
Dr A. B. Price **110**; **131** (bottom left); **131** (bottom right)
Dr R.V. Rege **109**
Saint Bartholomew's Hospital **92**; **108** (bottom right); **117** (top right); **117** (bottom center); **117** (bottom left)
Saunders College Publishing **10** (top left)
Science Photo Library **2** (bottom right); **7**; **25**; **47**; **48**; **60**; **62**; **71** (bottom right); **79**; **89**; **90**; **91**; **93**; **104**; **106** (top right); **106** (bottom left); **108** (top right); **109**; **125**; **136**
Tony Stone Worldwide **10** (center)
Telegraph Colour Library **21**
James C. Webb **19**
Zefa Picture Library **20**; **53**; **131** (top left)

**Front cover photograph:**
Barry O'Rourke/The Stock Market

**Index:** Sue Bosanko

**Illustrators:**
Russell Barnet
Andrew Bezear
Joanna Cameron
Karen Cochrane
Peter Cox
David Fathers
Tony Graham
Andrew Green
Grundy & Northedge
Kevin Marks
Gillian Oliver

Lydia Umney
Philip Wilson
John Woodcock
**Commissioned photography:**
Steve Bartholomew
Susannah Price
Clive Streeter
**Airbrushing:**
Paul Desmond
Roy Flooks
Janos Marffy